MORAINE VALLEY COMMUNITY COLLEGE LRC/LIBRARY
PALOS HILLS, ILLINOIS

CO-AVW-300

WITHDRAWN

LET'S Really MAKE LOVE

BY ROBERT RIMMER

Novels

That Girl from Boston
The Harrad Experiment
The Rebellion of Yale Marratt
The Zolotov Affair (also published as *The Gold Lovers*)
Proposition 31
Thursday, My Love
The Premar Experiments
Come Live My Life
Love Me Tomorrow
The Love Explosion
The Byrdwhistle Option
The Immoral Reverend
The Resurrection of Anne Hutchinson
The Way to Go (unpublished)
The Oublion Project (unpublished)
The Trade Off (unpublished)
Dreamer of Dreams (unpublished)

Nonfiction

The Harrad Letters to Robert H. Rimmer
Adventures in Loving
You and I . . . Searching for Tomorrow
The Love Adventurers
The X-Rated Videotape Guide (vols. 1–4)
Raw Talent: The Adult Film Industry as Seen by Its Most Popular Male Star,
    by Jerry Butler as told to Robert Rimmer and Catherine Tavel
Whips and Kisses: Parting the Leather Curtain,
    by Mistress Jacqueline as told to Robert Rimmer and Catherine Tavel

LET'S

Really

MAKE
LOVE

SEX, THE FAMILY,
AND EDUCATION
in the
TWENTY-FIRST
CENTURY

Robert Rimmer

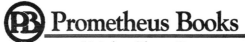 Prometheus Books

59 John Glenn Drive
Amherst, NewYork 14228-2197

Published 1995 by Prometheus Books

Let's Really Make Love: Sex, the Family, and Education in the Twenty-First Century.
Copyright © 1995 by Robert H. Rimmer. All rights reserved. No part of this publication
may be reproduced, stored in a retrieval system, or transmitted in any form or by any
means, electronic, mechanical, photocopying, recording, or otherwise, without prior written permission of the publisher, except in the case of brief quotations embodied in critical
articles and reviews. Inquiries should be addressed to Prometheus Books, 59 John Glenn
Drive, Amherst, New York 14228–2197, 716–691– 0133. FAX: 716–691–0137.

99 98 97 96 95   5 4 3 2 1

Library of Congress Cataloging-in-Publication Data

Rimmer, Robert H., 1917–
    Let's really make love : sex, the family, and education in the twenty-first century /
Robert H. Rimmer.
      p.   cm.
    ISBN 0-87975-964-X (alk. paper)
    1. Sex instruction—United States. 2. Family life education—United States.
I. Title.
HQ57.5.A3R56   1995
613.9'07—dc20   95-2877
                                                                                CIP

Printed in the United States of America on acid-free paper

Contents

Part Two: Where We've Been and Where We're Going

Glossary of Acronyms

Using acronyms to describe organizations became a way of life in the twentieth century. The problem was remembering the original names and what they stood for. In case you forget, here's a convenient listing of those used in this book.

A13er   Alternate 13-week work/study student in the GLUE program

Compars   Communal Parents. Graduate students who coordinate the Human Values seminars for Premars (A13ers who have chosen the ROSP option)

FFAC   Future Families of America Commission

GLUE   Originally GUE, the federally Guaranteed Undergraduate Education. With "L," for Loving, added, it became GLUE.

HARRAD   The original ROSP proposal appeared in the novel *The Harrad Experiment,* when HARvard and RADcliffe where separate institutions.

HV   Human Values seminar—a one-hour weekly gathering of forty-eight A13ers in the GLUE programs.

K-12   Education from kindergarten to the 12th grade

8 GLOSSARY OF ACRONYMS

NSME   New Sexual Morality and Education legislation

NSV   An arts rating—Not Sexually Oriented or Violent

PREMARS   A13ers taking the ROSP option

ROSP   Roommate of the Other Sex Program

SD   An arts rating—Sexually Devalued

SDH   An arts rating—Sexually Devalued Historically

SN   An arts rating—Sexually Natural

Part One

Transforming America: The New Sexual Morality and Education Legislation

Utopia is the *protest* against the status quo; the *anticipation* of the possibilities of social change; and *the insistence of realizing everything immediately,* which constitutes a refusal of defeatism. [italics mine]

—Ernst Bloch

The basic function of Utopia is to *maintain a project* for humanity in the face of meaninglessness. [italics mine]

—Paul Ricoeur

I'd like to take as a motto for my talk one of the inscriptions on the walls of the Sorbonne in Paris: "Let us be realistic, let us ask for the impossible."

—Herbert Marcuse

1

This Land Is Your Land

My working title for the first draft of this book was *Sexual Sanity Now.* The publishers weren't enthusiastic about that title, so I suggested *The Final Sex Revolution,* which expresses a thesis I have adhered to throughout the book. No—they wanted a title without the word sex in it. So I proposed *Let's Really Make Love!*

Late in 1994 Little Brown published a condensed version of *The Social Organization of Sexuality.* The original book had been co-authored by Edward Lauman, Robert Michael, Stuart Michaels, and John Gagnon, who are, mostly, active professors of sociology. It was published by the University of Chicago at a price of $49.95. But Little Brown's version of *Sex in America: A Definitive Survey* was, and still is, available at a much lower price. Courtesy of the book clubs, and with interrelated promotional help from *Time* magazine (October 17, 1994), as well as all the media, it may outsell the Kinsey studies and convince millions of Americans that questioning 3,432 citizens about sexuality offers the *definitive* answers on American sex habits. Sexual reality in the twenty-first century apparently can be determined from answers to numerous questions such as: How many sexual partners have you had since the age of eighteen? How many in a lifetime? How often have you had sex, masturbated, had oral sex, had anal sex, had extramarital sex partners in the past twelve months, rented porno movies, had group sex, forced someone to do something sexual? How do you feel about abortion, anal sex, and homosexuality?

Time was happy to confirm their mid-1970s feature article that the sex revolution was over. In their summation of *Sex in America,* in 1994, *Time* pointed out that 94 percent of married people were faithful, and twice-a-week sex was the average among monogamous couples, who actually had more sex and enjoyed it more than the unmarried. Garrison Keillor (in the same issue) was pleased: "There is an incredible amount of normality going on in America these days, and it is good to know that our country is not obsessed with sex." And *Time*, never very good at future prophecy, concluded:

> In 1994—Americans, it seems, have come full circle. It's easy to forget as recently as 1948, Norman Mailer was still using the word fug [*Time* won't print the word *fuck*] in his novels. There may have been a sex revolution—at least for those college educated whites who came of age with John Updike's swinging *Couples*, Philip Roth's priapic *Portnoy* and Jong's *Fear of Flying*, but the sex revolution turned out to have a beginning, a middle and end.

Thus *Time* continues to believe that we're all back to normal. The 1960s' sex revolution is really over. The premise of this book is that the sex revolution really began after World War I in America and has been, and still is, in progress. *But*—in America the final battle in the sex revolution with no bloodshed is not only possible but is inevitable, and sexual sanity *now* is within our grasp.

Some of the new statistics from *Sex in America* are obviously totally out of whack with American sexual reality. Take it from me—the homosexuals may have come out of the closet and dared to be honest about their sexuality, but no sane married (except possibly swingers, of whom there are at least two million or more, according to Bob McGinley, head of the North American Swing Association) will reveal their extramarital life to interviewers. Millions of Americans who have strayed beyond monogamy, and hundreds of thousands who are living in a ménage à trois group relationship or intentional community are not interested, or are simply very much afraid, to reveal their nonmonogamous lifestyles for fear of losing their jobs, which are often controlled by more religious, monogamous bosses. Nor do they want to battle with, or shock, conservative friends and neighbors, or try to explain their extramarital relations to their children until they are old enough to deal with them.

Amusingly, for the monogamously faithful, the second most popular sex activity, according to this National Opinion Survey, is "watching their spouse undress." (Better than oral sex, believe it or not!) Obviously, since 23 percent of the males and 11 percent of the females surveyed bought or rented X-rated movies in the last twelve months, a good 100 million Americans, altogether, are not only thinking about extramarital sex but enjoy watching people, other than their spouses, take off their clothes and cavort in their birthday suits. (Note that the numbers are well over one-third of their sample and probably more than half, since the younger people interviewed are much more likely to be "doing it" than watching on videocassettes.) One statistic that makes the others even more dubious is that 54 percent of males think about sex daily but only 19 percent of females do. The interviewers obviously missed the vast female audiences watching Oprah and other talk shows—women who for the most part think about sex as often as men but probably negatively.

The reality of books like *Sex in America,* and the innumerable sex surveys that have appeared since the Kinsey report, is that they leave it to others to weigh the truth and fiction, and no one ever deals with the consequences. Despite the so-called cooling of sex in America, the divorce rate isn't declining much, but today in a sickly, legal manner, divorce solves the problem of additional sex partners. Nor does this report deal with the problem of premarital sex before the eighteenth year, which is obviously a lot hotter than the marital rate and presages later marital problems of many kinds.

So, please keep in mind that my proposal—*Let's Really Make Love*—is really a complete, controversial, but inevitable reformation of some aspects of Christian, Judaic, and Islamic moralities, along with a completely new approach to public education for all Americans from kindergarten to grade 12 (K-12), continuing with a four-year federally guaranteed undergraduate education for all high school graduates.

Call it utopian, but my prediction is that the New Sexual Morality and Education legislation that I am proposing must eventually happen. When it does it will usher in the final sex revolution. It will incorporate four more years of public education beyond K-12, open to all high school graduates on a work-study basis. For computer buffs the password is: interactive K-16 and the Five Ls. The keynote to utopia is the Five Ls—Living, Loving, Learning, Laughter, and *Ludamus* (Latin for "all of us playing together"), and with the conviction that in a soundly motivated society the play ethic would ultimately replace the work ethic.

Taking the advice of my agent who told me that the book would reach a wider audience if, as I did in *The Harrad Experiment,* I would write some of the ideas as fiction but with a "here and now reality," I have just finished a novel. Called *Dreamer of Dreams* (and as yet unpublished), it is the story of a former porno film maker who has created a new religion, with a theology based on recent scientific chaos theories. His followers are called Wonderers and, with several thousand franchised churches dubbed "Love Dromes" throughout the country, they exalt human sexuality and offer not only a complete sexual education for Wonderers and their children, but also provide a rite of sexual passage for "Seventeeners." This is in addition to similar things that I have proposed in later chapters in this book—like the Harrad and the Premar Experiments in the education area. Wondering is a twenty-first-century religion that is an achievable reality in your lifetime. *Dreamer of Dreams* is a fast-moving novel designed, like this book, so that you can be the judge and jury.

I subtitled the first draft of this book "A Presidential Platform for 2000," and I envisioned a presumably living Senator Newton Morrow (long before Newt Gingrich) offering it, with my help, as a "white paper"—the reaction to which, if favorable, would give him the impetus to run against whoever might be president at the turn of the century. My reasoning is that unless we have a president who dares to use his "bully pulpit" to challenge old moralities and outmoded approaches to the education of a new generation, then, by the year 2050, when current predictions are that there will be 100 million more Americans than there are now, instead of leading the world, you will be one of nearly 400 million of us living in a democracy that is drifting to disaster.

Newton Morrow (you can play on the words New Tomorrow) is a character in my novel *Love Me Tomorrow*. He believes that he is a reincarnation of Edward Bellamy, who was once famous for his vision of a saner twenty-first century in his novel *Looking Backward*. I wrote the novel in 1975, and although it is out of print and envisions a unique new economics and sexual morality for the year 2000 (more likely 2050), it has become a "cult" novel appealing to thousands of readers today who are searching for new kinds of premarital and postmarital structures, which are still theoretically possible. I'll cover some of these later in the book.

Without going back to post–World War I and the so-called Jazz Age, when your grandparents began the rebellion against Victorian moralities, it's fascinating to look back and ruminate on what we have and haven't accomplished since the quiescent lull in the sexual battle during the Norman Rockwell–style 1950s. I will be doing this in subsequent chapters. But now, before I evaluate the whys and wherefors, the hows and whethers, and the painful past and present, making a new birth, a Renaissance 2000, a necessity; and before I show you how we could redirect America and create a sexually caring, fully employed, joyous world, with a large majority enjoying the self-fulfilling life of the Five Ls—here's a brief survey and listing of domestic problems that we are facing in the mid 1990s, all of which confirm the necessity of new leadership and daring new solutions. (I have left aside the major health-care problems, which at this writing, after a year of hectic inquiry, are in limbo.) I'm sure most of the following will be familiar to you personally or a part of your daily fare from the media.

1. A divorce rate that is still 50 percent of the marriage rate, creating a dangerous subsidiary problem of six million kids in the 1990s being raised by a single parent who, in most cases, has no strong family support.

2. A related problem of working wives and husbands (a phenomenon that few futurists of the 1960s anticipated and didn't exist a half century ago) creat-

ing the necessity of child care for ten million or more preschool children. Child care often costs more than the working wife can earn—and because of low wages paid in the child care industry it often endangers the child's welfare.

3. The problem of premarital sex in the United States which results in a million teenage pregnancies annually, with many of the mothers ending up as single parents. The 1989 census reveals that there are ten million women who are trying to raise children with absent fathers. Fifty-eight percent of them are receiving child support, averaging about $3,000 annually. Three million mothers were never wed—an increase of nonresponsibility of 11 percent. The Clinton administration tried to address this problem on a financial cut-off basis. In March of 1995, following Newt Gingrich's "Contract with America," Republicans passed a new Welfare Bill which, as I write this, still has to be approved by the Senate, and if so will probably be vetoed by President Clinton. Surveys of state laws reveal that trying to discourage young women from collecting additional cash benefits if they have another baby have mixed results and work only about 50 percent of the time. Frustrating the potential savings of $55 billion a year is whether reduced welfare will increase abortion demand. As for the additional $500 income-tax credits to make it easier for low income families to afford further education for their children—this, in view of the minor tax savings versus the cost of under-graduate education—is ridiculous.

4. The problem of a majority of young people experimenting with their sexuality between the ages of twelve and seventeen, endangering themselves not only with unwanted pregnancies, but the potential of contracting AIDs or other venereal diseases.

5. The problem the disappearing nuclear family of a husband and wife and two children with the husband providing the financial support, and the combined family presumably providing emotional and financial stability. Despite wishful political thinking, the Norman Rockwell, 1940s–1950s style of families no longer exists in reality or daydreams. Fewer than 35 percent of those now listed as families in the U.S. Census come close to this category and most of them are dependent on two working parents. Millions of these families are unable to provide any lasting kind of social structure. One out of four children now live with single parents, most of whom have little time to spend with them. Seven million children are living with stepparents, most of whom are also working parents.

6. The problems of drugs and more than two million drug addicts in this country. Politically the only solution still being offered is a continuing war on drugs. Many nationally known people, including George Schultz, former U.S. Secretary of State, economist Milton Friedman, conservative commentator William Buckley, and many others believe the only solution is the legalization of drugs. But when Surgeon General Joycelyn Elders suggested that legalization is worthy of study most of our political leaders, including President Clinton, were morally hor-

rified. Although there are close to a million people in prison, many for drug dealing, with no room for more, the solutions being offered are to build more and better prisons.

7. The problems of education—700,000 kids who drop out of high school each year and 27 million who are unable to read beyond a sixth-grade reader. And the even greater problem in secondary schools where Scholastic Aptitude Tests (now being questioned for their validity but with no solutions) reveal that American children are scoring at all-time low compared with young people in other nations. On top of this, for a majority of young people the financial cost of undergraduate educate is now beyond the earning/saving capacity of 80 percent of American families. Combined income of most working parents is less than $50,000 a year. Most parents are unable to support even one child in college with a year of undergraduate study now costing $25,000 a year or more.

The current political solution is National Service, which has now become law. A Democratic Congress created a Corporation for National Community Service funded with $700 million annually and rising to a total of $1.5 billion annually to loan to young people who presumably will repay it by doing minimum wage National Service work when they complete their education. In the initial years it will provide only enough money for loans to about thirty thousand undergraduates, the day dream assumption is that eventually all Americans (at least 10 million more who don't get further education) will be enrolled in National Service and will be able to continue their education. The new Republican Congress in March 1995 was contesting Americorp legislation, which Clinton in his Martin Luther King speech called his greatest first-term achievement. Republicans estimate that the federal costs will exceed $47,000 a year per student enrolled, and that covers only 100,000 students enrolled by 1996. Americorp still leaves millions of Americans who will never be able to afford any kind of continuing education after high school.

8. The problems of minority groups and racial and ethnic problems which will increase substantially in the twenty-first century, when one-third of school age children will come from poor and undereducated minority groups. Right now at the undergraduate level minorities as distinguished from "native" Americans are more than a third of the entering classes. But there is still very little assimilation of black and white students. Black students in most colleges and universities form their own enclaves, and neither blacks nor whites know how to break through and embrace each other. Despite religious moralities that we are all brothers, or the Constitutional morality that we are all equals, the new compromise is why can't we all live happily together extolling "political correctness" and the innate superiority of each of our separate cultures. The white melting pot (blacks excluded) that created America as we once knew it is now a dirty word.

But the basic concept is still valid. Unless we learn how to really integrate all Americans regardless of race, color, or ethnic origin, the dream of our nation— indivisible, with justice for all—will become a nightmare.

9. The problems of sexual sickness, sexual deviance, along with those who cannot live by the Decalogue, problems that are now exposed and overexposed by all the media as never before in human history, is making a K-12 generation certain that neither their parents, nor their teachers, nor their religious leaders are able to contain, let alone moralize about their own sexual drives or provide any sane guidance.

There's AIDS with condom distribution in high schools horrifying parents and religious leaders. There's *incest,* with a television comedienne, Roseanne, revealing the prevalence of fathers (and stepfathers) forcing underage daughters to have sex with them, or Woody Allen, accused by Mia Farrow of seducing their adopted daughter Soon-Yi.There's *date rape,* with William Kennedy Smith and Mike Tyson appearing in "did he or didn't he" television dramas. There's *sexual harassment,* with Francis Conley, a surgeon at Stanford State University, complaining about her fellow doctors; and the Clarence Thomas–Anita Hill imbroglio with sexual details on television and in the media, for parents and children alike; and the Tailhook scandal with U.S. Navy male officers harassing the female officers, leading to the resignation of the Secretary of the Navy; and Robert Packwood, a U.S. senator, who presumably sexually annoyed a sizable number of female constituents; and O. J. Simpson beating his wife, Nicole, more than once but never with any future thought that it might be a prelude to real mayhem. There's *adultery* with President John Kennedy's extracurricular sex life receiving detailed media exposure, and President Bill Clinton accused of adultery and proposed adultery by Paula Jones and Gennifer Flowers. Or, moving down to just plain folks, there's the Amy Fisher/Joey Buttafucco story told endlessly in the media and twice in television dramas. There's *prostitution* with Sidney Biddle Barrows, the Mayflower Madam, and Heidi Fleiss, her Hollywood sister, both read about by a majority of Americans, young and old. There's *pedophilia,* with the problems of priests, and Michael Jackson appearing endlessly in detailed media stories and courtroom dramas, along with clerical adultery (flaunting one of the Commandments) also receiving detailed exposure.There's *wife beating and marital rape,* with the Bureau of National Justice Crime Survey revealing that 25 percent of all murders occur in the home, with two thousand to four thousand battered women beaten to death every year by their husbands or boyfriends. There's a daily fare of *sexually induced murders* on television, topped off with total television and media exposure of Pamela Smart in New Hampshire and Vermont, who contracted with her boyfriend to murder her husband, or Charles Stuart in Boston, who murdered his wife and tried to make it appear as if a black rapist did it. And Susan Smith, who finally admitted to drowning her two boys apparently in a fantasy dream of marrying her wealthy young lover, who didn't want the responsibility of having children.

10. There are the problems of *birth control, abortion,* and *homosexuality,* all intertwined with Catholic and fundamentalist religious beliefs enlisting or indoctrinating young people from childhood to become pro or con activists.

11. All of the above problems are creating a K-12 environment of *sexual devaluation and sexual vulgarization* that ultimately affects all human relationships. The problem is exemplified in newspapers like *The National Enquirer* and its relative, *People* magazine (and its clones), along with the women's magazines, *Cosmopolitan, Redbook,* and many others offering the latest premarital and postmarital sexual panaceas. All of them are stridently displayed at supermarket checkout counters which, interestingly—to keep female shoppers happy?—do not sell *Playboy, Penthouse, Hustler,* or any of the "skin" magazines, evidently because women prefer the Harlequin or Danielle Steele romances in which the male finally sees the light and becomes a good lover and homemaker.

Spewing out of the same devalued sex volcano are the talk-show hosts and hostesses, Oprah Winfrey, Phil Donahue, Geraldo, Joan Rivers, Sally Jessy Raphael, and many others in local markets, plus the Howard Sterns and others on radio and television, all upstaging each other with accounts of sexual insanities.

If sick sex reality isn't enough there's R-rated movies in theaters and on cable, and a new variety without rating, labeled "Adult Only," that are being produced by the hundreds for rental in video stores. Produced by directors like the Dark Brothers (famous for X-rated films), they offer the same "recreational" mostly noncaring or noninvolved copulation that is the hallmark of X-rated films. All of these are available not only to adults (even hotels and motels now have "soft core channels" for their guests!) but for under eighteeners who can easily circumvent the R-rated restriction thus offering a neat form of rebellion against their parents. And whether you actually see the R-rated movies or not, widespread magazine and newspaper publicity informs both young and old about Madonna murdering an old guy for his money by screwing him to death in the film *Body of Evidence,* or Sharon Stone in a snuff murder in *Basic Instinct,* or Oliver Stone offering a combination of sick sex and violence in *Natural Born Killers,* and one film after another. Or *Boxing Helena,* which serves up a sickie to top them all: A surgeon is madly in love with a woman who ignores him, but he finally gets partial control of her body when she's in an automobile accident and he has to amputate her legs; then he completes the job by cutting off her arms, after which he completely owns her body and ultimately her mind. Then there's Internet, the international communication channel which, among a million other things, offers sexual discussion in every imaginable form—originating all over the world—plus hard-core pornography for those who learn how to download it or access it directly, or via other on-line channels. Nasty pictures can even be downloaded. A crime bill to censor Internet was introduced in Congress in early 1995—with many howls from those opposed to censorship. But pornography on Internet is small change compared to that available on the relatively low cost new RCA Direct Satellite TV. And at a slightly less sexually febrile level, there's cable TV with R-rated films that walk the thin line of X-rated, and MTV bringing popular teenage music to life and giv-ing it sexual reality, plus the Playboy Channel with endless soft-core sex, and the Adam & Eve Cable Channel (the company that sells sex toys and X-rated movies by mail) now going all out with live TV action. And, of course, rap music which, long before it was excoriated for violence against cops, thrived on the illusions it gave young males that they were cocks of the walk in sexual command of the female, which is also the basis of much of vocalized rock music. In contrast, coun-try music, appealing to the older generation, is more oriented to the sad male who has betrayed his loving wife or girl friend, or vice versa.

There's also a change in the style of television news shows and the news-media conviction that most Americans are bored by the "MacNeil Lehrer News Hour" and prefer news "entertainment" be it bizarre, bloody, tragic, or sexually juicy. Copying the style of syndicated shows like "A Current Affair" and "Hard Copy" which give you sexual insanity in detail, they sound bite the stories because in any one day there are so many of them. Freedom of expression on highly successful local news shows is following in the footsteps of the Hearst- and Murdoch-style tabloids, where catching Jacqueline Kennedy in her birthday suit or Princess Diana tossing her cookies makes the headlines of the moment.

For the younger generation and their parents, there's video games, with Sega and Nintendo revealing their Japanese origins (the Japanese censor *Playboy* and full-frontal nudity but are delighted with bondage and discipline sex—female breasts and asses showing,in tied-up and gagged situations, where the female gets her proper comeuppance. Video games like *Night Trap* and *Mortal Kombat,* tak-ing hours of playtime and featuring scantily clad women protected by good guys and chased by bad guys—all of whom are either eviscerated or end up with blood spewing out of their chopped-off heads and exposed entrails. Some toy stores are refusing to offer these games but like violent rap they are big sellers. And finally there are interactive CD-ROM discs in which the mostly sexually hung male can not only change the story direction but also discover female heroines who will with a few clicks of his keyboard or mouse happily undress for him, "talk dirty" and almost climb out of the tube to do anything he wants.

Meanwhile in December 1993 *Newsweek*, admitting that many clerics con-sidered "NYPD Blue" "a sinkhole of depravity," nevertheless called it "simply the best new show on television"—even though it has crossed the previously accepted boundaries of nudity and profanity. Raising the question not so much of sex devaluation and nudity as sexual vulgarization and accentuating our verbal inability to define another person in any depth except with words like "asshole," "pissy little bitch," "son of a bitch," and "scumbag" all being words approved by the network censors.

Turn eighteen, and not only can young women become porno stars, but they can offer their beautiful bodies and recreational sex as daydreams to males of all ages. Accounting for four hundred million rentals, in addition to unknown quantities of direct sale, there are more than fifty thousand, all presumably different, X-rated VCR tapes now available. Several thousand new ones are being filmed or videoed annually. Many women are as avid renters and viewers as their boyfriends or husbands. Almost all of the X-rated tapes extol recreational sex with many partners married or unmarried. The big-selling 1993–1994 variety were the amateur and "pro-am" (professionally guided) videos made by "swingers." According to Bob McGinley, president of the North American Swing Associations, there are more than a million Americans, married or not, who enjoy recreational sex with alternating partners. In essence the people who live next door, or in the same high rise with you, are making videos of themselves enjoying every conceivable kind of sex and selling the tapes to the porno distributors. Despite the fear of AIDS and other venereal diseases, the demand is for condomless sex action, and for anal sex displayed in graphic full-screeners. Watch them and you are convinced that thousands of women are begging for male cocks deep in their intestines, or so called "DPers," one cock in the lady's vagina and the other in her anus. By contrast, unless they rent gay male videos (there are thousands of them as well), heterosexual guys who can't wait to bugger a woman would most likely be horrified to have a cock in their intestines.

But topping either *Boxing Helena* or any X-rated fantasy in 1993 was the reality of Lorena Bobbitt (appropriate name) who, with her husband, John became instantly famous. In rage because John came home drunk and tried to force her to have sex, Lorena cut off his penis with a kitchen knife, stormed out of their bedroom, his prick in hand, and drove off in their car. Later she threw his cock out of their car window. Fortunately for John it was found. A few months later, after John was saved total emasculation by David Berman, M.D., who managed to sew the penis back on, *People* magazine's December 13, 1993 (among many others), featured Lorena on its cover and ran a four-page article (never mentioning the surgeon's name) but treating the episode humorously and wondering whether it might become a feminist way of life since one feminist group, along with many feminists, was supporting Lorena as exemplifying the new empowerment of women. Meanwhile both John and Lorena were offered plush book contracts, and John appeared on the Howard Stern show (and many others) to raise money to cover his medical and legal expenses. Happily wearing a sweat shirt marked "Severed Parts", he enjoyed his fifteen minutes of fame and hundreds of sick sex jokes spun off by Jay Leno and David Letterman. Millions laughed but a few wondered whether Lorena bobbing her husband's penis was really the grand finale—the destruction of sexual wonder. To top it off in 1994, an X-rated film called *John Bobbitt, Uncut,* directed by the porno sleaze master extraordinaire, Ron Jeremy, tries to retell the whole sleazy story and features John himself, in graphic sexual action, using his sewed-on penis with other women and a porno actress portraying Lorena before she excised it. The producers expect it will outsell Linda Lovelace's fantasy clitoris, in her *Deep Throat,* and earn several hundred thousand dollars for John.

12. The final domestic problems are *violence, crime,* and *underemployment.* More jails and police on the street, or better gun control, may give a small percentage reduction in violence and crime, but it will never stop the massacres in fast food restaurants, post offices, or railroads that have occurred in the past few years, nor will it stop serial killers, or thousands of senseless gang, "drug," and sex-related murders that are the daily fare of the media. The reality is that an economic system that accepts 6 to 7 percent unemployment as inevitable and benign, and an educational system that doesn't give all Americans a full know-thyself emotional and vocational education is headed for disaster.

Can we give millions of young people and their parents a new sense of national purpose? Absolutely! But it has to be set in motion with leadership from the top. In the following pages I offer you a New Tomorrow that could begin with the president, or a farsighted member of Congress—does Newt Gingrich qualify?— offering a New Sexual Morality and Educational Bill which would be guided and directed by Future Families of America—a new federal agency.

This approach to educational and sexual sanity now, which would resolve or ameliorate many of the problems listed above, will shock many people because it deals with the the vastly changing educational and sexual reality at the beginning of the twenty-first century. Neither parents, nor teachers in the schools, religious leaders, priests, rabbis, ministers, groups, associations or lobbyists, most of whom are working with conflicting philosophies and agendas, can resolve these problems. A new sense of values and a new American morality must be defined politically by a daring leader. Then as Bill Clinton and Hillary Rodham Clinton tried to do with health care but hopefully with more success, and no doubt with even more controversy from the Christian Right, we can not only define the problems but cut through centuries of religious miasma with sounder approaches to human sexuality and education and offer a national commitment on which the majority of us can agree.

But first, before detailing new educational and sexual legislation that would, as Bill Clinton insisted in one of his State of the Union speeches to Congress, "give people and especially our young people something to say yes to," let me, in the following pages, underline the necessity for a new sense of national purpose; let me show you how, and why, we are floundering, and why, if we don't find workable solutions that combine freedom of expression with a closer merger of church and state, we may well open the door to a kind of apocalypse now, an authoritarian government directing its version of sexual and educational sanity at the American people.

2

Searching for Tomorrow

There is no lack of solutions that may or may not solve the problems of our trillion-dollar debt, our balance of payments, and our underemployment problems. In his book *Work of Nations,* subtitled *Preparing Ourselves for 21st-Century Capitalism,* Secretary of Labor Robert Reich offers a scary analysis, not discussed much by either Democrats or Republicans, predicting that those who are employed in manufacturing and farming—"routine production services," 25 percent of the working population at present—will find fewer jobs as this kind of work goes global at lower hourly rates. "In-person service" employment will increase but not at comparable rates to those who were formerly engaged in manufacturing. This will leave those who provide "symbolic analytic services," coordinating information from databases and making new discoveries in all areas, only 20 percent of those working, who will earn above-average incomes.

Time magazine of November 23, 1993, asked in a cover story "What Ever Happened to the Great American Job?" The magazine pointed out that in addition to U.S. unemployment figures of the then 8.8 million officially counted as jobless, there were another 6.2 million who would like to work full time, but were trying to survive on part-time jobs. *Time*'s answer, with no national solutions in sight that would work for what may be as many as 16.2 million people who are underemployed, was: "Get as much education as possible . . . the future belongs to the knowledge worker."

How our economic and work problems are solved will affect all our lives. Not only America but the entire Western world must discover how to keep hundreds of millions of people employed. Unemployment, human lives with no earned income, nothing to do, day after day are lives that soon become meaningless, and prey to charismatic barbarians who will delude them with authoritarian solutions ending in police states. With global manufacture of every kind of material goods equal to or better than American made, the only area left for millions of jobs is in the information sector. Not the new daydream, the projected "information superhighway," which depends on humans interacting with other humans via satellites and fiber optics, but rather a totally *personally interactive teaching world* with old and young working and playing together in lifetime learning environments, in which education—teaching and learning and searching for answers to every aspect of life—provides employment and good hourly pay for millions more people than are now engaged in the education (and entertainment) industry.

But before I show you how a benign federal approach to morals, and a national funding of sex education (optionally available to all public schools) along with a guaranteed undergraduate education could, within a few years, solve the problem of underemployment as well as most of the problems I have listed in chapter 1, let's take a broader look at what our cultural gurus have been, and are still, telling us. They are reaching millions of educated Americans (you who are reading this book, and can redirect the future) via major news publications like *Time, Newsweek,* and the *Wall Street Journal* as well as many major local newspapers. There's much worry and dismay. But very few solutions—except a return to religion—are offered. Reading this chapter, you may agree that "Whistling in the Dark" would be a better title for it, since most of the papers are beating the bushes, and never getting a grip on the tigers burning bright.

In a feature article, "Whose Values," on June 8, 1992, *Newsweek* pointed out that the Democratic party platform made it crystal clear that the province of sexual morality was an area that politicians should leave to the family and church.

Joe Klein summed up Dan Quayle's attack on Murphy Brown (in case you don't know, she's a fictional TV character) for having a child out of wedlock as, "One of those lovely, loopy moments when American politics stumbles up against popular culture and careens off into the Twilight Zone." Whether you agreed with Quayle or not, unlike George Bush or Bill Clinton at the time, Quayle dared to move into an area of family values where, in the future, like it or not political angels will have to play their harps of gold. Interestingly, in a *Newsweek* interview on December 13, 1993, Clinton admitted, "There were a lot of good things in that Dan Quayle speech. The Murphy Brown thing was a mistake. It was too cute because this woman is not symbolic of the real problem in society. Would we be a better-off society if babies were born to married couples? You bet we would." But then Clinton carefully modified his views. "Just so long as we make it clear that we are not advocating that young people who become pregnant choose abortion over childbirth. But we are going to have to reestablish the conditions in which the family can flourish." Unfortunately, as yet, Clinton hasn't dared to spell out the basic details—thorough sex education, birth control, and planned parenthood.

As Klein pointed out more explicitly, "The solid, secure, two-parent family Quayle posited as an antidote to urban violence and moral decay is a symbol that cuts close to the bone. . . . An explosion in crime, child abuse, learning disabilities, welfare dependency, and many other social problems are the direct result of divorce, and out-of-wedlock birth rates in the United States, and some kind of valid family structure that cannot be achieved by a single parent."

Later Quayle dared to go a step further. "It sometimes seems that we have two cultures, the cultural elite, and the rest of us. . . . Many in the cultural elite sneer at the simple but hard virtues, modesty, fidelity, and integrity. . . . The elite's culture is a guilt-free culture. . . . It avoids responsibility and flees consequences. . . . Confronted with life's great moral issues, a sneer is not an answer."

In that speech Quayle sounded a deep-down American belief that we must do something to fend off the potential decline and fall of the American empire. But because he didn't have answers on how to fight moral decadence, he soon was hoisted on his petard. Responding to the hypothetical question, "How would you react if your daughter wanted to have an abortion?" Quayle answered, "She should make her own decision," which contrasted sharply with the opinion of his wife, Marilyn, that if their thirteen-year-old got pregnant she would make her bear the child.

Daniel Bell, writing in the *New York Times,* July 26, 1972, offers another point of view. "What may be happening is an unravelling of the middle class and the erosion of its comfortable expectations for the American future. . . . This generation may be the first in American history who will leave it's children poorer than itself. . . . We may be at the end of old ideologies, and old history, but there are no unified beliefs to take their place, only the splintering of culture."

The *Wall Street Journal* tackled the problems in an "American Civilization" series of articles and pointed out on July 27, 1992, that three-fourths of all Americans believe that the country is on the wrong track, with Peter Drucker seeing little difference "in the upsurge of tribalism occurring in America, dissolving shared values" from what was occurring in Yugoslavia. In a continuation of the series called "Future Imperfect" (August 11, 1992), the people of the thirty-something generation "fearing the loss of the American Dream are convinced that their parents had more cause for optimism." Later, John Updike (September 16, 1992) saw "a nation frustrated by its own dreams . . . an America turning inward . . . the extended family is gone, the traditional nuclear family is eroded by divorce and changing life styles. . . . What remains is self and its lonely quest for transcendence beyond self." Concluding the series Dennis Farney (October 28, 1992) discussed the continuing loss of middle-management jobs and various economic factors "forcing America to redefine its idea of America." Like the other worriers, he failed to show how.

Ultraconservative Irving Kristol, writing in the *Wall Street Journal* in December 1992, asked why the issue of "family values" fizzled so badly for the Bush/Quayle presidential campaign. Kristol's ostrich-style answer was, "There is no failure. Many of the changes in family we observe are simply the side effects of affluence. . . . Why this increase in sexual activity? You can't expect modesty (to say nothing of chastity) from girls who worship Madonna. Nor does public policy know how to discourage promiscuity. We provide these girls with a 'sex education' that is blandly nonjudgmental toward sexual activism. . . . Afterwards in the name of compassion, we offer food, shelter, medical care to the young mothers of illegitimate children with no hint of official disapproval."

What is Kristol's solution? He has none except to excoriate the public schools "which are securely in possession of an educational establishment that is infused with the counter-culture values of the 1960s, and there is no point of trying to inject family values into these institutions. They will debase and corrupt the very idea while pretending to celebrate it.

In a sexually sane society, teachers in the later grades of high school during courses in human sexuality would be encouraged to discuss not only Madonna but Anita Hill and Clarence Thomas, William Kennedy Smith, or any current problems of sexual deviance and sexual morality, and teachers would help young people acquire a sound value structure for their lives.

But first, to underwrite the necessity for the final sex revolution, here are a few more excerpts from those who moan and cry shame but don't dare to face twenty-first-century realities.

Lawrence Criner, associate editor of the *World & I* magazine, in the *Wall Street Journal,* July 23, 1993, discusses America's teenage pregnancy rate—the highest in the world with more than a million—and three million young people contracting sexually transmitted diseases. He lambastes Surgeon General Joycelyn Elders's "condom relief." "Many fear that she will use her position as the nation's chief doctor for sex-ed evangelism. They expected her to lead a charge for national 'comprehensive' sex education curricula, possibly including teaching masturbation, and making it a valid option in pre-marital sex education that stresses birth control, as well as school-based clinics, and the acceptability of alternate life styles." Criner's solution? "Every school district should be turned into a battleground over condom distribution, alternative lifestyles, school-based clinics, and the rights of parents to have a say in what their children are being taught. The recent explosion over sex education in the New York City public schools—in which a school's chancellor was soundly defeated—should serve as a warning." Criner ignores the fact that millions of parents, all by themselves, are simply unable to combat the anything-goes morality of the entertainment industry or the incessant lack of caring human values being exposed daily by the media.

William Bennett, former secretary of education, who followed that with a federal tour of duty solving the drug problem, is the author of many books, including his recent *Book of Virtues.* In a *Wall Street Journal* article of December 10, 1993, he encapsulated all the problems. The repetition is worth reading because Bennett has no solutions except a return to a daydream past which seemed to work because freedom of sexual expression, despite the First Amendment, was largely prohibited.

> There are places where virtue is taught and learned. But there is a lot less than there ought to be. Earlier this year I released the Index of Leading Cultural Indicators. It showed that since 1906 there has been a 560% increase in violent crime. There has been a 400% increase in illegitimate births, a quadrupling in divorce, a tripling of the percentage of children living in single parent homes, more than a 200% increase in the teenage suicide rate, and a drop of 75 points in the average SAT scores of high school students. Today 30% of all births and 68% of black births are illegitimate.
>
> The U.S. ranks near the top in the industrialized world in its rates of abortion, divorce and unwed mothers. We lead the industrialized world in murder, rape and violent crime. And in elementary and secondary education we are at or near the bottom in achievement scores. But there are other signs of decay, ones that do not easily lend themselves to quantitative analysis. There is a coarseness, a cynicism, a banality and a vulgarity to our time. There are too many signs of a civilization gone rotten. And the worst of it has to do with our children. We live in a culture that at times seems almost dedicated to the corruption of the young, to ensuring the loss of their innocence before their time.

"What can be done?" Bennett asks. After musing that the real crisis of our time is spiritual, he insists, "We desperately need to recover a sense of the fundamental purpose of education, which is to provide for the intellectual and moral education of the young. . . . As individuals and as a society we need to return religion to its proper place. Religion, after all, provides us with moral bearings." But Bennett said previously, "Our first task is to recognize that it is foolish, and futile to rely *primarily* on politics to solve moral, cultural and spiritual afflictions."

Bennett is wrong. Laissez faire economics never worked, and neither will laissez faire moralities or situation ethics for millions of Americans who, despite high school diplomas, are sadly undereducated.

George Will, in the same time frame, December 13, 1993, wrote in *Newsweek,*

> The sociology of virtue is more problematic than in Jefferson's day because our society is saturated by prompting to degeneracy. . . . We made it—are making it. Much of it comes from the top down, a trickle-down culture that begins with the idea that the good life consists in satisfying every impulse. Many intellectuals have helped to supplant the moral categories essential to civilized living, replacing them with a thin-gruel vocabulary of "lifestyles" and "values" and "self esteem" . . . and now there is the idea of "victimization." . . . The age has obliterated human magnificence by linking banality with a non sequitur—the observation that every one has flaws, and the conclusion that therefore no one merits emulation. Having denied the reality of human excellence, we have also, as Delattre [Dean of Boston University's School of Education] says, "obliterated the reality of human depravity by the doctrine of moral equivalence of all life styles."

Since the Catholic and fundamentalist right wing vote in the United States will throw roadblocks in the road to the inevitable, final sex revolution, a brief update from Pope Paul VI, the encyclical *Humanae Vitae,* issued July 29, 1968, and Pope John's tenth encyclical, *Veritas Splendor* (The Splendor of Truth), reflects a common ground of thinking among the cultural gurus and the right-wing Protestants. Commenting in the *New York Times* (August 1, 1993) on Pope John Paul's visit to Denver, Peter Steinfels pointed out, "Many critics believe that *Humanae Vitae* contributed to the breakdown of sexual norms by undermining the church's credibility on questions of sexual morality in general, especially among the younger generation."

Twenty-five years later a survey made by the National Center for Health Statistics shows that only 4 percent of Catholics follow the Vatican directives. A majority of Catholics may disagree with fundamentalists on the inevitability of premarital sex, but have a common ground on abortion, adultery, euthanasia, and homosexuality. Meanwhile, while not departing from Pope John Paul's thinking, Pope John II, in *Veritas Splendor,* tries to show why moderns no longer make moral sense to one another. Analyzing the encyclical, Father Richard John Neuhaus (*Wall Street Journal,* October 8, 1993) covers the familiar ground. "Making sense, assumes that there is some truth about the matter in dispute. But when it comes to morality, it is widely assumed that there is no such thing as truth. Indeed 'moral truth' is thought to be an oxymoron. You have your 'values' and I have mine, and there discussion comes to a screeching halt. . . . John Paul II argues that Pontius Pilate's question, 'What is truth?' should be a discussion starter . . . and puts it repeatedly, 'Authentic freedom is ordered to truth.' "

But the real truth is that while a majority of Americans, even the 60 percent who don't go to church, admit to some belief in God (according to a *Time* cover story, December 27, 1993, even more, 69 percent, believe in angels) but most only give lip service to Jesus' command to follow him: "I am the way, and the truth and the life" (John 14:6). Even the Confucians and Buddhists are looking for Tao, "the way," but most people agree with the Spanish poet Antonio Machado, who wrote, "Wayfarer there is no way to go. One makes the way by going."

Since my contention is that finding the way and making it work requires national leaders who believe, like B. F Skinner in *Beyond Freedom and Dignity,* that if you want better people you must create better environments, I'll wrap up this survey of those searching for tomorrow with the problems that Bill Clinton is facing when he tries to use his presidency as a bully pulpit to help create new family values and sexual sanity now.

Inheriting a "hands off" view of government initiated by Ronald Reagan and half-heartedly continued by George Bush, which the *New York Times* labeled the Reagan curse on Clinton, the philosophy extends beyond economics to whether the federal government has any right to meddle in American values and morality.

In his nomination speech at the 1992 Democratic convention on July 16, 1992, Clinton said, "I want an America where 'family values' live in our actions, not just our speeches. An America that includes every family. Every traditional family, and every extended family. Every two-income family, and every single-parent family, and every foster family." But Clinton qualified his "need for a new approach to government" by saying, "It's time for us to realize that there is not a governmental program for every problem."

I'm sure that Bill agrees with Hillary when in a speech in Texas, she stated, "We suffer from sleeping sickness of the soul ... we lack at some core level meaning in our individual lives, and meaning collectively, that senses that our lives are a part of some greater effort, that we are connected to one another." But as Anna Quindlen, writing in the *New York Times,* October 17, 1993, sadly pointed out, "Mrs. Clinton's remarks were ridiculed by journalists. ... Her speech sank like a stone in a swamp, largely unremarked and unremembered, inspiring no national debate or plan of action. In this speech, she spoke of a crisis far greater than any described by her husband in his call for universal health care."

I agree. Not since Franklin and Eleanor have we had a president and his wife who have tried to lead the way and give the country a new sense of national purpose. But for the Clintons it may be the equivalent of the Pilgrim's Progress and walking through "the slough of despond." Not only was he warned by the Vatican newspaper

L'Osservatore Romano not to open the door to a fresh discussion of "fundamental" moral issues, but the editors specifically referred to abortion and euthanasia.

Ultimately Clinton, or a future president, must challenge Catholic doctrine which refuses to make the connection between increasing abortions and a new generation who could easily be taught the complete whys, wherefores, and hows of birth control, including really "safe" periods in the menstrual cycle, along with the joys of planned parenthood. And eventually an improved version of the morning-after pill, RU 486, may eliminate the current choice and pro-choice insanities and make it a private decision.

In August 1993 the headline was: "The President Using His Bully Pulpit and Preaching Values." In addition to agreeing with Dan Quayle Clinton told an interfaith breakfast gathering on August 30, 1993, "I think the environment in which we operate is entirely too secular." At Yale University on October 9, 1993, he said, "I think God wants us to sit and talk to one another and see what values we have and how we can put them inside the millions and millions of Americans who are living in chaos." In *Time* magazine on December 3, 1993, Clinton dared to state, "I don't want to see society get in a position where the message is, If you get pregnant, it's better to have an abortion than have a child. What we need is an approach that recognizes the whole problem: the family breakdown, the moral breakdown, the total absence of traditional economic opportunity."

But, then, agreeing that crime, drug abuse, and violence are byproducts of the breakdown of the family, the community, and disappearance of jobs, Clinton once again puts the burden on each of us: "Some of this cannot be done by the government. We must reach deep inside to the values, the spirit, the soul, the truth of human nature. None of the other things we seek to do will ever take us where we need to go."

Dissenter James Carroll, columnist in the *Boston Globe,* on December 14, 1993, like many others, worried,

> The crisis of American violence has prompted President Clinton to mount the bully pulpit, despite the risk of falling from it. . . . In becoming an advocate of a new ethic of personal and family responsibility, Clinton dares to violate the liberal taboo against preaching in public. He bemoans "the great crisis of the spirit." He proposes to "counter violence with values." In a Memphis church, he invokes Martin Luther King, and a press aide cites the influence of Stephen L. Carter's book *The Culture of Disbelief.* . . . President Clinton knows that a recovery of American conscience requires the rescue of public moral discourse . . . but the President must not use talk of religion and values in the way so many politicians do. . . . We are right to distrust preachers who exempt themselves from moral judgment.

That was written before the *American Spectator,* a far-right magazine, printed an article titled "His Cheating Heart," in which two Arkansas state troopers, Clinton's security guards when he was governor told a lurid story about arranging sexual rendezvous for Clinton. Hopefully, true or not, millions of Americans will agree that presidents, too, would benefit from a new America where sexual sanity prevails.

But, alas, even the best known cultural guru of them all, Rush Limbaugh, vociferously spouting millions of words, and getting hundreds of thousands more into print in his books, *The Way Things Ought to Be,* and *See, I Told You So,* only offers the same "We gotta return to the good old days" philosophy. In his last epic, detesting liberals and Democrats and insisting "We, the conservatives are winning," Limbaugh offers a final chapter and "Prescription for the Future" for the Republican party, which, leaving aside his Reaganesque economic beliefs for better or worse, tells us: "We should vigorously promote educational choice and the voucher system to instill competition in our failing schools." And in the area of family values (covering all the problems I have listed), Limbaugh tells Republicans, "Despite the constant sermonizing by the media, Republicans did not lose the Presidency because they were 'co-opted by the right wing values.' The case for values simply was not made effectively and persuasively. Call it family values, traditional values, or whatever you want: what is important is that conservatives capitalize on this opportunity for them to explain that traditional values are what make the society work—what hold it together."

For Rush the traditional values etched in stone are the Ten Commandments, but search through his books and you'll find no answers on how to indoctrinate a new generation, or create new environments and better people. At the same time Limbaugh calls himself a fuzzball and his "pull yourself up your own bootstraps" economics are pretty fuzzy.

The Horatio Alger (Newt Gingrich) philosophy has some merits, if we create capitalistic environments where most people can carry it out. I recommend Limbaugh's chapters surveying "How to Win the Culture War" and "Dan Quayle Is Right" in *See, I Told You So,* which cover all the moral/values problems of the mid-1990s. But, interestingly, in the sexual values areas, he doesn't challenge the right-wing fundamentalists or the Catholic church, neither of which are dealing with sane sexual reality. Why? Because obviously Limbaugh knows that they are among the conservatives (including Ross Perot, who he dislikes), who he expects to triumph and return to power to dictate their version of twenty-first-century moralities,

Rush is the kind of Socratic gadfly (I'm surprised he doesn't use the term). But he's no longer declaiming an out-of-power point of view. I hope that he, and the Christian Coalition, and the New Republican Congressional majority get on board with me—the Last Puritan—and endorse the New Sexual Morality and Education legislation that I am proposing in the next chapter. Whether you are liberal Democrat or conservative Republican, it's the only long-term solution that will work.

3

The New Sexual Morality
and Education Legislation

Take a deep breath. In this chapter I'm going to give you a fast scan of some very limited federal legislation that would cost relatively little and wouldn't conflict with the First or Fourteenth Amendments to the Constitution.

Assume that ultimately I will convince some top congressional leadership that our basic social problems, which I have outlined, can be solved only by creating a sounder moral environment, and that this cannot be done by parents, teachers or clerics without help from the top, followed by majority American agreement at the polls. Let's also assume that a senator or representative—"Leslie Lovemore"—introduces the Lovemore bill in the House or Senate. Such legislation is more likely from a woman, and since seven million more women vote in national elections than men, I'm sure it will be more certain of passage. Without putting it in legal language, here's the essence of it.

It would create a new federal agency—a Future Families of America Commission—with a relatively small budget, $100 million to $200 million. The commission would be staffed by a carefully chosen group of male and female educators, clerics, and business leaders. They would have broad functions in the areas of family stability and education from kindergarten through a four-year undergraduate program (K-16). The FFAC would work closely with the Departments of Education and Health and Welfare.

Keep in mind as you read this brief survey of FFAC's functions that once the legislation was passed it would be put into effect gradually, over a four-year period. In the remaining chapters of this book I will expand the raisons d'etre, as well as the potentials in various areas. Obviously, as Hillary Rodham Clinton has done with health care, Ms. Lovemore would conduct a six-month-to-a-year interim assessment of all the public pros and cons in which you as the reader of this book are welcome to participate.

The Future Families of America Commission would not only consult with selected monogamous families, exploring and evaluating the reasons for the success or failure of particular families, but it would underwrite experiments in new-style extended family relationships in which carefully chosen couples could participate. They would discover and learn how to cope with interpersonal problems with and the potential of multilateral relationships such as *ménage à trois* (one woman and two men or two women and one man) or group marriages, all of which might be legalized, including a concept of corporate marriage and family corporations of up to three couples and their children. Merged families could not only provide health and nursing care for each other (thus reducing the need for external health care and nursing homes) but could offer alternating child care among the participants, as well as offer a wider variety of role models. In addition, they could increase the merged families' monetary viability.

Future Families of America would propose optional federal legislation and funding in all public schools for a one-hour-a-week course following the *Guidelines for Comprehensive Sexuality Education (Grades 1-12)* proposed by the Sex Information and Education Council (SIECUS—located at 130 West 42nd Street, New York, New York 10036). But the FFAC will go one step further and for grades ten thorough twelve will redesign the one-hour weekly courses so that trained teachers can unflinchingly teach a younger generation about the long history of pornography and devalued human sexuality.

Teachers in these later grades would deal with sex-related news stories such as the Anita Hill/Clarence Thomas conflict, the William Kennedy Smith case, and even the problems of presidents straying from monogamy. They would show X-rated videos and explore the many aspects of devalued human sexuality portrayed in the media, movies, television soap operas and talk shows, as well as the long history of pornography. The hour per week in the last three years of high school could be scheduled for early evening hours so that parents could attend with their children, if they wished. From the ninth grade, teachers of the weekly hour-long courses in human sexuality would try to convince all young people that responsible sex and loving was the greatest source of human happiness. But child bearing before they finished their Guaranteed Undergraduate Education (see below) would put them at the bottom of the economic ladder. And even though they would be fully cognizant and trained in birth control, they should delay sexual merger until their seventeenth birthdays with "petting," as it was once called, and masturbation alone, or together with a person of the other sex. For those who could not wait (which I'm sure would please Joycelyn Elders), masturbation is recognized as a temporary and recommended teenage behavior, during which two people can share the wonders of their genital responses, and the release of a mutually effected, caring human orgasm.

It should be noted that while this approach contravenes current Catholic and fundamentalist teaching, the federal funding would be optional and could be turned down by any local school board. The presumption is that gradually as the New Moral Sexual and K-16 Education program takes hold, and is encouraged by many religious leaders, along with a new approach to media ratings (see   ) that there will be many isolated groups who will object.

Future Families of America would also propose and campaign for a voluntary, new, self-imposed rating system for the arts. A "Sexually Natural" (SN) rating would include and permit all portrayals of naked human beings in movies, television, the arts, and all the media. The SN rating would also approve all caring one-to-one sexual mergers and oral sex between heterosexual couples past the age of seventeen. All Sexually Natural productions could be shown on national network television, on film in movies, and in the arts with no restrictions. A self-imposed producer rating of "Sexually Devaluing" (SD) would be required on all portrayals of what the Commission lists as deviational, or obviously non-caring sex. Productions with SD ratings could not be shown in movie theaters or national television (except paid cable). Like cancer warnings on cigarette packages, SD warnings would appear prominently, perhaps with the statement "May be injurious to your mental health."

"Sexually Devaluing Now" (SDN) and "Sexually Devaluing Historically" (SDH) ratings would permit, documentaries and fictional stories portraying the realities of devalued sex, as it may still be occurring nationally or globally, as well as historical portrayals of deviational and devalued sex on national television and in movie theaters, but accompanied by appropriate warnings that these productions reflect a time, and climate, of sexual sickness. Productions with SDN or SDH ratings must be accompanied by a foreword or afterword from the producer/ director or writer revealing his/her motivations in offering such a film or video. "Ultra Violent" (UV), another self-imposed rating, would indicate movies that also could not be shown on network television or in theaters but would be available as they now are on paid cable channels and through video rental. Since SDH and SDN films and programs with producer/director or writer raison d'etre observations, before or after the film or video, would be popular, and give wide audiences a chance to agree or disagree with the self-imposed ratings, there would be no lack of violent and sexually degraded portrayals, but they would be sharply contrasted with sane human behavior.

Ratings on all creations that might not be as sexually explicit as SN films and videos, and might depict some constrained violence, will carry a self-imposed "Not Primarily Sexual or Violent" (NSV) rating which would replace the PG and

PG-13 ratings. Keep in mind that all ratings would be appraised by FFAC, as well as all the media. Producers trying to bypass SD or SDH ratings with an NSV rating would receive wide negative publicity

A final rating would be "Gay Sex" (GS)—gays or lesbians naked and making love—which could not be shown on network television or theaters but would be available, as now, on videotape. The reason for the exclusion of graphic gay and lesbian sex-making is that it does not reflect the fundamental function of sexual merger—procreation, even if procreation must be limited to zero population growth (two children). In essence, caring, heterosexual sex and the naked human body would be liberated as a normal, wondrous aspect of life. While devalued sex would be available, as now, my guess is that it would only appeal to a small fringe group. Similar ratings to the above would be applied to books, all the print media, as well as photographs, recorded music, video games, ROM computer discs, and online computer transmissions.

Since display of the human body would be liberated from censorship, FFAC would propose that being naked where it was convenient to be naked on federal lands and seashores be permitted. Actually, at the moment, there is no federal law against this. Defining this as federal policy would lay the groundwork for state laws that would make it legal for anyone, young or old, who wished to enjoy the sun, air, and water naked in the out-of-doors, swimming, sunbathing, gardening, mowing lawns, or playing games together. Engaging in public sexual contact would be illegal, and being naked on streets, driving, public transportation, or at work would be prohibited.

At the same time that the human body and caring human sexuality comes out the closet, the Future Families of America Commission, in combination with the federally funded grade and secondary school course in human sexuality and many religious leaders, would advocate a national program to make caring sexual merger, which all young people have grown up watching on television and in the movies, a celebrated rite of passage on each person's seventeenth birthday, and after graduation from high school.

This would coincide with the Guaranteed Undergraduate Education legislation. Even before the GUE legislation is proposed it will be evident that the $1.5 billion National Service Trust Program that is now destined to continue through 1996 isn't going to work and will turn into a huge boondoggle. As a sounder alternative, and underlying the foundation of the New Sexual Morality and Education legislation, the Lovemore bill will offer an entirely new approach to education—K-16—public education in the twenty-first century covering the first twenty-one years of life instead of the first twelve. Such education is soundly based on new longevity statistics. Americans are living longer and during the first quarter of their lives have time for necessary, extended education.

Eliminating practically all federal educational subsidies costing billions of dollars, Congress would pass legislation that would underwrite a guaranteed four-year undergraduate education for all *unmarried and childless high school graduates with C grades or better.* The guarantee would be based on a thirteen-week work and study cycle similar to that being offered by Northeastern University and several other universities. Unmarried high school graduates who must continue unmarried and childless for four years (no summer vacations), based on their high school grades, could pursue a bachelors degree or several vocational degrees. All manufacturing and service businesses employing ten or more people would be required to hire a percentage of work study students, who would be paid an established hourly rate. All businesses employing work study students would receive tax credits against this segment of their payroll. Weekly wages, less 10 to 15 percent, for clothing and entertainment, would be paid directly to the colleges or universities at which the student/worker was enrolled. Employers would receive no tax credits for hiring young people who were still attending high school, or had not graduated from high school.

The federal subsidy would be available to all participating colleges, universities, and vocational schools for the costs of room, board, and tuition not covered by the earnings of students on the thirteen-week work cycle. On the financial side GUE would be controllable and the savings in billions of dollars in state and federal education expenses would keep the costs down. Education would become an industry that employed millions more people than it does now. Youngsters graduating from high school and jobless would be kept off the unemployment market. Even more importantly, every American would be given an opportunity to earn his/her own education directly, not through charity work, but as a valuable part of the mainstream market economy, with no loans to pay back after they graduate. At the same time the annual million teenage pregnancies would disappear as young people suddenly realized that if they were married, or unmarried and responsible for creating a child, they couldn't apply for the GUE program—or welfare. On top of that, the sex education program, coupled with the GUE program, would completely change the direction of secondary education. With the exception of ongoing, continuous, complete computer training, no vocational courses would be offered in secondary schools. The emphasis in high school would be totally on the liberal arts and expanding the mental horizons of all future citizens.

In addition to the basic Guaranteed Undergraduate Education, Future Families of America would also propose an optional Roommate of the Other Sex Program (ROSP), which would be available to all unmarried and AIDS-free high school graduates at selected universities and colleges. Exposing and conditioning young people to the possibilities of nonbiological extended families, the ROSP program would also function on a work study basis. Participating students would be assigned roommates of the other sex—four different roommates over the first two years—with at least one roommate of another race or ethnic culture. Called Premars (premarital), they would be encouraged to enjoy caring sex with each other, many for the first time as the entire program was in gear. Organized in groups of twenty-four couples, or forty-eight students, in addition to their undergraduate studies, they would meet daily in hour-long human values sessions run by graduate students during which they would explore all aspects of their sexual drives as well as their growing abilities in self-revelation and the confirming of each other as loving, caring humans.

So there it is. Is it all a wild daydream—an unachievable utopia? If you think so, then what are the alternatives? There's only one. America with a 50 percent increase in population by 2050, becoming a second-rate banana republic with diminished democracy and individual freedoms as it drifts into a class struggle between a totally franchised, but vastly uneducated majority, and the 5 percent who have the monetary power and who eventually will align themselves with a new breed of benevolent dictators.

Before you say impossible, come fly with me and explore a new way of living, loving, learning, laughing, and ludamus, a contract with America that would give all Americans a new sense of national purpose.

4

Being Naked with You Is the Most Important Thing in My Life

Many years ago I wrote a book called *The Love Adventurers,* in which "Being Naked with You" was the title of one of the chapters. I was referring to both mental and physical nakedness. Teaching the how to's of self-disclosure, and achieving mental intimacy with more than one other person, should be a basic concept of the K-12 course in human sexuality. Later, when teenagers are seventeen, it will become the joyous prelude to sexual intimacy. But first we must lay the groundwork and get rid of the biblical Adam-and-Eve association of shame and evil with being bodily naked.

In the coming chapters I will explore the completely new approach to K-12, public school education made possible by New Moral legislation that would legalize nudity, fund public school courses in human sexuality, free the depiction of caring sexmaking, and force a new, self-imposed rating system on all the arts.

I'm not going to detail the guidelines for a one-hour-a-week course on human sexuality that would be federally funded. The guidelines I have previously mentioned, published by SIECUS in a fifty-page booklet, are available to you for $5.75. They are organized around four age levels with key concepts and topics in each level that include human development, relationships, personal skills, sexual behavior, sexual health, and society and culture. In the new moral environment I am proposing, specific approaches for all grade levels could be changed to accommodate the changing sexual environment made possible by the Lovemore legislation. But, even now, the SIECUS guidelines for the primary grades are soundly developed. In later grades, the new sexual environment, combined with GUE, will condition teenagers to delay sexual merger until after their seventeenth birthdays.

As I write this only about twenty states have mandated that all school districts provide sex education in public schools, yet most of this education is a far cry from the SIECUS guidelines. There are many parents, groups, associations, and religious leaders who approve of only the most basic sex education. As we explore various areas such as being physically naked I will include their objections. They may reflect your own feelings. But you must keep in mind the larger perspective of achieving sexual sanity now, and not ending up with a police state and a "benevolent dictator" who resolves our moral problems his or her way. In the meantime, if you haven't seen the Children's Workshop production *What Kids Want to Know About Sex and Growing Up,* intended for children eight years old and up, borrow it from your video store (some stores offer free rental). This hour-long tape with children of all races, colors, and religious backgrounds participating is a partial preview of what could be accomplished.

Early in the twenty-first century, when the Lovemore bill becomes law, Americans, young and old, can, on their own option, be happily naked together where it is convenient to be naked, thus defusing the female body as a sexual come-on. In *Becoming a Sexual Person,* which is widely used in undergraduate courses in human sexuality, but will now be used in the tenth to twelfth grades, Robert Francoeur offers a letter from a Norwegian who was raising her teenagers in the United States. She wished her children could have grown up in a saner sexual environment. Her letter gives a little perspective on the final sex revolution in United States.

> At the age of ten, we learned all about our bodies, and those of the opposite sex. This provided no thrill or titillation for us because almost everyone in the town swam and sunbathed nude and many families were nude at home. We learned about boy's erections, and masturbation for both sexes and how it is pleasurable. We learned exactly how intercourse occurs, and how each partner arouses the other by foreplay.

In the federally funded courses on human sexuality, the K-12 generation will learn the history of human nudity. They will discover that humans, as distinguished from other animals and monkeys, began covering their bodies with animal skins and cloth, not from modesty, or shame of their genitals or mammaries, but to keep warm. Gradually humans discovered that clothing and furs, feathers, beads, tattoos, juices from berries, colored earth, and later metals (armor and helmets) could give one a distinct individuality. Change your image, and you could convince friend or foes, visually at least, that you were superior to others. Females decorating their bodies were sure they were more sexually attractive. Males, with their not-too-impressive bobbing penises, wearing bristling uniforms covering their genitals, looked more powerful. Properly clothed, kings and priests, insisting they were descendants of deities, expected to be praised, rewarded, and obeyed. Later generals, presidents, and prime ministers, without a direct pipeline to God, expected the same. Imagine Napoleon or Hitler naked, or any one of their contemporaries naked, trying to convince their people to go to war. Maybe the ultimate freedom of expression in the twenty-first century will be to use computer imaging techniques, as was done in the film *Forrest Gump,* and recast our leaders and cultural gurus haranguing us with their genitals dangling.

Young people will learn that in the past their parents believed that children being naked together with adults was linked to child pornography and encouraged pedophilia. Being naked after puberty was even worse and was not only shameful but sexually titillating, or in the vernacular "down and dirty."

Very few children, growing up or in old age, ever saw their parents or other relatives, including grandmothers and grandfathers, naked. We knew our friends and relatives by their faces, and we never saw them as complete persons with genitals, buttocks, and breasts (firm or sagging). By the turn of the century female beach wear for young women permitted display of naked buttocks and partially revealed breasts, and daytime elasticized miniskirts covered but sexually accentuated female behinds. Many women, displaying their butts, crack and all in Lycra, would be horrified to be told that God, or whoever designed their bodies, fully intended her swinging derriere to be a sexual come-on for the male, and *she* may be guilty of sexual harassment.

Because live or pictured human nudity is such a constant monkey on the back of saner approaches to human sexuality in the United States I invite you as a dubious futurist who must vote for a new sexual morality to take a fast look at the past fifty years of sexual insanity.

Male or female, today, if you should answer your doorbell naked (God forbid the caller might be of the opposite sex) you would be instantly categorized as morally loose—even a dirty old man, or a bit whorish, as the case might be. Local chapters of Morality in Media are incensed at many television shows, or R or NC-17 movies shown in local shopping malls. Most of these films offer quick glimpses of female nudity, and sex-making with no graphic views of genitals. A 1972 movie version of my novel *The Harrad Experiment,* in which several of the Harrad students are shown swimming naked together (including Don Johnson and Laurie Walters frontally naked), has never been shown on network television. But along with hundreds of R-rated movies, it is often run on paid cable television.

If you are male and were born before World War II, the only way you could discover what a mature female looked like naked was to go to a burlesque show. But you never saw a hairy female delta, or, God forbid, an exposed female vulva.

Your only hope in seeing a naked lady was in *National Geographic,* and she was black, usually with nose and lip ornaments, and had a decorously covered pubic bush. Or you could sneak into the stacks in your public library and look at plump, naked mythological ladies painted by Rubens, Tintoretto, or some Italian painter defying the Vatican. They all had pretty titties but, like Venus de Milo, no pubic hair.

Early in the 1940s a Baptist minister, Isley Boone, plump and way past middle age (proving that there is lots of potential encouragement in religious areas for sexual sanity) helped establish the American Sunbathing Association at Mays Landing, New Jersey. He made it clear that alcohol and being naked together was a no-no, but he extolled the benefits of family nudism, and as an unsung feminist insisted that a naked woman was a reflection of a loving God, and not Eve the seducer.

The American Sunbathing Association won the famous *Sunshine* case over the question of whether it was against the law to publish photographs of naked men and women revealing penises and female pubic hair. Prior to this time nudist magazines that published pictures of their members, many not young—with sagging bellies and breasts—were forced to airbrush pictures of both male and female genitals. The Supreme Court finally ruled that the human body was not obscene. But currently the court isn't too sure. In *United States* v. *O'Brien* (1990) the justices agreed that being naked in public places (nude dancing) was not protected by the Constitution.

The *Sunshine* decision made it possible for Hugh Hefner and Bob Guccione to publish pictures of completely naked women with unshaved deltas, but, even today, the only way that you can see live humans naked is to join a nudist camp. Also in the 1960s Broadway shows like *Hair, Jesus Christ Superstar,* and *Oh! Calcutta* drew huge audiences largely for the shock and amusement of seeing naked people on stage. Also in the 1960s, a new genre of films, "tits and ass" movies, flourished, making many producers like David Friedman, Kroger Babb, and Dan Sonney millionaires as American males flocked to rundown movie theaters to see nudist films and sexy stories (often with tacked-on morals to prove they had literary or artistic merit). During these films you could see not only beautiful female bodies but "soft core sex"—no visual merger of erect males into female vaginas.

Isley Boone didn't live to see the Pandora's box that the *Sunshine* case opened. The basic premise of social nudism is, and was, to enjoy the freedom of walking, playing, and swimming in the fresh air without the constraints of clothing, and at the same time to appreciate the miracle of the human body, young or old, and to desensitize children to nudity-as-sexuality, to show them that being naked with young people of the other sex need not be a prelude to sexmaking.

Obviously that is not the belief of Hugh Hefner or Bob Guccione, who became multimillionaires with their magazines and R-rated videos featuring glamorized, naked females in their twenties. In neither magazine will you ever find a naked woman past forty*—and never any naked guy with his penis showing. *Playboy* restrains itself from the so-called "beaver and crotch shots," that would totally reveal a woman's labia and vaginal opening, but *Penthouse* and the "skin magazines," including *Hustler,* go the full route with spread-legged women happily enticing male viewers. Teasing shots of complete female nudity (and sex with no graphic view of male penetration) have become the raison d'etre of R-rated films and videos. The male's neverending interest in the female body is encapsulated in an amusing book, *The Bare Facts Video Guide,* put together by Craig Hosda as a hobby. It lists several thousand R-rated movies in which your favorite Hollywood actor or actress has revealed some part of his or her anatomy never seen before. As I write this, *Playboy*'s 1994 mail-order promotion offers an official male survey of *"Playboy*'s perfect woman" and concentrates on her "body parts" and "sexual attitudes," with some generalizations about "her brains." Using new guidelines for human sexuality courses, grades ten to twelve, teachers will use *Playboy* and *Penthouse* with SDH ratings to show how prohibition of sexual wonder and curiosity turns to sick sex insanity.

Reading this chapter you may get the impression that I am envisioning a world where everyone walks around bareass, and as a byproduct everyone loves everyone else. No way. Most of the time sane people will wear clothing, but when there is complete freedom to play together naked in defined public play areas, and around one's home, one step on the road to sexual sanity will have been taken.

If you're still hung up on being naked alone, or with another person where it's convenient to be naked, you are not alone. A good example of muddled American reaction appeared in the *Grand Rapids Press* in 1993, which published an article, "Stripped of Pretense," about a local Forest Hills Club with 180 nudist (many prefer to be called naturists) members of all ages enjoying life sans clothing. The paper actually ran pictures in color of a naked mother with her three-year-old baby and a plump gentleman playing volleyball naked (with clothing he could have passed for president of a local bank). Calls and letters to the editor were outraged. Here are a few reactions. From a forty-two-year-old man: "You people are supposed to guide the community. People put a lot of stock in what you are portraying. You owe this community an apology—particularly families with children." From a thirty-year-old man: "You brought that nudist club into my home in front of my kids and wife. They were embarrassed. You should be, too. You are an

---

*Happily, for the first time, in the May 1995 issue of *Playboy,* Nancy Sinatra proves that forty-years-plus ladies can be pleasingly and erotically naked.

absolute jerk." One woman, age not given: "I wouldn't walk indecently clothed from the bedroom to the bathroom, if my children could see me. I have a real concern for what you are teaching our young people—so should you."

By contrast, the world-famous architect Richard Neutra pointed out in an article titled "Some Notes on the Complex of Nudism":

> We revere the early Greeks who portrayed the gods in their Pantheon in the nude ... but we cannot understand their acceptance of nakedness on almost all public occasions ... to them nakedness was natural. Today nudism is an "ism." It is something that separates nudists from the rest of society. Until it can assume the place it had in ancient Greek society nudism will remain outside the pall of general society ... the fact that clothes cover up the body offers a serious problem, worthy of consideration. *We need to understand the pathological consequences and threats to sound mating and matching and to general social balance that clothing creates in our society today.* (Emphasis added)

The church, mosque, and synagogue, in conjunction with the New Moral and Education legislation, can sacramentalize human sexuality and exalt the human body. The following excerpt from *The Seduction of the Spirit* by Harvey Cox, a professor at Harvard Divinity School, shows a religious path toward the final sex revolution. After experiencing the hot sulphur water tubs with a mixed group of people at Esalen in Big Sur, California, a place famous in the 1960s and 1970s for its explorations of the human potential, Cox wrote,

> It reveals that nakedness with other human beings can unite people spiritually ... Jesus wisely foresaw that once we accept others' ungainly parts, following his command about foot washing, and accept our most removed members, our spiritual separation from one another would already be in the process of healing. ... Dan Berrigan once expressed the theological meaning of flesh ... "it all comes down to this ... whose flesh are you touching and why? Whose flesh are you recoiling from, and why?"

In a later chapter I will cover the late twentieth-century activities of the American Sunbathing Association, the Naturist Society, and the Elysium Institute, all activists for a new generation who will discover that being naked together is not a prelude to sex orgies, but rather that naked men can calmly view naked women, and interact verbally with them, without getting an erection or wanting to have sex with them.

But, at the turn of the century, forty-seven states in the United States have varying laws prohibiting public indecency. The courts in seven states have upheld laws to prevent nude dancing, mostly female. Women dancing alone or in groups naked, or with men will be legal under NSM legislation, but would carry a self-imposed rating of SN or SD, depending on the style and intent. In 1993 the Indiana nude dancing prohibition was challenged by a nightclub owner and three women who said they wanted to dance without wearing panties and the G Strings required by law. A federal appeals court reversed a trial judge's conviction of the plaintiffs for indecency and concluded quite sanely that, "Nude dancing is inherently expressive." However, the judge failed to deal with the sleazy, nightclub environmental reality. A man or woman dancing naked in a nonalcoholic setting can be one of the many ways of exalting the human body, and like the appreciation of a beautiful sunset, embody a cosmic or religious feeling.

The case ended up in the Supreme Court, and in June 1991 Judge David Souter cast the pivotal negative vote. He deemed the Indiana law constitutional because it serves "the state's substantial interest in combatting secondary effects," meaning that repression and suppression of nudity is one way to minimize other potential evils such as prostitution, sexual assault, and presumably related violent crimes. Amusingly, in September 1994, the New York Transit Authority, in the case of two women who were contesting the double standards that allowed men to appear on subways bare chested, ruled that so far as they were concerned women could ride topless in the subway. Equal rights for sure, but the New York subway is not a place where it is convenient or practical for women to be even half naked.

The American sexual muddle over nudity and sex climaxed early in 1994 with Stephen Knox, an honors graduate student of Pennsylvania State University sentenced to five years in prison by a federal district court for violating the anti-child-pornography law. He had possessed videotapes of girls aged ten to seventeen dressed in bathing suits, leotards, and underwear in which the camera zoomed in on their pubic and genital areas, which were covered by clothes. Knox appealed, but the appeals court upheld his conviction and the Supreme Court returned the case for further hearing. Meanwhile, both Congress and the president got into the act. President Clinton told Attorney General Reno to draft new legislation. Accused of being soft on pornography he wanted "the Federal Government to lead aggressively in the attack against the scourge of child pornography." Reno responded with a proposal that would define as unlawful "the lascivious exhibition of the genitals or pubic area of any person, whether clothed or unclothed." The law would say such a display was illegal "if its purpose is eliciting a sexual response in the intended viewer even if the child did not know that the depiction is designed for such a purpose." But then more than a hundred Republican and Democrats joined the battle insisting that present laws were adequate and no new law was needed.

Reno's law would knock the props out of much of the sexual come-on advertising that sells American products. Writing in the *New York Times* on December 4, 1993, Marjorie Garber points out the reason for congressional interest. "It is everywhere evident that the high pop culture of the 1990s flirts with the most forbidden of all topics, the borderline between adult and child." She points out the prevalence of baby doll dresses, the current popularity of waif models; Nabokov's *Lolita* being a runaway bestseller in the 1950s; Elia Kazan's film *Baby Doll,* with a screenplay by Tennessee Williams; Amy Fisher being labeled the "Long Island Lolita"; the Coppertone kid losing her bikini bottoms to a frisky pup. "We eroticize the look of youth but are made nervous by sexy images of children. . . . If national attention is to be focused on defining child pornography what we need is not hasty legislation . . . but an informed conversation about the power and ubiquity of such images. . . . It ought to be possible both to safeguard children from exploitation and to acknowledge the importance in both high and popular culture of images of erotic youth."

The Comprehensive Crime Act was passed by Congress and signed by President Bush on November 29, 1990. Buried in that legislation is a clause that makes it a felony to knowingly possess books, magazines, videos or other matters that visually depict persons younger than eighteen engaging in sexually explicit conduct real or simulated. Previous legislation made it a crime to photograph, film, or videotape people under seventeen who were naked. The Lovemore bill and the New Sexual Morality legislation would resolve the problem by forcing a self-imposed SN or SD rating on child pornography, with the media and all concerned giving wide cease-and-desist publicity to lascivious sex exploitation of anyone young or old.

Before I wrap up this chapter with some of the effects on education at the K-12 level, take a look at a book called *Show Me.* It is now totally banned in the United States, and reveals American hangups about nudity and sex education, and young and old being joyfully naked together. First published in Germany in 1974, it was a coffee table book consisting of joyous photographs by Will McBride and a text explaining some of the mysteries of sex for young children. St Martin's Press published it in United States in 1974 and was forced to withdraw it within a few months. If it were republished today both the authors and publisher would be convicted of producing child pornography and would be serving time in prison.

In a saner world, books like this will be used in levels 1 and 2 of human sexuality courses. The 140 pages of pictures and text in *Show Me* begin with a naked three-year-old boy and girl talking to each other as they look at their penis and vagina (I'm sure that, like me, most of the readers of this book grew up "playing doctor" with the opposite sex). "I've got a penis and you don't!" the boy exclaims.

"So what? I've got a vagina." And the little girl lying on her back displays it. "Your penis is out where you can see it. But my vagina is inside. Isn't that great?"

The following pages, all with young children and their parents naked together, show a new baby nursing on her mother's breasts while the younger children watch. Growing up, the children are happy to see that a penis gets erect and a boy can also urinate through it. Pictorially, you see a girl grow up and become a young lady whose breasts are beginning to develop. Now older both the boy and girl are beginning to grow pubic hair. They play and wrestle together, and as naked children they talk about making love together someday. They spy on their older sister (she's sixteen) making love with her boyfriend. You see the three-year-old later as a fourteen-year-old examining a young naked pregnant woman, and you see kids who grow up playing games with each other naked, tumbling naked together with their parents.

In essence it's a sexually moral picture book for twenty-first-century children who grow up in a no-longer-sex-inundated society and no longer listen and hear daily about AIDS, and condoms, and rapes, and sex murders but instead learn about themselves as incipient caring sexual human beings.

Author, Dr. Helga Fleischauer-Hart points out, "Through these sensible, visual sexual processes taking place in their bodies, adolescents experience new situations with particular intensity: the transition from being a child to an adult. But on no account must the non-repressive sex education be equated with the recommendation of indiscriminate indulgence in sex." As Alex Comfort comments in his book *Sex in Society,* "It is virtually impossible to persuade a child by lecturing that sexuality is a perfectly worthy component of life, and that its exercise calls for some reasonable restraint as does other social conduct—if we ourselves are inhibited and irresponsible."

New federal laws permitting nudity on public lands and seashores, gradually spreading down and changing state laws, are sure to evoke moral shock, but like the SN (Sexually Natural) ratings in the arts which I will explore in the next chapter, the overriding message is that the human body and a man and woman making love is reverential. Long before Judaic, Christian, and Islamic beliefs the seeding ground of religion was sex wonder and worship. Eros merged with agape in the twenty-first century, is sitting on the church door steps waiting to be invited back in. Along with their religious leaders Americans can create a wholesomely naked and American nation, and restore the word "wholesome" to a loving American vocabulary, as defined by Webster: "promoting spiritual or mental health and well being; conducive to moral or mental soundness—beneficial to character."

The New Sexual Morality legislation is one giant step for all mankind that exceeds any steps in the future on the moon or in space. It will create a wholesome world where, in addition to the bedroom, a natural, wholesome place to see female breasts, vulvas and anuses, or a man's bobbling penis, is not in X-rated videos or men's skin magazines, but when they are playing together—tennis, golf, swimming, sailing, volleyball, soccer, basketball, bowling, or even simple croquet. In the process, naked sports will gradually lessen interest in the armored, all-male sports of hockey and football, because men battering each other to win artificially created goals will no longer be as interesting as a mixed team of lithe, physically fit men and women playing together clothed or unclothed. As for coed baseball, which would require testicle and female breast protection—joyous home runners could wave their jock straps or bras at the cheering crowds.

In this new world of sexual sanity, K-12 children, taking the federally funded course in human sexuality, will, in their gym activities, if approved by their parents, play together naked. Teachers would not discourage body tumbling or touching. By the sixth grade these young people would be fully aware of themselves as incipient sexual creatures, with the boys occasionally revealing unplanned erections and the girls developing breasts.

From the seventh grade to the twelfth, again on the option of the participants, coed sports could be played together naked on school grounds. Lockers and shower rooms would be combined, and neither the boys nor the girls would be embarrassed by natural body functions, including menstruation, during which the girls might wish to withdraw from physical activity. Teachers would emphasize, along with continuous conditioning by the media, parents and religious leaders, that sexual merger before one's seventeenth birthday is against all social values. Teenagers who think they are in love, or are simply testing their new found sexuality, should express it in the school areas with a friendly hug and defer sexual merger until after graduation.

On their own, graduating high school seniors will quite likely exchange naked pictures of themselves, and not only enjoy looking at them in later life but show them to their children, reminding them that physically there is little or no difference between the generations. Facially homely young people will discover that their bodies as a whole compensate for shortcomings in one area or another. They will discover, too, that *Playboy* and *Penthouse* were wrong. Small-breasted women, often with pear-shaped behinds, are just as physically attractive as their bigger-busted friends.

Ultimately, unlike John Kennedy and Lyndon Johnson, who swam in the White House pool naked, but alone or in male company (presumably Kennedy never swam naked with Jackie, but she did with Aristotle Onassis and he did with various other ladies), the president will often be seen on television swimming naked with his family, or jogging or sailing on the Chesapeake wearing nothing but a smile.

5

Educational Reform

Before I pursue the saner premarital and post-marital values, and happier sexual byproducts of the New Sexual Morality Education legislation, and show you the hows and whys and benefits of the self-imposed rating system on all the arts, along with the general acceptance of the naked human body, occurring in the same time frame as the K-12 Comprehensive Human Sexuality seminar, let's take a breather from from the sexual aspects of the final sex revolution, which may continue to horrify many readers but are the only feasible solution to our current malaise.

I want to show you how, ultimately, the additional four years of undergraduate education on a work study basis, guaranteed by the federal government, will give Americans a new sense of national purpose. GUE will not only recreate and revitalize public education with an entirely new sense of direction, but it will give all parents, and their children (families with children, both those below poverty level and the middle class), a new conviction that America is the land of opportunity, and all of us, rich and poor, are equals when it comes to achieving a full education.

So here's a fast survey of the failures public education from the primary and secondary grades through the undergraduate years during the past thirty years. It will give you perspective and show you how the Guaranteed Undergraduate Education feeds all the way back to K-12 education and resolves many of the problems listed in chapter 1.

When the Soviet Union launched Sputnik, the first manmade space satellite, in October 1956, followed by Sputnik II in November, Americans woke to the fact that in the realms of mathematics, science, and engineering the United States was no longer the world leader. During the next twenty years math and science courses in high school and as majors in colleges and in universities got a new lease on life. Sociology, psychology, and even business majors took a back seat.

Thanks to trillions of dollars spent on defense and presidents who were either determined to get to the moon first, or save the world with "Star Wars" techniques, we soon led the world militarily. The "evil empire" collapsed and was supplanted by a frenzy of nationalistic behavior. I've written a fantasy novel, *The Oublion Project,* showing how to resolve the ethnic and nationalistic war-making potential, but thus far it is unpublished.

Despite the Sputnik prod, during the next twenty-five years we didn't make much progress in the area of public and private education. Because of cutbacks in the defense budgets and arms manufacture (actually minuscule thus far in the mid-1990s) engineers have become a dime a dozen. Scholastic Aptitude Tests were showing no startling signs of improvement. The Japanese were showing that they might not excel in basic research but their high school graduates were far smarter and better educated than ours in the areas of math and science, and they knew how to move faster and turn our undeveloped research into profitable products. On top of that, a biotechnological revolution was plunging us, and the world, into sexual moral problems such as the potential of cloning, or "designer babies," with doctors proposing to use ovarian grafts from aborted fetuses to generate eggs to be used by infertile women, creating a world of children whose mothers were never born.

In April 1983 the National Committee on Excellence in Education panel, set up by Terrel Bell, Ronald Reagan's secretary of education released its report: "A Nation at Risk." It warned against "a rising tide of mediocrity" that threatened our future as a nation, and as a people, if the public schools and the education of the younger generation wasn't vastly improved.

The solutions offered combined parental commitment, new student motivation, and technological immersion (computers in every classroom) along with federally established national curricula in English, math, and science, plus new national SAT achievement standards. Bell also called on the states to pass Parental Responsibility Acts obliging parents to become actively involved their children's schooling.

President Reagan wasn't too interested. He had previously indicated he wanted to abolish the Department of Education. No one paid much attention to the reality. A decade later *we remain a nation at risk.* Meanwhile, although teachers' salaries have jumped 22 percent over the rate of inflation, rising from $22,000 annually to a national average of $33,000 in 1993, Scholastic Assessment Tests (a new name that hopefully takes a broader view of mental aptitudes) stopped falling but still haven't shown a significant upward turn as of the mid-1990s.

In 1991 President Bush told us, "We must transform the public schools. . . . We must not only challenge the methods and the means used in the past, but also the yardstick we have used to measure public progress." William Bennett, Bush's secretary of education, proposed a voucher system and school choice to force public schools to better themselves. He also advocated nationally standardized college entrance examinations, similar to those used in Japan and France, which high school graduates would have to pass before admittance to colleges and universities.

Writing in *Time* magazine on September 16, 1991, Walter Shapiro noted, "No issue cuts closer to the core of America since, of itself, the character of its public schools for education is the function of government closest to the people. Failure of the schools is a failure of the State—different in degree, but not far from, food lines in the Soviet Union."

The failure of the states and our federal government continues. School choice is no solution to the problems of primary and secondary education. As Shapiro pointed out, "Those assailing the public schools as a self-staffed monopoly that needs to feel the hot breath of free market competition raises the question is America fast becoming an Ayn Rand universe in which everything is measured by its price?"

In his America 2000 Education Strategy to Improve Elementary and Secondary Schools, Bush went all out for the voucher system, with individual states giving parents substantial sums (but less than the current annual per-student state cost of public school education) so that parents and children could choose their own private school . . . even if run in American style, of course, for profit. Part of the America 2000 proposal was that the federal government would offer $30 million in grants to design school choice experiments. It would also provide $200 million to help disadvantaged students participate in school choice programs, and allow them to change schools without losing federal aid.

Bush's tempest in the educational teapot generated the New American Schools Development Corporation, and the Edison Project (a byproduct of Chris Whittle's television in every classroom program) and in late 1993 Proposition 174 on the California ballot. In brief NASDC is a private, non-profit, tax-exempt organization "formed by American business leaders to support the design and establishment of new high performance learning environments that communities across the nation can use to transform their schools for the next generation of children." By January 1993, Nazzdec, as it is sometimes called, based in Alexandria, Virginia, raised initial capital of $40 million with direct donations from American industry. Eleven design teams are presumably developing and refining their prototypes for the best schools in the world. From 1993 to 1995 the designs will be tested in communities throughout America. The Clinton administration hasn't given the effort much publicity, With our $200 billion annual deficit, future Federal funding is unlikely. But on December 17, 1993, NASDC, which had been struggling to raise money, got a new lease on life. Billionaire Walter Annenberg made the largest gift ever to education, $500 million. NASDC will receive $50 million of the gift. The Coalition for Essential Schools located at Brown University will receive $50 million. They are committed to restructuring schools so that students are more engaged and taught in smaller, more personal settings. Annenberg's gift is to be made over several years and no doubt many other futurist educational groups will be funded, for better or worse.

Then there is Chris Whittle, super education-for-profit promoter, who conned many of the nation's 110,000 public schools into letting students listen to his Channel One, a daily 12-minute classroom news program with two minutes of commercials, by giving the schools free television sets. Whittle quickly moved on to a bigger and more profitable mixture of education and business. His new daydream, the Edison Project, would create a national chain of innovative public schools for profit that would totally revitalize American education. He sold the idea to Benno Schmidt, the former president of Yale University, who elaborated on it in a *Wall Street Journal* article (June 5, 1992), and in subsequent brochures from the Edison headquarters in Knoxville, Tennessee. "We are going to create a new conception and model for education for children from the earliest years through what we now think of as high school. . . . The aim is to provide a laboratory of educational innovation, new models of schools that the public schools can emulate if they wish . . . but the Edison Project will not rely on public funds, and takes no position on the wisdom of vouchers."

Whittle's original plan was two hundred "campuses" serving 150,000 students, the first to open by 1996. By 2010, two million students would be attending Edison Schools. But American investors had more sense. The Edison Project ran into deep financial problems. Whittle quit. The company was unable to raise the $2.5 billion needed for the first one hundred schools. Whittle Communications was supposed to invest $3 million in each school, which would then offer heavy emphasis on academics, art, and music and would be in session longer than public schools.

In the meantime, although their Edison Project "for profit public schools" was dying a noisy death, the debate whether public schools are obsolete goes on. In its October 31, 1994, issue, featuring "New Hope for Public Schools," *Time* surveyed the "grassroots revolt, parents and teachers seizing control of education" as a result of state subsidies to the charter-school movement. In Freeland, Michigan, Northlane Academy gets an annual $175,000 from the state lottery and Ron Helmer, a former school administrator, and two other teachers are using his garage and living room to teach students in grades 6-12, who are now enrolled in Northlane but no longer have to attend public schools.

Northlane is only one of many charter schools. Noah Webster Academy, a charter school that opened September 1994, has no classrooms. According to the *Wall Street Journal,* September 16, 1994, it is a network of two thousand students throughout the state who are taught at home by parents—many using a religious curriculum. Eleven teachers work out of a cabin in Ionia, Michigan, manning toll-free telephone help lines. The Academy plans to install a state-of-the-art computer network for text transmission, video lectures, and assignments.

The New Puget Sound Community School, a so-called "virtual school," among many other things, teaches its students to submit their homework by modem and communicate with other students by E-mail.

On a much larger scale Education Alternatives, a Minneapolis-based company, whose stock you can buy, in September 1994 signed a five-year contract with the Hartford public-schools board to manage Hartford's thirty-two public schools. The company has agreed to invest at least $20 million in Hartford schools, including $15.6 million during the first year for new computers and building repairs. Education Alternatives expects to make a good profit by splitting their saving per pupil with the city of Hartford.

Americans will have to learn the hard way that American schools cannot be operated the Ayn Rand/Newt Gingrich way as a profit-making business, and neither can education reform be mandated back to the states with block grants. Total education of all Americans is a national/federal responsibility, which can rekindle all Americans with a new sense of national purpose.

To top off the insanity, in March of 1995, the school board of Wilkinsburg, Pennsylvania, voted to turn over their public schools to Alternative Public Schools, a company recently formed by two Nashville, Tennessee, businessmen who have never operated a school before, but will be paid $5,400 per pupil to run the Wilkinsburg schools.

Meanwhile, in late 1993, vouchers and school choice became a state and ultimately national issue, when Proposition 174 appeared on the California ballot. If Proposition 174 had become law in California, parents would have had the option of using $2,600 in vouchers—less than half of what an average California public school spends—to send their kids to private schools. Conservatives and right-wing church groups spent millions to get the votes for Proposition 174, but teachers' unions spent more—$15 million—and it was defeated. While neither the teacher unions nor those in favor of vouchers and school choice have any sane solutions to the problems of public schools, vouchers are not a dead issue. As a *Wall Street Journal* editorial of October 25, 1993, scarily pointed out, "California's Proposition 174 is only the latest battle in a crusade to allow parents without extraordinary knowledge or resources to have some of the educational freedom of choice that insiders and the better-off already have. Anything less will perpetuate the caste system and the bottom rungs of opportunity will be cut off for children living in the wrong zip code."

Those who still extol school choice point to the success of choice in District

4 in East Harlem, where instead of vouchers a business-oriented teaching company was paid to take over District 4 schools. After a long battle the new Board of Education finally approved the program, which has brought vastly improved SAT scores and quality of schools to the area. A Carnegie Foundation report pointed out that while quality schools would be strengthened, weak schools would vanish entirely, leaving an unfilled educational vacuum. But the real problem, as I will show, is that K-12 education lacks the total liberal arts focus that GUE will make possible.

As an aside, in an article I wrote for the *Wall Street Journal,* I outlined my alternative GUE proposal, which would completely eliminate the "caste system." The paper refused to publish it.

So we arrive in the mid-1990s. In addition to the National Service Trust, Americorps, which I will cover in a moment, instead of America 2000, Clinton renamed the Bush educational proposal, and more than five years later Goals 2000, the Educate America Act, was passed by Congress, on March 26, 1994, after a bitter struggle over school prayer initiated by Sen. Jesse Helms.

With a billion dollars pumped in annually through 1999 by the federal government, the money is to be used by the states in their own programs with no overall federal guidance. The goals are: (1) all children in America will start school ready to learn; (2) students will leave grades four, eight, and twelve having demonstrated competency over challenging subject matter; (3) teachers will have access to programs for the continued improvement of their professional skills and the opportunity to acquire the knowledge and skills needed; (4) Students will be the first in the world in mathematics and science achievement; (5) every adult American will be literate and possess skills necessary to compete in a global economy, and exercise the rights and responsibilities of citizenship; (6) every school in the United States will be free of drugs, firearms, alcohol, and violence and will offer a disciplined environment conducive to learning; and (7) every school will promote partnerships that will increase parental involvement and participation in promoting the social, emotional, and academic growth of children.

It is interesting to note that while these goals are all directed at secondary schooling that will presumably prepare millions of high school graduates for further undergraduate education, the professional skills and math and science achievement will somehow be acquired without the additional four-year education. Other than Americorps there was no solution as to how these better-educated young people can afford the $100,000 cost of the additional four years. Unresolved also are the fourth-, eighth-, and twelfth-grade competency tests that will require a federal commission of some kind to determine.

Amusingly, and a far cry from the twenty-first-century GUE programs, is that the education act was passed at the same time as the annual spring undergraduate vacations. An estimated million or more undergraduate students were taking a "spring break" in Florida and Mexico, which becomes an anything-goes alcoholic saturnalia during which, according to one student, "All the girl/guy tensions get thrown out the door. The girls can get naughty before they go back to their regular lives, and the guys can go crazy and don't have to worry about getting into trouble—a free-for-all."

Unlike Goals 2000 and Americorps, NMSE legislation will create a secondary school liberal arts educational environment for all students that can be readily measured, and the K-12 sexual education, with one's seventeenth birthday as a rite of adult sexual passage, the GUE, human values seminars and work study programs (all of which I will detail in coming chapters) will give all young people a personal sense of purpose that is totally lacking in either Goals 2000 or Americorps.

Ultimately, like Americorps, the results of the revised Goals 2000 will be ephemeral and largely unmeasurable. Goals 2000 will not get to the heart of the problem. Nor has the 1994 education secretary, Richard Riley, formerly governor of South Carolina, put much fuel onto the dying embers of failed solutions to our education problems.

William Bennett and Lamar Anderson (who announced in 1995 that he was a presidential candidate)—both former secretaries of education—along with Newt Gingrich, are urging the abolition of Education as a cabinet position. Bennett's 1994 book, *The Devaluing of America—The Fight Over Culture and Our Children,* should be required reading for parents of high schoolers, particularly pages 51–64, in which he describes a sound approach to secondary education.

But it soon becomes apparent in the book that Bennett is an enthusiast for the voucher system. His reasoning seems to be that this is the only way to control the National Education Association, which actually is a power lobby with more money than the National Rifle Association, and perhaps even more dangerous. Bennett points out that NEA practically runs and controls the education department and its policies, and he is the only one who ever dared to challenged some of its policies.

Bennett was probably the best secretary of education ever. He may not approve of NSME legislation but when it's passed, the Federal Families of America Commission should insist that whoever is President, Republican or Democrat, reappoint Bennett as secretary of education. With a revitalized cabinet position and with these new approaches to secondary education, Bennett could force Albert Shanker, or whoever is in charge of NEA, to straighten up and fly right. And I'm sure that no one would object if Bill's *Book of Virtues* became required parental reading, at least!

Before I move into the current fiascos in undergraduate education, I recommend that you read *School's Out* by Louis Perelman, a corporate planner. He offers the ultimate science, no-fiction, fantasy to top them all. "Hyperlearning" is the future of education and, according to him, will resolve the problems of vouchers, school choice, public schools, and even undergraduate degrees, "which don't matter." Firmly ensconced on the "information highway" roller coaster, daydreamer Perelman is convinced that "school" is obsolete. In the future anyone can learn anything and everything better from the electronic media and teachers on your computer/television tube, and do it at a faster pace than you can ever do it in public or private schools at any level of education. And it will be big business with home schooling, and "micro vouchers" available (state or federally financed) to provide pay-per-view telecourses in every subject imaginable.

In Perelman's future world live teachers don't inspire kids, they learn without live peer group interaction. They do not compete for grades. They need none of the socialization that schools and college provide as they mature, but somehow with the "ghosts in the machine," superior teachers as role models, they will acquire a sound moral ethic to live by. "For most adults and many youth, school will not be identified with any distinct building or location, but rather with a brand or franchise of media through which services are accessed. Home technology—video, audio, computer, telephone—is far more adroit at meeting diverse life cycle needs for entertainment, information, work and learning than is the technology of conventional academic structures."

In November 1991 the Census Bureau released its report on school enrollment and the economic characteristics of students as of 1989. You can be sure there has been little or no change since then—except for the worse. Of the 13.2 million students enrolled in the nation's colleges and universities, 40 percent, or five million, were twenty-five years old, and three million were thirty or older—showing that relatively few older people are trying to remedy their lack of education beyond high school.

Of these students, according to the *Boston Globe* in September 1993, 41 percent are part-timers, which means they are pursuing college degrees at colleges, universities, and community colleges, and acquiring credits toward a degree that may take many years, or they finally give up due to economic pressures and lack of time. Actual figures are hard to come by, but in Massachusetts there were 71,000 part-time students in the 1990, out of a total of 333,546 students pursuing undergraduate degrees, presumably full time. In any case thousands of students were priced out of full-time study, and had to go at it part time or not at all. Projections for 2002, nationwide, are that 5.7 million of the 13.7 million students will be working part time.

When President Clinton announced his National Service Plan with direct student loans from the federal government, which would replace the guaranteed student loan program, which is the basis of the business of Sallie Mae (Student Loan Marketing Association—with 47 billion dollars in assets), there were screams of dismay from the nation's bankers. Sallie Mae reinsures low-interest bank loans made to students by the nation's banks. Total federal student aid in 1992 was $21 billion with over $15 billion in loans. The default rate, students not paying their loans, was $5 billion annually. As Robert Andrews, a New Jersey Democrat pointed out, "It's free lunch for people making money off the program." As one example, the CEO of Sallie Mae was paid a million-dollar annual salary. According to Sen. Paul Simon, who was the sponsor of the direct-lending legislation, "The evidence is overwhelming that the federal government will save money [Clinton claimed a billion annually] and we'll make college more accessible to more people and reduce paperwork massively."

As I mentioned previously, it will be several years before the insanities of the National Service Trust legislation become apparent. Thousands of high school graduates are anxious to join the National Service Corp, before or after graduation from college,and presumably are eager to work as teachers, tutoring the young, helping the elderly, caring for the sick or cleaning up neighborhoods at "roughly minimum wages" in return for college benefits, which will include up to $9,450 in educational grants. Participants must compete 1,700 hours of service work a year and would receive $4,725 a year for up to two years to apply to college tuition. Students in Americorps, as it is now called, can also borrow money directly from the government at savings about a half percentage point below bank rates, and will have the option of volunteering for national service and take low-paying jobs to pay off their debts, but only as their income will allow.

While the direct costs were far below Clinton's original proposal of a five-year effort and a 7.4 billion dollar budget and will surely be cut back by a Republican Congress, the new law will, at the maximum, take care of about 47,000 students, assuming a $15,000 annual cost per student. On top of that, direct student loans must still be available, and will most certainly increase if college costs continue to rise 6 percent annually, as they have in the past twenty years. Predictions are that by 1997 $27 billion will be needed for student loans. What will the default rate be then? How many students will finally become involved in Americorps?

Straws are in the wind. In twelve of sixteen states surveyed by the American Council on Education in 1993, colleges and universities reported a sharp decline in enrollments. It's not because of the slightly reduced pool of eighteen-to-twenty-year-olds, but rather increased costs are making undergraduate education a comme-ci, comme-ca choice. Combine the declining college enrollments with an increasing percentage of part-time undergraduate students who can't afford to study full time, and must work days to pay for night courses, along with a larger majority who give up after high school and don't try to learn anything on their own, and within the next fifty years it will become apparent that "national service" will have to become a peacetime draft to keep millions of high school graduates off the streets and the unemployed rolls.

The national census report on poverty revealed that 13.55 percent of Americans, or 33.6 million people, are living at the poverty level. More than 10 percent of those, are on the edge of starvation. They can still procreate and recently the problem of the homeless has been accentuated by the discovery that many homeless people are actually families. Another recent, disconcerting statistic from the Department of Health and Human Services is that in the mid-1990s there has been a sharp rise in birth rates to unmarried white mothers. In 1991, 29 percent of all births were by unmarried women. The unwed-mother birth rate has soared by over 50 percent between 1987 and 1993. As Sen. Daniel Moynihan, who has long been pushing for welfare reform, pointed out, "In communities with a large portion of families without a father, you ask for and get chaos."

Worse is a future with millions of half-educated children. Before he was elected president of the United States, Bill Clinton was, from March 1990 to March 1991, president of the Progressive Policy Institute. Composed of seven hundred Democrats, in late 1992 the group published *Mandate for Change*. Americorps is the current result, but beneath the surface and spelled out in the book is another proposal, which in essence resurrects a dream of William James, the famous psychologist. In 1910, he proposed that national service to one's country was "the moral equivalent of war." That kind of sad future is in the offing, if only to siphon off and subdue a hopeless, partially educated younger generation.

Prior to a Citizen Corps, spelled out in *Mandate for Change,* and now in embryonic form, the larger plan was to budget millions for a Youth Apprentice Demonstration Project, with the belief that this would ultimately grow into a working relationship between schools and business. The theory is that a school-based apprenticeship program would not only improve student grades of non-college youth, but the enhanced education opportunities would eventually curb early sexual activity, drug use, and, with greater earning power, would stabilize family opportunity. It would also create an American caste system of which the *Wall Street Journal* would probably approve.

By contrast with the small number of high school graduates who may benefit from Americorps, in the coming years at least twenty million young Americans will reach the seventeen-to-twenty-one age bracket annually. Right now there is a shortfall of ten million or more who will never receive any formal education beyond high school, with a million or more of these high school dropouts. Once it is in place and functioning, the Guaranteed Undergraduate legislation will solve the problem. It will give all Americans, except a relatively few million who, because of too early parenting, or marriage, or lower mental capacities, are not eligible, a complete liberal arts and vocational education.

Benno Schmidt went down the wrong road with Chris Whittle, but he sums up what the GUE legislation will accomplish. "New approaches will have their roots in the great purposes of liberal education . . . to develop critical autonomy; to encourage rigorous intellectual standards; to lay a solid foundation of knowledge in math and science, the arts and humanities, and the varieties of human culture; to develop creativity and individuality; to build civic virtue and capacity for freedom."

It is within our grasp. You can make it happen!

6

Guaranteed Loving
Undergraduate Education

First, let's take a look at the surface functioning of the GUE legislation and what it will accomplish. Later, I will examine many of the side effects in detail. You should keep in mind that many aspects are socially interlocking and the transition for a complete redirection of American education will take about three years. But the stimulus emotionally and economically will be immediate. Since the legislation accentuates "a new and loving America," you will note that I have expanded the acronym GUE and from now on will call it GLUE. A Guaranteed Loving Undergraduate Education that instead of a melting pot will glue all Americans together with a common objective and a new sense of purpose. These are its elements:

1. The federal government will not be guaranteeing the complete costs of undergraduate education for every high school graduate, only the shortfall between a student's earnings during his thirteen-week work cycle and the complete costs of a four-year undergraduate education. Six months before graduation, all high school seniors, regardless of family income or ability to pay, can apply to the GLUE headquarters in their state asking to participate in the alternate thirteen-week work/study program. They will be quickly known as A13ers. All qualified A13ers must be unmarried, childless, and not previously parents. Young women who have had abortions will be disqualified as will the aborted child's father. All A13ers must agree to continue childless and unmarried through their four undergraduate years. Pregnant students will be immediately terminated. All potential A13ers must have a minimum C grade average in their senior year. They must also agree that during the entire four years of undergraduate study that they will accept whatever jobs they may be assigned during the thirteen-week work cycle, and at whatever minimum wage for A13ers is determined annually by

60

Congress. A13ers will be fully aware that there are no summer vacations, and their alternating work/study education continues year round for four years.

2. Coordinating GLUE headquarters staffs in each state will try to assign students to participating colleges and universities in locations which are at least one hundred miles from their home, the premise being that A13ers are embarking on an educational adventure. They no longer should have home or parental distractions or the necessity of providing income or support for parents. During their undergraduate years they will be actively involved in learning with their peer groups.

3. Students who require no financial aid including scholarships or grants, which will have largely disappeared, may join the program or not as they prefer. Some private universities may decide not to participate but many private colleges for economic reasons may decide to become GLUE affiliates. Yale University, for example which once managed to run on endowments, in 1993 ran a $10 million deficit and needs about $1 billion for repairs to its physical plant. Students who are financially able to pursue their undergraduate studies without becoming A13ers will be housed separately on campus, since they will not be in the work/study program. But they will be intermixed in classrooms.

4. Students with C grade levels through high school will automatically be assigned to undergraduate vocational courses and study. During their four undergraduate years, they will have their choice of studying and becoming thoroughly proficient in a minimum of three vocations. To expand their vocational teaching abilities, all participating colleges and universities will coordinate their teaching with certified local vocational schools and community colleges, or develop new courses in specific vocations. Students with B grade averages or above will have the choice of studying for bachelor of arts or bachelor of science degrees, but if they prefer they can chose the direct vocational degrees. Of course, most public universities offer many varying vocational degrees, and a large student majority will prefer the three vocational degree course of study since acquiring specific vocational skills is, for them, the raison d'etre of undergraduate education. Also, because a total liberal arts education will be the focus of all K-12 education, the number of students pursuing bachelors of arts may decline rapidly. But, as I will point out later, all A13ers will continue to have their undergraduate courses integrated in required human values seminars.

An outstanding example of the basic change that has occurred in undergraduate education in the past fifty years is City University of New York (CUNY), which has twenty-one senior and community college campuses in the five boroughs of New York City, with 207,000 students, mostly part time. Anne Reynolds, chancellor of CUNY, recently tried to eliminate nearly two hundred baccalaureate and associate degree programs that duplicated each other. GLUE will gradually eliminate part-time students and lower the age level of all students nationally. A13ers will fill colleges and universities beyond their present capacities, but many military installations previously closed, or due to be closed, can be transformed into new seats of learning. At the same time college and university administrators will have to revise their vocational degree courses extensively and without unnecessary, nationwide duplication, and offer degrees in many new occupations from automobile mechanics, carpentry, and construction to zoology, many of which were formerly the province of vocational high schools.

A13ers pursuing vocational degrees will be fully aware that their undergraduate studies will not qualify them to pursue graduate degrees in law, medicine, engineering, and other professions, or specialized doctorate degrees. A13ers who are specifically pursuing BA or BS degrees, which would qualify them for graduate study, must pay for graduate study at their own expense. But if they have high undergraduate grade averages and are accepted for graduate study, they will be able to obtain low-interest loans direct from the federal government. They will also have the option of teaching undergraduates, at minimum wage levels, to augment their income while pursuing higher degrees.

In passing, it should be noted that CUNY, like most public universities, is dependent on public spending. Total CUNY operating costs in 1993 were approximately $678 million, with tuition payments providing $409 million—a shortfall of well over $250 million, which is currently made up by state and federal aid.

5. There will be two different roommate programs for A13ers. The first is similar to most dormitory programs. Students will be given room assignments with members of their own sex. Whether they call themselves African Americans or blacks, Hispanics or Latinos, or Asians with specific national identities, no ethnic or racial enclaves will be permitted. The coordinating GLUE staff, working with the participating colleges and universities, will thoroughly intermix all roommates. An optional Roommate of the Other Sex Program (ROSP) will be available to all high school graduates who qualify. I will detail this later.

6. It should be kept in mind that GLUE is not a "free trip to ride." All GLUE students will be earning their own undergraduate education. Working with state governments, GLUE headquarters will organize minimum wage public service and community work for A13ers. But mainstream business organizations will provide most of the jobs. A major provision of the legislation is that *all* businesses employing ten or more people are required by law to hire A13ers at the Congressionally established A-13 minimum wage rate. The number of A13ers working for a particular company will be in ratio to the company's total full-time employees. Not only will employers quickly discover that young people can be easily trained to do particular jobs, but once trained, if the A13ers agree, employers may reemploy them continuously on their continuing work cycles, thus effec-

tively training future full-time employees. All business organizations will receive compensatory tax deductions for wages paid to A13ers. Cities and states employing students would also receive a proportionate federal subsidy based on wages paid to A13ers for public service work.

The legislation will make it illegal for business organizations to hire any teenager under age 17 who has not graduated from high school. This will free millions of jobs now being filled on a part-time basis by high school students who are under seventeen. At the same time it will restore a saner environment for tenth- to twelfth-grade students who are dissipating their energies in supermarkets and fast food franchises instead of studying or participating in sports or extracurricular learning groups.

According to the Simmons Market Research Bureau, more than five million kids between the ages of twelve and seventeen now work part time, and in their senior high school year, many put in more than twenty hours a week on the job. A feature article, "Too Old, Too Fast," in *Newsweek* of November 16, 1992, explored the sad phenomenon. Lawrence Steinberg, a psychology professor, summed it up, "Everybody worries why the Japanese, German and Swedish students are doing better than us. One reason is that they're not spending their afternoons wrapping tacos." In a study made by the University of Michigan, professor Harold Stevens pointed out, "74 percent of the high school juniors in Minneapolis worked compared with 21 percent in Sendai, Japan. Indeed, almost half the public schools in Tokyo prohibit students from working."

7. Keeping in mind the huge federal deficit, the thrust of the GLUE legislation is that the shortfall between a student's earnings on the work cycle will be made up by savings in other areas. To cover as much of undergraduate education costs as possible, the guaranteed A13 minimum wages may be higher than the national average. Assume a minimum wage of $7 an hour. Based on a five-day work week, each student would earn $280 a week, or a total annual wage of $7,280 during his or her two thirteen-week work cycles during each of the four years. Employers, whether they be private or city and state, will pay the student's wages directly to the college or university that the student is attending, less $25 a week that will be paid directly to the student for personal expenses, or an annual total of $650 for transportation, clothing, and entertainment. It won't be much, but more than many families have for these expenditures, and most families, freed of any support for undergraduate education, will be able to supplement this. The balance of the money earned by an A13er, $5,630, will be applied to nationally averaged costs for room, board, and tuition and books. In 1994, the Massachusetts Educational Authority estimated the average national cost of an undergraduate education at a public university, which included these items, was $8,562, and at private colleges and universities was $17,846. They also project-

ed for a child born in 1994, with the 6 percent annual increases in education's costs continuing as they have in the past, a four-year college education at a public university will cost $100,000 and more than $200,000 at a private institution, topped by $300,000 at an Ivy League School.

8. Obviously the minimum wage assumptions given above will have to be adjusted upwards, if this sorry kind of inflation continues. But using the 1994–95 public education costs of $8,600, and with the certainty that GLUE can sharply control the rising costs of education, there would be a shortfall of about $3,000 annually for each student's education. This would be paid under GLUE legislation by the federal subsidy. In total with a doubling of the number of students between seventeen and twenty-one now in college, the annual shortfall would be $100 billion to a $150 billion. Don't gasp—more than $150 billion is now being expended, and creating a going-nowhere educational wasteland.

9. Recognizing that major, competing team sports were a twentieth-century unifying activity for most colleges and universities, GLUE will permit payment, at the established minimum wage, for one thirteen-week work period, annually, to students who excel in and are chosen to play football, basketball, baseball, and hockey, competitively against other participating institutions. The cost of paying individual athletes for one thirteen-week period each year would be factored into the average undergraduate annual cost, and covered by the subsidy. Every effort would be made to cover the costs of particular sports by parent donations and broadcast income, or they could be discontinued. Individually competitive sports, for those who excel, could be pursued as one vocational option but not on a work/study basis assumed by a particular college or university.

10. GLUE will force a complete reorganization of federal and state aid to education, which now tops $100 billion annually, much of which goes to undergraduate education. The incentives, to get a complete education, provided by GLUE will practically eliminate the problem of teenage mothers and single mothers ending up on welfare. A substantial portion of the $68 billion dollars spent by state and federal governments annually for welfare and aid to dependent families will provide many additional billions. Eventually, with millions more Americans job trained for more than one kind of work, not only will welfare costs be reduced, but GLUE will also take millions of high school graduates off the unemployment rolls and will effectively reduce the unemployment rate, thus saving billions of dollars in unemployment benefits.

GLUE will also eliminate the Federal Job Training Program, which was established by law in 1985 to retrain people on welfare and food stamps, and hopefully get them new jobs and reduce the need for government aid. No great reduction was ever accomplished. On December 16, 1993, the *Wall Street Journal* exposed the current government agency as a pork barrel boondoggle, and pointed out that the Clinton Administration "would like to eliminate 150 different education and training programs that drain $24 billion out of the Federal coffers each year, and concentrate the funds on those job training programs that work." The *Journal* listed the fourteen agencies that are running these job training programs, which include the Education Department: "Laying out Federal loans to train 81,600 cosmetology students a year—but the job market is only creating slots for 17,000."

Writing in the *New York Times* on January 4, 1994, Gary Esler points out: "American business says schools are not producing enough skilled workers, and according to Phyllis Eisen, an official of the National Association of Manufacturers, industry is spending $40 billion a year training employees, much of it in remedial education."

"In 1988," Esler wrote, "the U.S. spent 5.7 percent of gross national product through government expenditures exclusive of grants, tuition and endowments on education. But Vance Grant, a specialist in education statistics for the Federal Department of Education, calculates that in 1992–93, total spending on education, including expenditures on private schools, is now 7.8 percent of the gross national product."

11. Take that percentage of a $5 trillion gross national product and you'll see that the shortfall costs of GLUE are not only manageable, but considerably less than current educational costs. If any shortfall exists in the federal subsidy guaranteeing all Americans an additional four years of education, it will be totally balanced by an educational environment that will lift America by it's bootstraps. And it will cover a few additional costs built into the GLUE legislation, including the additional costs of limited federal funding to rural areas to assure that busing is available to primary and secondary schools, and that the quality of a new liberal arts education is equal to high schools in major city areas. In addition, the $3.3 billion currently being spent on Head Start will be increased to the $5 billion recommended by Jonathan Kozol in his book *Savage Inequalities*. At the present time Head Start is helping about 721,000 children and their families whose incomes are below the federal poverty level of $14,550 for a family of four, but the program is still reaching only 35 percent of the eligible children. In essence the quality of liberal arts teaching anywhere in the United States should be comparable. As a byproduct, continuous national achievement tests at different grade levels of potential A-13 qualifiers should also be comparable anywhere in United States.

There are many economic byproducts of the Lovemore legislation, all of which are based on going far beyond the information highway concept and making the in-depth education of future generations the biggest industry in United States, and the world. As a result, not only will more Americans than ever be employable, but jobs, with all of us educating each other, will multiply exponentially. Since GLUE headquarters wail be moving A13ers to different parts of the country to pursue their undergraduate degrees, and employing them in every area of the United States, building construction for new campuses, and rehabilitating old ones, will be a major industry for years to come. Top companies will spend billions setting up branch work locations in cities and towns where A13ers will be studying, and in the process revitalizing areas that have previously lost manufacturing or service companies. Multibillion-dollar computer companies and book publishers will top the *Fortune* listing of the top 500 corporations, and, unlike new-style manufacturing companies, will be major people employers.

All of this is based on primary and secondary schools being able to concentrate completely on the liberal arts. In 1990 President Bush called a Governor's Educational Summit in Charlottesville, Virginia. The governors of all the states agreed with the National Assessment of Educational Progress report that "achievement tests are essentially flat." In the areas of science and mathematics, young people in most age groups did better than similar groups in 1973, but hoping for some kind of miracle Bush announced new educational goals. In the next ten years (by 2000) the predictions were, every child starting school would be ready to learn, the high school graduation rate would rise to 90 percent, and students in grades four, eight, and twelve would demonstrate competency in basic subjects. United States students would be the first in the world in science, and every adult would be literate and skilled enough to compete in the world democracy and assume responsibilities of citizenship. On top of that all schools would be drug-free.

Four years later, President Clinton hasn't been able to pull Bush's rabbit out of the hat, and he has announced somewhat similar education goals for 2000. Proclaiming dreams of the future, without creating the environment to realize the dreams, is a typical political maneuver. Unfortunately, none of these goals are underwritten with programs that might achieve this magical alchemy and turn lead into gold.

The GLUE legislation will do this. Once all vocational training is moved forward to ages seventeen to twenty-one, there would be no vocational subjects taught in the first twelve grades except typing and computers. There would be no high school vocational degrees in automobile repair, how to be a carpenter, electrician, cook, or you name it. All of these vocations and thousands more would be available to A13ers. But it should be kept in mind that in a society like ours, and in many Western nations, all young people grow up getting some basic vocational abilities. No longer eligible for part-time employment in the business world, many of them will earn money during summer vacations doing community work, and millions of parents, no longer having to pay for undergraduate education, will be able to send their children to summer camps to enjoy a respite from their high school studies in fun, games, and sports, and, incidentally, create another huge industry.

A few contrasts between present directions in vocational education and the future will show the validity of GLUE and a revised K-12 education. Project ProTech in Boston, Massachusetts, funded by the Department of Labor for $900,000 (the department funds five similar projects nationwide) takes high school students, who are chosen by teachers and officials, to spend one day a week at six participating hospitals, where they are taught by the hospital staff. They are picked up during summer vacations to work in labs and in demanding medical work. The program was developed in response to the urgent need to prepare young people for careers in the health field, where major shortages of skilled workers are expected in the future. Nationwide it is expected to encompass a variety of professional fields and industries.

Commenting on the program, the *Boston Globe* wrote, "Organizers of ProTech hope to change the image of vocational education, which had traditionally been a dumping ground for the less academically capable students who are trained in fields like cosmetology and baking, for which there is a decreasing demand . . . and to awaken young people to the possibilities of higher education."

And that's our present caste system problem in a nutshell. Teaching vocational subjects in high schools separates students into different educational environments and is the foundation of a dangerous divided class structure that endangers a democratic government. The GLUE premise is that young people who have acquired a broad general education are better able to learn vocational skills between the ages of seventeen and twenty-one, especially in a work/study undergraduate environment when lifetime goal seeking becomes more apparent to students as a way of life.

In the following two chapters I will examine some radically different approaches in this new K-12 liberal educational environment. But basically the function of all elementary and secondary schools will be to educate *all* citizens and make sure they are competent in reading, writing, and mathematics, and one other language. They will also study language roots and the problems of communicating with people whose languages express their realities differently. All of these areas will be taught historically, giving students exciting overviews and perspectives on past lives and problems of all our ancestors—average human beings who gradually subsumed the power of their self-proclaimed military leaders and royalty who traced their lineage and responsibilities to gods and all-powerful deities. Books such as the five-volume *History of Private Lives* (1987, Belknap/Harvard), and Charles Mancreon's *Age of the French Revolution* (1972, Touchstone) which describes in detail the changing mores, religious views, and insanities of wars, will be studied in grades nine to twelve with no difficulty for most students, since *reading, reading, reading* will be a way of life for K-12 education.

Science would also be taught historically, with young people rediscovering with their teachers the wonders of early scientific discoveries, and learning not only how the things that are a part of their lives work, but how they developed into their present forms. Story telling via written novels, short stories, and plays would be continuously contrasted with visual story telling by movies and television, which can only indirectly express the myriad aspects of human emotions and thoughts. Teachers would also show students how the act of reading engenders a mutual creativity between an author and his readers that is usurped or can never be fully realized by filmmakers trying to capture an author's ideas with visual images. Young people would not only be given a thorough background in the arts, music, and comparative religions, but would discover the continuous lifetime need for every person to be able to express himself or herself in creative ways.

You can compare this approach with the federally funded National Standards for United States History (a 271-page document funded by Goals 2000 legislation), which outlines what students from grades 5 though 12 should know about the American past. Along with a parallel guide to world history, these federal approaches have created a storm of protest and bitter intellectual skirmishings. Lynn Cheney, who headed the National Endowment of the Arts (also fighting impending Republican cutbacks to its relatively small funding), called the history standards "a politically correct fare thee well"—and both outlines most certainly reflect the overworked "multicultural" approach to teaching history.

By contrast the GLUE approach to secondary education would give all high school graduates a comprehensive survey of the past, not just in a specific history course but in all the subjects from literature to chemistry, biology, mathematics, and physics, as a continuing facet of specific studies.

The GLUE approach may not appeal to Newt Gingrich, who in January 1995 announced, "The great challenge of our lifetime is to imagine a future that is worth spending our lives to get to. The old order is gone. The only question is how long it takes to get rid of it."

Gingrich is an admirerer of Alvin and Heidi Toffler but probably not the chapter in *Future Shock* where Toffler admits to the possibilities of Proposition 31 and my proposal for merged corporate families. The Tofflers believe that humans have moved through two waves of civilization, agrarian and industrial, and we are now in a third computer-communication wave. But I'm sure they'll agree, unless a new generation really understands the raison d'etre for past human motivations induced by the previous waves, we will probably go backwards and try to relive the past. It doesn't make much sense that Gingrich, a former history teacher, emphasizes the past and the value of orphanages and poor houses.

The thrust of GLUE is that a completely educated citizenry with a sense of its own past and history will be able to communicate with each other on all levels. This kind of holistic K-12, liberal arts education will eliminate the communication gaps between those who pursue so-called higher education and become either doctors, lawyers, scientists, teachers, engineers, or leaders in business and manufacturing. A vast majority of undergraduates would be A13ers getting their education on a work/study basis. Rooming assignments will mix students studying for vocational degrees with those studying for BA or BS degrees, most of whom would be planning to go on to graduate school. Since they all would have had a wide K-12 liberal arts education, a gradual leveling would occur in their later lives. The huge gap that exists in income and prestige between those who have had an additional two-year or four-year professional education would disappear. The lawyer, doctor, or scientist who could not repair his or her automobile, or fix his or her computer or television, would quickly discover that the auto mechanic or the electronic repairman was as broadly educated in the liberal arts and the ability to think as they were, and they would all discover that that their K-12 education had not only taught them all how to engage in a continuous search for sound universal human values, but taught them how to care for each other no matter what their level of vocational expertise or financial rewards.

Everywhere you turn in the middle 1990s various groups, mostly on the wrong track, are worrying about K-12 education or undergraduate education. At $14.95 a copy you can buy *An American Imperative: Higher Expectations for Higher Learning.* The basis of the report, sponsored by various foundations including Johnson, Lilly, Pew and the Hewlett Foundations, is: (1) finding a way to instill values that will make students better able to contribute to society; (2) reorganizing educational institutions for the benefit of students rather than the convenience of education; and (3) integrating colleges with other teaching institutions, libraries, museums, and business to create "a seamless system that can produce and support a nation of learners." This report, supported by numerous educators, is a straw with no wind blowing.

On May 10, 1993, an editorial in the *Wall Street Journal* praised the formation of a new organization, the American Academy for Liberal Education, headed by Jacques Barzun and Edward Wilson. The group wants to establish mandatory undergraduate courses in sciences, math, languages, and literature and ensure that students get a solid grounding in Western civilization. Unfortunately, the association is in the wrong pew. Changing the direction of undergraduate education is too late in the game. Multicultural K-12 liberal arts education, for everyone, followed by GLUE and integrating human values seminars for all A13ers will create a new kind of American who, twenty years later, will wonder at the stupidities of "political correctness." To see how all this ties into the final sex revolution, read on!

7

Teaching Human Sexuality, Grades 9–12

Keep in mind as you read this and the following chapter, that the federally funded course on human sexuality is optional. And even if local school boards approve, parents can still decide whether their children should take the weekly hour course or not. Also keep in mind that, based on the self-imposed rating system on the arts, most children, unless parents restrict their television and movie viewing, will have watched men and women making love in SN (Sexually Natural and caring) situations, and most young people will be comfortable with human nudity.

Although in this and the following chapters I will explore the how-to of teaching human sexuality in depth, you should also note that the comprehensive K-12 course on human sexuality in all grades represents a very small portion of K-12 liberal arts teaching. All students in grades nine to twelve will be taking courses in history, government, psychology, sociology, comparative religions, and world literature in print and film (story telling), along with math and the sciences. In these courses teachers will have many opportunities to discuss and evaluate problems of life and world problems along with the long history of sexual devaluation. At the same time, as I will show, the self-imposed rating of the arts will be accentuating and creating an environment with an upbeat new morality and value structure.

Despite the present-day claims of parents, religious leaders, and our elected representatives that teaching morals is the province of home and church, no one seems to know, in a democracy that extols freedom of speech, how to deflect the continuous sick sex barrage that young people encounter every day. As it stands, the young must try to make some sense of it, but mostly on their own. Articles

70

and books like *Culture Wars,* by James Davison Hunter, explore our almost-any-thing-goes moral pluralism versus the rigid fundamentalist views. *Moral Values and Higher Education: A Nation at Risk* offers a collection of essays, pro and con, arguing whether teaching morals and values is a university and college responsibility. In their book *Sex and Morality,* Dr. Ruth (of television fame) and Dr. Louis Liebermann examine in detail the Catholic, Jewish, and Protestant religions and their varying moral beliefs and sexual norms. They ask, "Who should teach morals, ethics and values? . . . We hear this controversial question raised almost daily in the press, courts,and on the floors of Congress. Should the schools teach morals, or should we leave it as always to the churches and synagogues? Should it be left to those closest to the children—their parents?"

In his *The Culture of Complaint,* Robert Hughes, who is on the opposite side of the fence from Rush Limbaugh, exposes the double-talk of Republican and fundamentalist morality. Stephen Carter in his book *The Culture of Disbelief* points out that religious faith once gave us a sense of common purpose, but today even the politicians trivialize religion, and "We err when we presume that religious motives are likely to be illiberal, and we compound the error when we insist that the devout should keep their religious ideas to themselves—whether good or bad."

The books, sans solutions, keep coming. Paul Knott, in his book *Remaking America: The Value Revolution,* reveals that millions of Americans are seeking values and a sense of purpose that any culture must have to survive. In his book *Why Johnny Can't Tell Right from Wrong* William Kirkpatrick points out that character development was an integral part of secondary school education until the late 1960s, but then the onus was put on the student in a process called value-free decisionmaking. "In the middle 1960s many people thought we had squandered our moral inheritance. They thought something was morally wrong with us, that our moral ideas were not worth transmitting. We had to start from scratch, and let the young decide what our values should be." Amatai Etzoni, in his book *The Spirit of Community,* notes that we have done away with the old forms, connections, and rules, but as yet have put nothing much in their place. "Moral transitions often work this way," he writes, "Destruction comes quickly. A vacuum prevails. Reconstruction is slow. This is where we are now. It's time to reconstruct."

And that's exactly what the New Morality legislation will accomplish. I will come back to new and more prosaic approaches to K-12 liberal arts education. But let's take a look at some other teaching aspects of the final sex revolution that will occur in grades nine through twelve. Again, it should be noted that all students will be in their fourteenth and fifteenth years, and for the most part are no longer boys and girls, but young men and women. They will have been conditioned to delay final sexual merger until their seventeenth birthdays, when the potential of sexual merger becomes a joyous rite of passage, after which they can choose to have caring sex with a friend, *but not have children,* if they plan to become an A13er either in the regular GLUE program or the Roommate of the Other Sex Program. In this saner sexual environment seventeen-year-olds will have been thoroughly trained in birth control, and wherever possible, and privacy permits, parents will encourage their seventeen-year-olds to enjoy caring sex with a friend in their own homes.

At this point, I'm sure that many readers will think I'm overemphasizing human sexuality and that there are many other more important aspects of life, even as basic as getting a good education and being able to earn adequate food, clothing, and shelter for oneself and family, and all this should predominate in secondary education.

But you must face reality. While we have come a long way economically since the beginning of the industrial age, young people grow up in a deeply frustrating emotional and sexual environment. Not a week goes by that some major magazine doesn't try to assess the situation and offer solutions. In its January 10, 1994, issue, *Newsweek*'s cover story, "Growing up Scared: How Our Kids Are Robbed of Their Childhood," points out the underlying causes: changes in the family—single-parent homes doubling since 1970 from four million to eight million, and producing 70 percent of juvenile crime offenders, along with children watching eight thousand televised murders and one hundred thousand acts of violence before finishing elementary school, and 26 percent of all girls age fifteen being sexually active as compared with 5 percent in 1970.

Looking back on what seems to have been a sexually saner past, we forget that less than a hundred years ago, before the industrial revolution took hold, there was no long sexual waiting period. Young women were commonly married early in their teens. Often, with limited contraceptive knowledge available, they were pregnant out of wedlock but male responsibility, with or without a "shotgun" wedding, provided the safety net. Women who refrained from early sex, and were passed by, became spinsters and maiden aunts and often remained virgins for their entire lives.

In those days most women got little formal schooling and most men, after graduating from grammar school, went to work on the farm or in mills and factories. There were few universities and many of those were for future ministers and teachers. Graduate schools, inspired by Johns Hopkins, didn't exist until the 1870s. Self-education was the rule. Doctors, lawyers, ministers, and teachers were in business after high school, which in urban areas gave a better liberal arts education than most colleges do today.

Today, marriage is delayed, premarital living together on campus is a way of life, and the safety net of male responsibility for procreation is no longer a way of life. But now we refuse to face the fact that, even if kids didn't grow up in an eros-driven society, there are always about twenty-four million teenagers between the ages of thirteen and nineteen who are experiencing a hormonic/harmonic surge in their bodies. Too many Americans are so trampled by religious moralities that no longer work that we don't dare, or know how to create, a sane sexual environment for teenagers. On January 16, 1994, the *New York Times* headlined, "Sex Educators for Young See New Virtue in Chastity." The story explained that about 180,000 children in a California program devised by the Grady Memorial Hospital in Atlanta were learning the rewards of postponing sex. The program relies on conditioning twelve-year-olds and up to remain virgins—"abstinence makes the heart grow fonder"—and instilling a fear of single-mother poverty, AIDS, and Sexually Transmitted Diseases. Costing California $5 million annually, the program has presumably reduced teenage pregnancies 10 percent, and perhaps delayed sexual merger. Gayle Wilson, wife of Pete Wilson, governor of California, hopes, "If we can just get them to wait until they are sixteen, we will have accomplished something."

Whether they are trying to create their own version of 1990s realities or are actually reporting existing phenomena, *Newsweek* and *Time* are well aware that premarital and extramarital sex are circulation builders, and with their enormous circulations are guides to political thinking for the middle class. In its October 17, 1994, issue *Newsweek* reported: "A lot of kids are putting off sex, and not because they can't get a date. They've decided to wait, and they're proud of their chastity, not embarrassed by it. Suddenly virgin geek is giving way to virgin chic." On February 27, 1995, *Time*'s feature story was "For Better or Worse," and told about the growing movement to strengthen marriage and contain divorce. But in an earlier, August 15, 1994, issue, *Time* featured "Infidelity" and their findings were, "It may be in our genes, but the good news is that they aren't designed to stay there."

Nor are they basically monogamous. The New Sexual Morality and Education Legislation deals with the basic reality. Premarital sex is an inevitable way of life, but we can design and create new environments that will not only eliminate out-of-wedlock childbirth but will lead to soundly based, long-time monogamous marriages where the door is left open to adventure and loving more than one person without creating grief or jealousy or the problem of fidelity to the original partner.

To qualify for the GLUE programs, kids at thirteen will know they have eight more years of education and will lose it all if they become fathers or mothers, or get married. Kids grow up knowing they have a sexual coming of age incentive—something to look forward to, like getting a license to drive a car at sixteen, and it gives them adult and parental acceptance, that at seventeen they are sexual adults. Now, at seventeen, and for the next four years of their lives as an A13er, during their undergraduate years, they may enjoy more than one sexual partner in the regular GLUE program, or without any attendant STD and AIDS risks, in the ROSP program (see ahead) enjoy a new-style sexual and mental growth, a safety net that will totally transform their lives and America, too.

It must begin in the schools, and an overall agreement that teachers are no longer afraid to probe all the moral and human value aspects of current sexual insanities and sexual devaluation. This must be done in the later grades of high school. In the ninth grade, human sexuality seminar teachers will not only move in rapidly on current examples of devalued human sexuality, but, with their students explore the sexual sickness of the fading 1990s, and encourage the students to evoke their own moral consensus. At the same time they will constantly show how the real wonder and ecstasy of our amazing bodies and sexual needs were being trampled in the mud because too many people had been indoctrinated with religious conditionings that were no longer valid, and because too many people had never learned how, or were unwilling, to make the effort to step into another person's shoes, and discover that the joy of becoming the other person is the seeding ground of caring love.

Many of the sexual insanities exploited by the media in the 1990s will be topics of discussion. Was Mike Tyson, who insisted that he didn't rape Desiree Washington after he invited her back to his hotel room, innocent or not? What motivated both of them? Was Magic Johnson, who finally revealed that he had lived a hit or miss, noncaring sexual life, and now had an HIV infection, really a hero in the fight against AIDS? And what about Madonna, the heroine of millions of teenagers? Should Time Warner have published her book, *Sex*? Teachers will show Madonna's two videos in the classroom, and discuss the advice that she gave young women. Calling herself Dita, "a love technician," Madonna insisted, "Some women want to be slapped around. You can learn to play S/M games and not let someone hurt you. Wearing panties is a turn on." She also warned, "Sex is not Love. Love is not Sex," a point which Madonna underlined with photographs of simulated bondage.

Or the Bobbitts. What kind of marriage did Lorena and John have? What kind of society was it that gets two hundred members of the press, including Gay Talese writing the story for the *New Yorker* (presumably the best literary magazine in America), jammed into the courtroom to listen to two people who didn't have the faintest idea of what loving another person was all about? Why? Because they, and ultimately the Bobbitts, will reap millions of dollars feeding this sad, sick sex story back to avid, if tongue-clicking, readers. Nor did the Bobbitts make any dent on people like Phyllis Schlafly, who insists that "the facts of life can be told in fifteen minutes" and "saving sex until marriage is the only safe sex." They were the people boycotting teaching young men and women how to confirm each other as sexual human beings.

Ninth-grade teachers will be unafraid to discuss Woody Allen and Mia Farrow's world—not just incest (noting that, based on bloodlines, Soon-Yi isn't Woody's daughter) but the larger aspects of narcissism and Allen's attempt via his movies to reflect on, and satirize, middle-class Americans and their sexual hang-ups in films like *Husbands and Wives,* which can be shown in classrooms.

The problems of Princess Diana and Prince Charles can provide classroom discussion on the interpersonal problems of love and marriage for royalty and famous people whose sex lives were grist for the mill of too many people who couldn't cope with their own unfulfilled sex lives.

Teachers will not only analyze current films and television offerings but also the incessant stories of rape, wife beating, sexual harassment, murder as a byproduct of adultery, men and women hiring "hit" people to get rid of their spouses, and Catholic priests and Protestant ministers involved with boys or young women parishioners.

And the classes will be made aware that Future Families of America (see ahead) is underwriting experiments on new-style families which may include two and three couples in a group marriage with a caring exchange of spouses as a solution for both adultery and the problems of long, monogamous marriages that lead to divorce. The classes will study the question of whether loving more than one person during a long marriage is possible without destroying the original pair bonding. And teachers will show in classrooms the no-holds-barred questioning of Bill Clinton by Steve Krofft on January 26, 1992, and whether Clinton had an affair with Gennifer Flowers, and possibly other women, after he married Hillary. Classroom discussion will raise the question, Could Clinton have had sex with another women and still loved Hillary? If he did why was it obvious that Hillary still loved him? And if Clinton did have sex with a woman other than his wife, as Franklin Roosevelt and John Kennedy and other public figures have, did it affect his or her abilities to perform in public office? Teachers will explore the reality that now in the 1990s, nearly 50 percent of American men and women have affairs, or a sexual encounter with another person in addition to their husband or wife. And they will discuss a growing possibility that in the twenty-first century, many men and women will discover how to incorporate one or two other caring sexual relationships, during a long lifetime, into the original marriage without hate, jealousy, or divorce as byproducts.

And they could raise the fascinating question of Henry Cisneros, former mayor of San Antonio, and now secretary of housing in Clinton's cabinet. In 1994, although Cisneros was married with children, his long-time relationship with Linda Medlar, another woman with children whom he supported, made national headlines. Essentially a bigamist, Cisneros denied that he used state or federal money to support his "wives." He is now reconciled with his original wife. A worthy subject for discussion in Grade 11 of 12 sex-education courses would be whether, as occurs in thousands of American families, a multiple sexual relationship within an approving marital structure might be much better than divorce for all and might even lead to friendship among all concerned. If Cisneros could have brought Linda and her children home to an accepting first wife, they all could have used most of the $200,000 he spent supporting Linda separately for better purposes.

And, of course, teachers will explore sexual devaluation in all of the arts, including heavy rock music and rap with lyrics that extol the derring-do of the male phallus and the throbbing female vagina. Teachers will actually play the music of Madonna, the Beastie Boys, Ice-T, Run DMC, 2 Live Crew, or whoever else comes along, exploring their continuous putdown of human loving, and also why practically all of rap and rock music is written and played by men, who have been conditioned by the male power syndrome that women are sex objects designed for their pleasure. By contrast, also played will be the gushily romantic, silly love songs of the 1940s and 1950s and the country music of the 1990s, in which the lyrics of love constantly ask, "Will you be mine—and you belong to me," along with conviction that owning your wife or husband was the basis for living happily ever after.

There are innumerable approaches to sane sexual values education for young teenagers, and these will grow in sophistication. But let's take another look at how teachers will explore the Bobbitt case, the Clarence Thomas/Anita Hill Senate inquiry (October 11, 12, and 13, 1991), a thirty-three-hour sexual tell-all soap opera, and the William Kennedy Smith trial. All of these offered a complete education on sick, devalued sex, which, far more than condom distribution and advertising, exposed an estimated seventy million Americans, and millions of teenagers, for the first time to every aspect of human sexual hangups and insanities. These, of course, were never evaluated in classrooms.

During the afternoon after school at four o'clock, Jenny Jones, one of the female talk show tribe headed up by Oprah Winfrey and Sally Jessy Raphael, with a full studio audience listening avidly, probed every aspect of John and Lorena Bobbitt's sex life—that he had had sex everyday, some times twice a day, more than nine hundred times in their short marriage, and that he had had sex with twenty-nine other women prior to their marriage, and a few after their marriage. Tenth graders will be amused that Jones was so fascinated with John Bobbitt's erectile abilities that if she could have, she probably would have had him unzip his pants and show whether his stitched-on penis was still capable of action—maybe with a blow job which she implied, but didn't dare actually say.

A few years before, during the Hill/Thomas hearings, teenagers learned about the charms of Hill's big breasts, or were told of big penises, oral sex, sex with animals, and pornography in detail. My fifteen-year-old newspaper boy at the time, collecting for deliveries, told me that he had to get home "to hear what was going on television." Like many young people, he must have been bewildered to hear Patricia Bowman tell how she struggled to keep Smith's penis from going into her vagina.

Like it or not, in the 1990s young people are getting a distorted view of human sexuality. Sex without caring, or loving—sex, dirty, nasty—laden with guilt feelings, seems to be the natural, expected way of life. Mothers, fathers, teachers, ministers, priests, and rabbis, along with senators, lawyers, and future judges have no common ground of beliefs and very few answers that would make much sense to teenagers.

Using videotapes, much more sophisticated teenagers, who have taken the comprehensive K-12 courses on human sexuality, will find it amusing that senators Orrin Hatch and Arlen Specter were so shocked, and were almost unable to discuss Anita Hill's allegations that Judge Thomas had talked to her about big breasts, and big penises, oral sex and group sex, or that the senators seemed to be unaware that these aspects of human sexuality were common fare in most women's magazines, letters to sex advisors in all the newspapers, as well as in men's magazines. Was it possible that Sen. Hatch didn't know that in 1986 his former page, Eliza Florez, a very pretty young woman, actually appeared in a porno movie, *Behind the Green Door, A Sequel,* during which she participated in almost every sexual act under discussion during the hearings, or that later she told reporters, "I decided to make one porno film because of Edwin Meese [U.S. Attorney General at the time]. Meese is strangling the Republican party, and he's hacking away at the Constitution. He's threatening First Amendment rights."

Was Florez any sexually saner than Orrin Hatch, who, in all probability, saw the X-rated film long before the hearings with nowhere near the shock he evinced during the inquiry? In the last phase of the human sexuality seminar, concentrating on pornography (see ahead), twelfth graders can watch Florez in action and decide.

Young people will know all about sexual harassment, a nonissue once the new sexual morality becomes a way of life. But they will learn about the sad spectacle of a man being evaluated for the Supreme Court based on whether he had harassed a woman with sexual remarks. In the twentieth century men weren't supposed to think about women as sexual objects, but many women encouraged them by dressing in clothing that accentuated their breasts and buttocks. In the 1990s the advertising industry was geared to using women as a metaphor to enhance male sex power in everything from automobiles to X-rated videos.

Young women in their early teens and later will be happily aware that they, as well as the guys, enjoy watching the other sex. They will have grown up seeing them naked, and they won't be ashamed of being titillated by the other sex. Both guys and gals will be romantically lusty with each other, and be well aware that half the fun in life is sexual attraction to another person. They will applaud Jimmy Carter, the first national figure who ever admitted that he, a married man, occasionally lusted after women. And they will understand in the larger sense that lust can easily be translated into love.

Teachers will point out that before the hearings became public, the committee could have investigated the charges against Thomas in a closed session with Hill, and avoided the intense and often sickening probe that occurred on television. They can also offer for student response a more likely scenario than emerged from the inquiry. Wasn't it quite likely that Clarence Thomas, thirty-three years old at the time, separated from his wife, and a normally sexual man (nothing to do with his race) was driven by his genes? During the hearings many women testified to "his decency, and to clear his name," but they might not have been as sexually appealing to him as Hill was. At twenty-six Hill was, and still is today, a very beautiful woman, and would attract many men who might fantasize about her as a sexual companion.

Most men and women fantasize sex with other persons, but in the past didn't dare to verbalize it for fear of being rebuffed. In the crude way of many older men, which is rapidly disappearing in the twentieth century, Thomas may well have been, in what seemed to him a laughing way, testing Anita's potential response as a bed partner. Dean Kophe of Oral Roberts University and Thomas's friend reiterated that Thomas was a "laughing man."

Thomas mentioned to Hill that he had watched a porno tape. Teachers can show it to their class (*Electric Blue 003,* released in 1981) and point out that it was a sad example of America's Barnum-style willingness to pay and see sexual freaks. In the video, Seka, a well-known porno star at the time, plays a Southern maid. She's delighted at the return of Long Dong Silver, a black male with a penis so long that it hangs below his knees. (Teenagers will be laughingly relieved to know he couldn't get an erection, although the video implied he was fucking Seka.)

Putting this up for classroom discussion, teachers will evoke the female response. If they had been Hill, would they have laughed or shrugged? At fourteen and up they will know how to deflect a sexual invitation and their peer boyfriends will not only expect it but approve. They will know, too, that in later life, at twenty-six, like Hill, Thomas wasn't harassing her but simply trying to discover whether, with common beliefs in other things they might have a sexual rapport—and a sexual merger that might have led to marriage. Both female and male teenagers will be well aware that the video is Sexually Devaluing, on the sick sex side.

But as teachers will point out, without the caring sexual sophistication of their generation, in those days Anita Hill, who had been raised as a Southern Baptist with very strict views on sexual behavior, was horrified. In those days, 60 percent of the women in a *Time* magazine survey agreed that a man telling them about pornography constituted sexual harassment, and the entire nation was determined to eliminate sexual harassment forever largely by denying that men and women could ever find a way of expressing their sexual attractions for one another without creating a sick sex atmosphere.

Students will be aware that power, and conquest of the female was an underlying conditioning of the American male in the twentieth century. Thomas denied his sexual interest in Hill, but William Smith admitted, inadvertently, that all he was interested in was a "quickie" with a woman he had known only an hour or two. Several other women in his life who were not permitted to testify indicated that Smith never had much mental rapport with any female. Interestingly, both men had strong religious conditioning, which obviously didn't include an ability to step outside their skins and really identify with a woman, or perhaps any other person, in situations that challenged their own egos.

Teachers will evoke a future William Smith, and the women they meet, for their ninth- to twelfth-grade students. Unlike the twentieth-century Smith, this young man will have been molded by the new sexual morality. He goes out for an evening with male friends and meets Ms. Maybe. The future Smith has completed his GLUE education, but not in the Roommate of the Other Sex Program. He's now in graduate school, unmarried, and hasn't had sex with a woman for a month or so. Ms. Maybe, who is divorced and has a young child, discovers that Smith and she are able to talk about many things together, and they seem to be on the same intellectual level. She quite frankly admits, pensively perhaps, if the right man came along, and could love her and her young child, she'd try marriage again. Smith is equally frank. He'd like a female friend to go to bed with, but he wants to travel and see the world before he settles down—and, he admits with a grin, he's not even sure that he could be monogamous forever. In the next hour or so they both dare to really share their most intimate feelings with each other (see, ahead, the ability to self-disclose taught in the K-12 liberal arts environment), thus, very quickly Smith and Ms. Maybe have learned a great deal about what motivates each other sexually.

If Ms. Maybe goes back to Smith's apartment, it will be because she has already decided that it would be nicer to spend the night with a loving friend than sleep alone. They tell each other that they know they aren't HIV carriers and will show their recent blood test credentials. He tells her that he would prefer to have sex without a condom. They both agree that "bare back" is more fun, and that they enjoy oral sex but she tells him that until they are more monogamously inclined, and perhaps, one day, might get involved in one of those "corporate marriages" that FFAC is experimenting with (see ahead), she'll be happier if they enjoy a lot of foreplay, and a condom-covered sexual merger. They both know from experience that the real joy of sex comes *after the orgasm,* and the continuing joy of discovery of each other as they fall asleep talking, and later wake up again to a flesh-to-flesh embrace that floods their brains, and they know that daring to be totally vulnerable and self-revealing with each other, is the key to their sense of fulfillment and the great sex that they shared.

Smith and Ms. Maybe, unlike too many people in the twentieth century, have had a complete liberal arts education, and can easily discover many common driving interests that enhance their sexual merger. They have learned the ability to completely surrender their minds and bodies as they make love knowing their efforts will culminate in a momentary, total loss of self, a peak experience, and a fleeting merger with infinity, God, or whatever may be beyond human comprehension. Their night together may be a prelude to a need for each other as complex persons, but it is not a come and go encounter. For a moment at least they became the other person.

As the rape trials revealed, and teachers will point, this was not the kind of sexual encounter that occurred in the William Kennedy Smith case. Why? Because Smith, like millions of younger and older men, had never learned how to be sexually honest with a woman, or accept rejection with loving laughter, if she didn't respond to him emotionally and intellectually. They will point out that in the twentieth century, when a man or woman kissed each other fervently, whether they believed it or not, they must murmur something about love, or presumably have some feeling of love that would persist beyond the sexual merger. The Smiths and Ms. Maybes of the twenty-first century are not interested in quickies or one night stands. The joy of discovery, mental rapport, self-revelation, and wealth of common interests were all byproducts of their education, which taught them how to share another person's emotional and mental needs and laid the foundations for them, and millions of other Americans, to create the final sex revolution.

8

New, Self-Imposed Ratings: Movies

The self-imposed rating system as defined by Future Families of America and approved by a majority of Americans will define many sexual values and give a new perspective on what is sexually moral and what is not. It also comes to grips with reality. Whether we like it or not, from the first moving pictures to ubiquitous television, in one way or another, movies and television define and create moral values for young people. And they do it on many levels with dynamic, visual story telling that parents, teachers, and religious leaders can never equal.

While both families, religious leaders, and the media will be the watchdogs over self-imposed ratings, teachers during the human sexuality seminars in the last three years of high school will be appraising some of the SDH (Sexually Devaluing Historically) and SDN (Sexually Devaluing Now) ratings. They will encourage students to evaluate these offerings and determine whether or not particular producers, directors, or writers were deliberately trying to cross the exploitation line, and whether preceding or following their productions they offered valid comparisons between the sexual sickness of the past and the SN (Sexually Natural) and caring environment that the NSME legislation has brought into being.

It should be noted that while the law permits much more graphic portrayal of SN sexual mergers on film and television than in the 1990s, it prohibits the viewing of live action between consenting adults, unless it occurs in a stage presentation as a part of the story line. In the 1990s, live sex shows were available in the fringe areas of many large cities in the United States and widely available in Denmark and Germany as well as Thailand and Latin American countries. *Exotic Dancer* magazine, in its 1995–1996 issue, lists two thousand so-called Gentlemen's Clubs where porno actresses travel the circuit, and along with local women, earn thousands of dollars a week exposing their breasts and vulvas, as they dance and talk intimately to sex-hungry men. Their sole purpose was tourist shock, or solitary male sexual arousal, and the action as well as the environment was sexually devaluing. The premise is that SN, SDH, and SDN presentations on television or film, except for educational purposes, are a part of a story line and can be viewed in relative tranquillity, and the viewer can watch alone in rapport with the actors, and in most cases can share the sexual joy and laughter with other persons, including family.

So what is sexual devaluation? It should be emphasized that in no case will an SN rating be applied to story situations in which either sex is portrayed as sub-servient or the underdog in a relationship. Story lines revealing problems of inter-personal relations sans sex will be given self-imposed NSV ratings—Not Primarily Sexual or Violent. Although sex problems might be an underlying cause, and there might be anger and some violence, bad language, or even nudi-ty in these stories, the overall inability of particular people to resolve their exter-nal or ego problems would be apparent. Except for nudity, NSV offerings will parallel current PG offerings, which tend to be known in the 1990s as family "feel good" films. A few from previous years which would have self-imposed NSV rat-ings would be *City Slickers* and *When Harry Met Sally,* both featuring Billy Crystal and offering a blend of wry comedy and believable sexual dialogue; *Trust Me,* with many sad insights into human sexual behavior and which currently has an R rating; and all of Spike Lee's films (*Do the Right Thing, Mo' Better Blues,* and *Jungle Fever*). *Dances with Wolves* would have an SDH rating, which would have permitted more SN sequences, as would *Robin Hood.* I will explore this rat-ing in detail just ahead. Before you read them, keep in mind that they are partic-ularly weighted against female sexual devaluation. Surprisingly, some women, like Sallie Tisdale, a young mother in her thirties with three children, might dis-agree. In her 1994 book, *Talk Dirty to Me,* Sallie, admittedly bisexual, analyzes her own thinking, and other than outright sexual brutality, would probably admit that some of these sexually verboten sequences would turn her on, and she might enjoy them.

Great! I'm sure that Nadine Strossen, a lawyer and president of the American Civil Liberties Union, isn't rowing in the same boat with Sallie. Strossen's 1995 book, *Defending Pornography—Free Speech, Sex, and the Fight for Women's Liberation,* is actually campaigning against the totally negative approaches of Catherine Mackinnon and Andrea Dworkin. But Strossen's realistic and sensual view of women will probably shock many male conservatives. She's determined to protect women against "powerlessness and paternalism." But aren't they the basic theme of most X-rated films?

In any event, if either lady objects to the premise—which isn't complete censorship—all of the sick throw-up sex for the totally sexually hung up will still be available in video stores that offer X-rated videos. Does sexually hung up include Camille Paglia, who calls her approach in her 1994 book, *Vamps and Traps* "drag queen feminism"? Don't ask me? But it might be fun to go to bed with Camille and talk sex all night.

Rather than view the ratings as fait accompli reality, let's assume that the following listing of sexual devaluation guidelines proposed by FFAC has a majority approval reflected by national polls and the situations or portrayals can never be shown in movie theaters or on network television:

1. No sadistic or masochistic portrayals of any kind, including consensual bondage and discipline.
2. No male ejaculation into a woman's mouth, or anywhere outside a woman's vagina.
3. No group sex, or sex with more than one person.
4. No nonconsensual sex, rape, or violence during or preceding the sex act, or as its byproduct.
5. No sex with anyone under the age of seventeen. Reinforcing GLUE, stories or teaching films showing young people thirteen to sixteen avoiding or holding back from sexual merger in loving ways will be a popular new area for filmmakers. No sex between seventeen-year-olds and any person who is more than four years older. In later ages May/December SN mergers are acceptable. Since under seventeen sex avoidance and seventeen-year-old coming-of-age stories will be popular, all SN ratings in this area will widely monitored.
6. No body disfigurement, including tattooing, breast augmentation, or shaving the pubic area to create the illusion that a particular woman is underage.
7. No picturing women or men naked or partially naked who are using implied sexual action or dialogue as potential sale stimulators in any advertising.
8. No picturing of men or women naked that graphically emphasizes a person's genitals to the exclusion of his or her entire body (except for teaching sex films). In this category, unlike *Hustler* and other skin magazines, *Playboy* and *Penthouse* would probably be able to qualify for SN ratings, but since being naked will be a common way of life, most men will lose interest in glamorized photographs of naked women, and such magazines may not survive.
9. No sex with animals or urination or defecation in a sexual context.

Many of the above are familiar offerings on X-rated videotapes, which I will discuss later (see ahead). The self-imposed guidelines offered by FFAC will also state that visual presentations of any of these prohibited actions, even though they may be historically accurate and carry SDH ratings, or reflect current reality, cannot be graphically included in films or videos with these ratings. If any of these prohibitions are a part of the story line, or current reality, they must take place off screen with some limited dialogue explaining or implying the action.

Both the SN, SDH, and SDN ratings are controversial, and in the early years will be the focus of much public discussion, pro and con, and they are subject to modification. For example, based on these ratings all late afternoon soap operas, and evening variations following in the footsteps of "Dynasty" and "Knots Landing," along with many of the weekly hour series similar to "L.A. Law" and "NYPD Blue" would have an SD rating and could not be shown on network television. But the SN ratings will permit the visualization of many new kinds of sexual relationships that can be explored in an SN environment. This SN action could include adultery, consensual incest, or caring sex between married participants with a partner other than their spouse, in stories revealing the problems of people who have gone beyond monogamy, for good or bad in their particular lives.

But the NSME legislation is not dictatorial. There will be no attempt to rewrite the history books. There will be general agreement that the depiction of past or current sexual devaluation in films, books, videos, and other media is not being produced for monetary gain, but, like memorial museums, are vivid reminders of past human insanities. Forgetting, an out-of-sight, out-of-mind mentality, would provide the seeding ground for history to repeat itself. The value of SDH and SDN creations, which must offer their own raison d'etre, is to contrast the immoralities of the past with the saner, life-sustaining moralities of the twenty-first century. Some SDH ratings may also carry a UV (Unnaturally Violent) rating when the subject requires. For many years the demand to see the past recreated as it really was sexually, and the insistence on more historically accurate films with believable story lines, will guide all Americans morally, and provide much better dramatic possibilities than fantasy junk like *Batman* and *Dick Tracy* while at the same time giving all Americans much better historical roots.

Here are a few potential SDH historical remakes that would entrance audiences with their sexual maneuverings, such as the story of Queen Christina of Sweden (once played by Greta Garbo) and the nature of the warring world of Europe in her day, when politics and sex were continuously intermixed. Or an SDH film featuring Catherine of Russia, who lived during our own Revolutionary War era, could, along with SN and many SD motivations, draw huge audiences. A recent movie, *Young Catherine*, shot in England and Russia, is one of the better films of the 1990s, and could under this rating have explored, in even more fascinating detail, the reason Catherine, a German princess, following the empress of Russia's suggestion, took a lover, to provide succession to the throne. Peter III, Catherine's husband, who didn't love her very much anyway, was sterile, but not impotent. Before Catherine, in all probability, conspired in his murder, Peter issued a ukase that adultery should henceforth be exempt from official censure: "Since in that matter even Christ had not condemned men." The continuing story about the older Catherine, who wrote her own memoirs, and who Voltaire considered a truly great woman, can explore both the motivations of a highly sexual woman, and her attempt to make Russia the greatest nation in the world. It offers plenty of potential SN and UV action. Catherine never married again, but in her long lifetime, from age thirty-two to age sixty-seven, she had twenty-one lovers. The last was twenty-five when she was sixty-one. And none of her lovers resented the next one—no jealousy, and, amazingly, no unwanted children. Catherine was not only a feminist but was far better educated than most of peers.

There are thousands of stories from the past that are not only fascinating historical revelations but make the hoked-up television mini-series and improbable soap operas pale by comparison with past realities. These are stories that will reinforce the new sexual morality. In passing I'll toss in Anne Hutchinson's story, which I retold in the 1990s in a novel that resurrected America's first feminist. Not Anne, but the Puritans believed in resurrection. They were sure that they would be among that number when the saints came marching in. Why was Anne slaughtered by the Indians at the age of fifty-two? Why was one of her fifteen children saved by the Indians, after they murdered her? Were Thomas Dudley and John Winthrop involved in her murder? Why was she put on trial with Dudley and Winthrop acting as judge and jury for the Massachusetts Bay Colony? Why was she later banished by her church? Why did John Cotton, the minister she loved, betray her? Were her last two children his?

Or watch a film like *Caligula* again. It is currently X-rated. How close was it to the realities written about by Suetonius? Both *Caligula,* and the eight-hour-long "I Claudius" series, which appears intermittently on PBS, could have SDH ratings, and if they had been made after the NSME legislation, could have been much more sexually graphic, and reveal in bedroom detail the patriarchal control of women and the sexual devaluation that was endemic in Roman times. Or, for a current SDH example, a movie like *The Doors,* exploring the sexual insanities of the 1960s, would have an SDH rating. But all movies and other art forms complying with the prohibitions on sexual devaluation could also offer sexually natural situations counteracting, along with the required raison d'etre, the sick sex relationships inherent in these stories.

Michael Crichton's novel *Disclosure,* which was made into a film, and Armistead Maupin's *Tales of the City,* provide two current examples of SDN and

SDH ratings. While Crichton's story is a novel about a woman sexually harassing a male, Crichton, who is a preacher at heart, and writes thesis novels, provides the required explanatory afterword: "The episode related here is a based on a true story," he writes. "Its appearance in a novel is not to deny the fact that the great majority of harassment claims are brought by women against men. On the contrary: the advantage of a role reversal story is that it may enable us to examine aspects concealed by traditional responses and conventional rhetoric."

That, in essence, is the basis of the SDH and SDN self-imposed ratings. As Crichton said in an interview, "We need to make new rules about what is acceptable and what's not." While, as I have pointed out, sexual harassment will be a nonissue with a new generation who have had the K-12 moral/value sexual training, this kind of story in print or film reinforces the present by exposing the past.

"Tales of the City," a six-hour drama, is a good example of an SDH story that also has a GS rating. The show ran on PBS on three consecutive nights in January 1994 and portrays a slice of life in San Francisco in 1976. It is one of the few 1990s network dramas that offered casual female nudity as well as romance coupled with the sicker side of gay life—"cruising," as well as Anna Madrigal (played by Olympia Dukakis). She's a loving woman, a former transsexual who has had her testicles removed. The series also offers a wealthy woman whose husband is gay but who manages to get pregnant by her Chinese grocery store delivery man, and a child pornographer exposed by the naive female who has chosen to live in the Bay Area rather than back home in Ohio, in a moral environment of friends and family who don't approve of fringe people who happily share each other's sexual idiosyncrasies. Maupin, who is gay, appears at the end of the series and explains that the incidents are based on true life events that he experienced or heard about. The presumption is that these sexually screwed up people were as happy, or happier, than most people in the mid-1990s, which will amuse a younger generation who enjoy a heterosexual environment of wonder, joy, and laughter, and would lead to a discussion—whether Maupin should have provided a raison d'etre as a requirement of the SDH rating.

Here's one final example of the value of SDH films or videos which would come to realistic grips with the sexual sickness of past eras and at the same time provide new sexual morality insights. A film loosely based on William Kennedy Smith's encounter with Patricia Bowman could use Smith's own words, "We had sex," correcting his attorney's interpretation that their actions were "an act of love." The fictionalized movie could explore Bowman's need to be loved, and her overtures when she knows that she's being "picked up." The way she dances with Smith, moving her body suggestively, indicates to him that she is available. She's pretty and he'd enjoy sex with her. For him it's a one-night stand, but he tries not to be too overt in this attitude. Nevertheless, he's obviously not interested when

Bowman tells him about her failed marriage or that she's had a baby. He doesn't want to be brain-intimate with her. So you watch them in this SDH version of their story sitting on the deserted beach as they kiss and slowly strip each other, showing him caressing her breasts, and she playing with his penis. This is sexually natural, but she's dubious—especially when he wants to go back to the house, where they can make love more comfortably. So he goes for a swim to cool his throbbing cock. "That doesn't sound too romantic," the prosecuting attorney actually told Smith. "It doesn't sound like two people in the throes of passion."

Of course not. Both Smith and Bowman were in a moral stand off. She wants the warmth of sex and loving that equals her fantasy, but she's aware of what he may be thinking. In the male vernacular, she's not much more than "a piece of ass." Their mutual nonmental involvement is written in stone when he has two climaxes within a half hour with a woman that he calls Cathy at the moment of orgasm, and she keeps calling him Michael. Her later cry of rape is not realistic. She has somehow lost her dreams, her quintessential self, and tries to throw the blame on Smith. The sad truth as the SDH drama would reveal is that we were all to blame. Only now are we rediscovering ourselves in a sexually sane society.

Let us turn to the self-imposed GS rating, which accepts male kissing, and caring male sexual embraces such as occur in *Philadelphia* and other currently R-rated, gay-oriented films. As mentioned previously, visual presentations of men enjoying oral sex and anal sex, although they may be accurate facets of gay sex life, cannot be shown on film or video in movies or network television. The line drawn, in this case, faces the larger reality that the basic thrust of gay and lesbian sex is entropic. It doesn't reflect the reality that men and women were designed by God or Gaia and were either brought into being on the sixth day, or have evolved. If we have any purpose at all, it is to copulate with a member of the other sex and to perpetuate ourselves. If we don't, gay men and lesbians will soon vanish, and leave the planet to the saner fish, flesh, fowl, and insects, who, before they overpopulate manage to get eaten by their enemies.

It should be emphasized that the self-imposed ratings do not limit artistic creativity. Writers and filmmakers can join forces with the new morality. Past history or real life stories that portray sexual devaluation and violence will let writers and filmmaker reveal the sexual fears and dishonesty of the participants, in their particular times and environments, along with underlying new moral comparisons that will evoke positive responses from many viewers: "Thank God that today—at last—we live in a world where men and women, from their early teens, have learned to deflect their burgeoning sexual compulsions for a about four years until they are seventeen, with the certainty that for the rest of their lives they will really know how to enjoy their sexual drives and share them with caring friends, lovers, and spouses.

The need for a self-imposed SN, SDH, and SDN rating system following the FFAC guidelines is underscored by Michael Medved's book *Hollywood vs America: Popular Culture and the War of Traditional Values*. Medved points out that in film after film—many of them receiving top Oscar Awards—such as *Bugsy* (about a ruthless gangster), *Cape Fear* (a murderous psycho), *Silence of the Lambs* (a serial killer), *Prince of Tides* (suicidal manic depressives), *Fisher King* (a delusional psychotic), and *Home Alone* (kids who don't need adults and are smarter than they are, anyway)—in all these films Hollywood, unrestrained, is helping cut loose the moral anchors and moorings of the past.

"Did you ever notice how few movies there are about happily married people?" Medved asks. "Those that are made tend to portray marriage as a disaster, as a dangerous situation, as a battleground." There's been long series of murderous marriage movies, such as: *Sleeping with the Enemy*, where Julia Roberts eventually kills her husband; *Mortal Thoughts*, in which Bruce Willis beats up his wife; and *Thelma and Louise*, with a brutal, insensitive husband motivating the story.

Here are a few more 1992–1994 movies that would have an SD rating and never would appear on network television, or in theaters, and when they were shown on cable would be preceded with SD warnings or combination SD-UV warnings: *Drugstore Cowboy, Basic Instinct, Bad Lieutenant, The Hand That Rocks the Cradle, Body of Evidence, Rising Sun, Serial Mom, Pulp Fiction, True Lies,* and *Natural Born Killers*. There are hundreds more. Whether the authors or producers insist that these films are fictionalized versions of reality or not the premise is that they can be better portrayed in actual SDN versions that will satisfy whatever need people may have to witness sexual degradation along with the required comparison between a sick sex era and the present, where caring sex predominates in human relationships.

Medved's book covers all bases, including unnatural violence, which in the 1990s was even more popular than sex at the box office. His book was excoriated by the media and other film critics, who accused Medved of a "nervous breakdown," "puerile populism," "cultural fundamentalism," and the kind of Republican values expounded by Dan Quayle. But the naysayers refused to face reality. Millions of Americans for the past seventy-five years have been morally conditioned not only by the movies that they watch but by an additional fifty years of television, creating an American value system. In the 1920s, only a few years after moving pictures were invented, it became apparent that some film producers were going beyond the accepted sexual morality of the times. Gloria Swanson, Theda Bara, and even Rudolph Valentino appeared naked in films like *Intolerance* and *Blood and Sand*. To save themselves from the onslaught of shocked religious leaders, who were led by the Legion of Decency, in 1922 the producers themselves established the Will Hays office and what amounted to a self-imposed rating code. Although there were no ratings as such, the Hays office proclaimed, "The sanctity of the institution of marriage and the home should be upheld; low forms of social relationships should be avoided; adultery must not be explicitly treated, or justified, or presented attractively, films should not be presented to stimulate the lower elements of society, and rape or seduction is not the proper subject for comedy." For more than twenty years self-imposed codes made bad language an absolute no-no, and if you watch many of the oldies you'll never discover a man and woman in bed together. Even married couples had to sleep in twin beds.

In the tenth to twelfth grades, students will be encouraged to watch some of the American Movie Channel's releases of movies made during the years that the Hays Office and later the Motion Picture Rating Association supervised the moral structure of films. Practically every sordid aspect of human sexual behavior was presented in famous films from *Little Caesar* to *Peyton Place,* but the moral overtones of the times prevailed and the bad guys and gals got their comeuppance in vivid endings showing that God was watching, and not until much later were *Never On Sunday* prostitutes glorified. More on this in part 2.

As in the past, criticism of the NSME legislation and the self-imposed ratings will be based on the belief that you can't legislate morality. Perhaps not when it comes to drugs and alcohol or other brain escape mechanisms, probably because in many cases these have been allied with religious experiences and are not condemned by the gods or their prophets. By contrast, restraint of human sexuality is embedded in the major Western religions. In the mid-1990s a vastly undereducated majority, and a voluble, educated, and presumably liberated minority, often combined and tried to equate any sexual expression, degraded, devalued, or not, with First Amendment rights and freedom of speech. The NSME legislation exalting human sexuality and defining sexual devaluation provides the balance on the see-saw between the left and right. Like all common causes, top leadership at the federal level can lead the way, as it has done with smoking, and promoting condoms to prevent AIDS and sexually transmitted diseases (and, unsaid, to contain the growth of welfare mothers). In the coming years the federal government will most certainly be legislating morality in environmental issues and the many marriage and family problems raised by in vitro fertilization and our continuing biotechnological discoveries.

Unlike past and present movie rating systems the SDH and SDN self-imposed ratings are not the final decision of the producer or writer. All Americans will pass final judgment on whether the premise of the new ratings has been violated.

9

New, Self-Imposed Ratings: Television, Books, and the Arts

During June 1993, all the major networks began posting what amounted to self-imposed advisories, or warnings, on programs that contained violent material. Meanwhile, federal lawmakers, not satisfied with the results, drafted a plan to create a new rating system with independent monitors who would police the results. Afraid of this kind of censorship, cable companies (as distinguished from network broadcasters), whose vast audience of paid subscribers presumably prefer uncut R-rated movies, sexy and/or violent, countered with their own guidelines, which included restricting shows with graphic material (both violence and sex) to later hours. They also approved legislation which would require television manufacturers to insert a "V" (for violence) chip into new television sets. The chip would make it possible for the home user to block out programs unfit for children or for themselves.

During the 1990s citizens' groups appealed to the broadcasting industry to adopt a "voluntary code of socially responsible practice standards to counteract mounting evidence that the socially insensitive mass media is contributing heavily to societal crises." George Gerbner of the Annenberg School of Communications pointed out the basic reason: "Learning about the world is increasingly the byproduct of mass marketing. Most of the stories about life and values are not told by parents, grandparents, teachers, or clergy, but by a handful of distant conglomerates with something to sell." His point was well documented in the mid-1990s when broadcasters began to build their story lines around theme parks like Treasure Island, and, in a not too subtle way, tried to hypnotize parents into bringing their children to the actual site of the story action they have watched.

The self-imposed movie codes analyzed in the previous chapter, plus the K-12 comprehensive sexual education seminars, resolve the problems by confining

SD and UV showings strictly to cable. The so called V chip control would then make it possible for a rapidly diminishing cable audience to control underage viewing of programs that are prohibited on network television. Note that I predict a rapidly diminishing audience for SD and UV programs. Young people in the last four years of high school taking K-12 sex seminars, in addition to their twelfth-grade studies of pornography on a historical basis (see ahead) will act as a third force of young people who will denounce sexual devaluation. They will monitor the older generation, who are addicted to UV or SD showings. As has been shown with smoking and drunk driving, a disparaging minority can create new, majority opinions in a relatively short time, as well as new social conditioning on all levels. At the same time SDH and SDN programming, with its required raisons d'etre, balanced by SN (sexually natural) content will reveal the sickness and folly of past human behavior and create a total revulsion against sleazy, demeaning sex and slice and dice, hoked-up horror presentations.

In the mid-1990s Planned Parenthood estimated that teenagers watched nine thousand scenes annually on television of suggested sexual intercourse and sex comments. The group didn't include sexual innuendo, the sick sex content of most of the video talk shows, soap operas, and verbally sexual music presented visually on MTV. MTV video awards are often won by contestants like M.C. Hammer, Mike Patton, Michael Jackson, and others who grab their crotches suggestively, or Madonna and Janet Jackson, swirling their behinds in orgasmic ecstasy while they jiggle partially exposed breasts. Sexual come-ons, except in SN environments, will carry SD ratings and cannot be shown on network TV, but they will be available for those who think they are sexually deprived on paid cable, since complete censorship is not advocated and is impractical. Better to laugh sick sex out of existence with loving, joyous sex.

In addition to SDH, SDN, and SN story-related programming, Future Families of America will recognize that the new approaches to both sexual and liberal arts education in secondary school should be reinforced by substantial funding of public television, which, according to many critics in the mid-1990s, had lost its way, and was being effectively replaced by the Learning Channel, the Arts & Entertainment channel, and the Discovery Channel, all of which are dependent on commercial advertising.

In this environment if the Public Broadcasting System survives the cutbacks in the Contract for America, it can offer its own SDH and SDN presentations, and also create a backup New Sexual Morality network for parents, students, and teachers. Publicly funded television on Wednesday nights from 6 P.M. to midnight could offer actual classroom experience in K-12 education. The programs would be aimed at improving teaching in various subjects in all grades, and teachers could interact with parents and the young over open phone lines. Teaching ethics, new moral values underlying the NSME legislation, philosophy, psychology, economics, discussing environmental and regional and national problems, would get parents and young people involved in the joys of lifetime learning. World political leaders and their people would be interviewed, and religious, ethnic, and cultural differences of people in every part of the world could be explored in detail, as well as how religious indoctrination creates long-lasting internal conflicts with civil wars and hatred, as exemplified in the former Yugoslavia.

Hundreds of sex teaching films were available in the 1990s from the Institute for the Advanced Study of Human Sexuality and Focus International. Here are a few titles that could be shown on a PBS human sexuality series: "Breaking the Language Barrier—Sexual Slang"; "Sexual Anatomy and Physiology—Male and Female"; "The Naked Breast"—a study of the female breast in evolution; "Exhibiting the Male Genitalia"—picturing multiracial penises, flaccid, urinating, erect, ejaculating in both art and life; "Grand Opening: The Female Genitalia"—picturing the vulva in detail and examining the clitoris, labia, vaginal opening, and KV; "Male and Female Masturbation"—portraying masturbation in terms of realistic gratification and tension release.

While in a sane sexual society, defying the law by appearing naked in public won't make the headlines, television won't ignore the past heights of the ridiculous such as "streakers"—guys and gals running naked across campus in the 1970s to the chagrin of the authorities, as a protest and a form of sexual freedom that they believed was denied to them. Or the Princeton University officials arguing in December 1991 whether the famous twenty-one-year-old Nude Olympics, when several hundred young students felt compelled to run naked through the streets on the first snowfall, should be prohibited. Or Andrew Martinez, six foot three inches tall, with a muscular body, who as a junior was expelled from the University of California at Berkeley because he was determined to defy Western, sexually repressed traditions and go everywhere (weather permitting) totally naked. Martinez made national headlines as the Naked Guy, and was the subject of a long article in the *Wall Street Journal* weighing the pros and most cons of exposing one's body. Martinez said he got the idea in high school, when he was smoking marijuana and started asking the big questions: "What is the meaning of life?" "What is the big question?"

The big question young people brought up in a sane sexual environment where they've seen naked people of all ages from childhood will ask is: How did Americans get so horrified by their bodies that a young man achieved fame simply by exposing his? In this new environment, adding to Marshall McLuhan's words: "The medium will become the upbeat sexual moral message."

A few months before Lorena Bobbitt made penis a household word, school officials in Eugene, Oregon, were concerned about a television program that revealed the penis of Michelangelo's David, which had been covered for many years. John Wayne Bobbitt was offered $15,000 to show the reattachment of his organ, but refused. By contrast, the horror of revealing sexual areas of the human body is not so deep-seated in Europe. In the mid-1990s sex with laughter and nudity on television in Canada and England was commonplace. Even more surprising was Italy, whose broadcasters, defying religious moralities, offer full frontal nudity and spicy sexual conversation as a way of life after 10:30 P.M. *Newsweek* reported on December 1991, "Men in Italy don't bother to go to hookers any more. They just watch them on television." Italian TV offers programs like "It Pays to Make Love Well," during which every aspect of sexmaking is discussed. "Colpo Grosso" offers a weekly strip tease program, in which contestants must take off clothing if they give the wrong answers. A female member of the Italian Senate shrugs at the huge popularity of such programs: "Most Italian men are sadly ignorant about women. . . . Sex and sexuality would be much more useful on television . . . if it were presented in such a way that it helped lift the taboos, and let us understand the causes of repression." Illona Staller, a part time X-rated actress elected to the Italian Parliament, agreed and quite often showed her breasts to Italian lawmakers in response to their lewd gossip about her breast size.

During the first years, as SN presentations become a way of life on network television, there will be a conflict over whether sexual silliness, or sex with laughter, like some of the Italian programs, isn't also, basically, sexually devaluing. Writers and producers will walk a thin line, but will be well aware that the K-12 education of a new generation will eliminate millions of contrived "dirty jokes" that once were the conversational entrees in Western culture, but won't suppress natural, loving sex tease, or flirting by either men or women. The difference between demeaning sex and sex with laughter will be lemon tree obvious.

Past worries about how television, video games, and the inevitable merge of computer monitors with direct television access will affect the younger generation will be minimized once primary and secondary schools are totally focused on a liberal arts education. The broad, value-based education of the younger generation, including an ability to read rapidly with full comprehension, along with an education that gives a new generation deep historical roots will make children immune to "sound bite" dramas and newscasting. A better-educated people will challenge the shock values that once prevailed in much television advertising and on a political level will demand more programs of the MacNeil/Lehrer type, which attempt to present both sides of every kind of controversy in depth, impartially.

The self-imposed rating systems will apply to all video games. The SD- and UV-rated games so prevalent in the mid-1990s cannot be broadcast on interactive television. Like X-rated movies, games that feature kidnapped women, and games that Marsha Kinder, in her book *Playing with Power in Movies, Television and Video Games,* insists are underscored with "phallic empowerment or penis power," will still be available for rental but not for people under seventeen. A majority of Americans will have become aware, as Eugene Provenzo has pointed out, "These games do little or nothing to help a child develop an inner culture, a sense of self, and an awareness that while the world provides challenges and problems, personal resourcefulness and the use of one's own imagination are the important parts of being able to confront these challenges."

Learning via video games and CD-ROMs on computer tubes will enhance learning but will never replace the printed word. Despite the vast accessibility to all knowledge, transferring that knowledge to one's individual brain and making it usable is a slow process. Reading and rereading the printed word—digesting it, thinking about the meanings, and achieving the final distillation into one's brain, is not a tube-gleaning process.

The sad fact is that a majority of video games that created a multibillion-dollar industry in the 1990s offered a dangerously simplified world of good guys and bad guys that a finger-skilled child operator can zap out of existence. They also create the illusion that easy-to-come-by handguns can do the same thing. The self-imposed SD and UV ratings, along with K-12 comprehensive sexuality education, won't censor such games out of existence, but will gradually eliminate them as a saner sexual morality prevails.

The same thing will happen with many books and magazines. In the world of art, SD labels, like cigarette warnings, won't immediately deter many readers or viewers, but will remind them that they are no longer Sexually Correct, with SC becoming a more valid label than the ambivalent PC, or politically correct, that guided some educators in the 1990s.

In the mid-1990s the National Endowment for the Arts came under crossfire from the religious right headed up by Pat Robertson and Sen. Jesse Helms. Helms was so shocked by Robert Mapplethorpe's photographs, and the fact that Mapplethorpe had received federal money to pursue his photographic careers that he asked women and adolescent pages to leave the Senate chambers before he displayed them.

There were others: Karen Finley, who had her fifteen minutes of fame doing a strip act that presumably revealed male defilement of the female body; Andre Serrano, whose photograph "Piss Christ" cast aspersion on Jesus' divinity; and Annie Sprinkles (her name indicates her joy in urinating on men she's having sex with), a veteran porno actress who never received any government funding for her "Post Porn Modernist" program, during which she maneuvered her large breasts for laughter, not seduction, inserted a speculum in her vagina, and invited people in the audience to look at her cervix. All were a part of a fringe group of self-proclaimed artists following in the footsteps of Andy Warhol, for whom nothing was sexually devaluing if it was sexually honest by their standards.

Under the self-imposed rating system many of Mapplethorpe's photographs of men pissing on each other or enjoying anal intercourse, along with all of the above, would be labeled SD or SS (Sexually Sick) but, totally avoiding censorship in the printed book area, could be published with ratings prominent. Always keeping in mind that the NSME legislation is preventing men like Jimmy Baker or Jimmy Swaggart or many of those in the Christian Coalition from emulating Adolf Hitler, who wrote, "Theater, art, literature, cinema, press, and window displays must be cleansed of all manifestations of our rotting world. Public life must be freed from the stifling perfume of modern eroticism . . . the right duty recedes before the duty to preserve the race."

In the realm of erotic art there are thousands of paintings, drawings, and sculptures that portray nudity and human copulation which will be classified SN and will be widely available in school libraries. Teachers from the ninth grade on can use books like *The Erotic Arts* by Peter Webb, *Erotic Art of the West* by Robert Melville, *Primitive Erotic Art* by Phillip Rawson, and the two-volume *Erotic Art* by Phyllis and Eberhard Kronhausen, and they point out that in most cases the artist's sexual frustrations and hang-ups were the source of their sexually devaluing art.

Ultimately, once erotic art is freed of censorship, and future young artists grow up in a sane sexual society, a new-style Pre-Raphaelite brotherhood like Dante Rossetti, William Holman Hunt, and John Millais may develop a new narrative-style art embodying many aspects of human sexuality. Younger artists following Andrew Wyeth and Robert Brackman's lead can now go much further and paint graphically or impressionistically the joy and wonder of sexual merger.

As Judith Langer, who heads a market research consulting firm, pointed out in the 1990s, "We are a society going in different directions at the same time. Sexual behavior is, now, more conservative because of the AIDS epidemic . . . but even if people are becoming more monogamous, their fantasy lives, their desire to act out vicariously, will be even greater. We at least want to flirt with the idea of leading a risque life." Probably grinning a bit, Langer also stated that; "Nude men appeal to a lot of women. . . . It's not just homoerotic, but heteroerotic women are recognizing that they like the shape of men's bodies. Now men have to be on their toes and keep in shape. They can't allow themselves to go to pot."

Book publishers will conform with the self-imposed rating system, as will newspapers and magazines, who will confine SD news stories and features to a defined section. There will be no censorship or limitations on what can be printed in books or magazines. In passing, it's interesting to note that in 1994, Golden Book, famous publisher of children's stories, began to publish new, nonviolent versions of "Chicken Little," "The Three Little Pigs," and "Little Red Riding Hood"—proving, if nothing else, that publishers can censor themselves.

Widely circulated newspapers will avoid printing sexually devaluing photographs. The assumption, true or not, is that the sexual words, devaluing or not, are not so inciting to sexual action as pictures. Readers of pornography will be safe in their fantasy world. But where the approach in words or pictures is sexually devaluing, the books and magazines will carry the SD rating prominently and in the process reinforce the new sexual morality.

In June 1993 I was pleased to be on a Sex for the Librarian panel at the annual convention of the American Library Association in New Orleans. The Intellectual Freedom Roundtable, which sponsored the panel, was established by the ALA in 1973 to create a united front against censorship. One section of the Library Bill of Rights states, "Libraries should challenge censorship in the fulfillment of their responsibility to provide information and enlightenment. Libraries should cooperate with all persons and groups concerned with the abridgement of free expression and free access to ideas."

This, of course, opens a sexual can of worms. In the mid-1990s, depending on the location of a particular library—those in major cities were less inhibited by the local school boards and religious groups—the problems of what books, magazines, and video cassettes might be purchased and loaned and to whom, was and is a subject, in the area of sex, in which there were no nationally agreed upon standards. On the next page is a petition to the Library of Congress by the Intellectual Freedom Roundtable.

As I suggested to the librarians in some detail, they could immediately resolve many of their problems by using the NSME self-imposed rating system on all sexually oriented material. I have outlined above and announce nationally the following addition to their Library Bill of Rights:

> In the final years of the twentieth century, recognizing that there is a great diversity of opinion about sexual values and how they should be expressed in print and visually, and recognizing that freedom of expression carries social responsibilities, we are classifying sexual material in a way [on] which a majority of Americans can agree. . . . It is our belief that Sexually Natural pictures, videos, [and] magazines, as well as the printed word and material that extols and sacramentalizes human sexuality, will, with the endorsement of religious leaders and educators, lead to a healthier and more caring sexual society and will ultimately eliminate, or drastically reduce, the amount of deviant, brainless, voyeuristic sex that is undermining all our values. [We believe] that this approach will work much better than censorship.

While the proposal seemed quite utopian to librarians at the time, once the NSME is functioning, all that librarians will have to do is join with all Americans in policing the self-imposed ratings, and working with teachers in the human sexuality seminars to make SD material, past and present, available for research.

of men and women tried to find friends and sexual companions of the other sex through classified personals in many newspapers and magazines. The more flagrant weekly newspapers, like the *Boston Phoenix*, the *Village Voice*, and the *Los Angeles Free Press*, all with adult sections often larger than fifteen pages, featured porno actresses and wannabees offering verbal masturbation services by calling 900 phone numbers. Extended calls by sexually distressed males ran fifty dollars or more. In these weeklies you could also find advertisements for escorts, many of whom were professional prostitutes, and people of all races and colors ready and willing to participate in all kinds of deviational sex. All of these newspapers would label themselves SD or SS.

It should be noted that the K-12 comprehensive human sexuality seminars do not end with GLUE. All A13ers in the work study program pursuing either vocational degrees or bachelors degrees, whether they take the Roommate of the Other Sex Program option or not, will continue with a one-hour weekly human values seminar (see ahead), which, in addition to integrating their studies and examining all the values of modern civilizations, will, in equally mixed male/female groups, be encouraged by graduate student leaders to explore their first mating experiences and sexual problems, in depth, with each other. The weekly, coed, deeply interpersonal, undergraduate human values sessions will make it easier for all young people to find friends of the other sex with whom they can share caring and responsible unmarried sex, or, if they are in the ROSP Program do this in a nonthreatening sexual environment that in later life may show them how to reinforce monogamy with satellite relationships.

Stress Relief Clinics—legalized prostitution made possible by NMSE legislation (see ahead)—will help resolve the problems of both men and women who are deprived of sexual companionship.

Finally, in the area of materials that are sexually devaluing historically, once the new sexual morality prevails, teachers of tenth, eleventh, and twelfth graders can raise the question of whether some of the advertisers, using sexually natural situations and almost nudity to sell their products, might have been heralding a saner sexual morality. After NSME, using sex to sell products will require an SD labeling. Actually, in the mid-1990s some of the sex come-on advertising was sexually humorous and natural. The basic change under NSME is that such ads will no longer work, or have prurient appeal, because newspapers, magazines, and television, with no advertising sponsorship, have all embraced human nudity and caring sexmaking

But, in retrospect, Joanna Lipman's report in the *Wall Street Journal* of September 30, 1991, offers interesting comparison between past and future: "Ads with naked bodies and leering innuendo seem to be pushing the envelope of taste ever day. Calvin Klein's controversial jeans program, with barely clothed women and men fondling each other and themselves, is the latest in a long line of sex-centered ads for everything from Sansabelt pants to Camel cigarettes. . . . The old saying 'Sex sells' still prevails."

Roy Anderson of the Bozell Agency tried to qualify that point: "But it has to be done with taste." At a seminar on the problem run by Bozell, beer advertisers were considered Neanderthal in their attitude toward women, particularly when Old Milwaukee's was offering a gaggle of women they called the Swedish Bikini Team with the punchline: "It doesn't get any better than this!"

Writing for the *New York Times* on December 15, 1991, Stuart Elliott also offered interesting vignettes:

> Lever Brothers uses a peek-a-boo shot of a man and woman lathering their stomachs, chest and legs to promote 2000 soap; Calvin Klein pushing Obsession with a naked man and woman standing face to face in a swing; Teledyne ogles a muscular man from a variety of angles to promote their shower massage; Calvin Klein promotes their jeans in a supplement to an issue of *Vanity Fair* with a 116-page insert of Bruce Weber's photographs, among which was a young man taking a shower naked with his jeans clutched in a strategic position over his genitals; a young woman drawing a young man toward her by pulling down his unbuckled belt; a woman leaning against a tree, her hand on her breast; and a young man urinating, looking over his shoulder smiling.

And *Vanity Fair,* which offered a nude cover photo of actress Demi Moore pregnant, was paving the way for the final sex revolution and sexual sanity in the twenty-first century.

A new generation that has been educated from childhood to revere the wonders of their bodies and each other's sexual drives, a generation with many people who have learned how to share their lives with one or two people of the other sex, will enjoy magazines that run pictures or men and women of all ages, in all shapes and conditions, playing together—and, past seventeen, making love together. In a century in which the baby boomers will outnumber the younger generation, there will be much more emphasis on health and longevity, with many accolades for older men and women who have, as a result of their genes, or, more likely, careful eating, and nonstressful, caring love for each other, been able to maintain attractive and sexually appealing bodies. From seventeen to seventy and beyond there will be much media glorification, and advertisers, hailing the joys of sound minds and bodies that can still enjoy sexual merger.

10

Teaching Pornography,
30,000 B.C. to A.D. 1500

Before the passage of the New Sexual Morality Education legislation it wasn't possible to teach the history of human sexuality as a separate subject in high school, and it rarely happened in undergraduate studies except as a byproduct of other courses.

Now, with NSME and a totally liberal arts approach to secondary education made possible by GLUE, it will become accepted teaching practice in require courses in all of human history, literature, arts, and comparative religions to accentuate the ordinary lives of men and women and contrast them with their power-grabbing leaders—royal, military, and religious—who have dominated history books in the past. Thus, young people fourteen to seventeen will discover how Americans have come full circle from primitive times and once again are, without sin or shame, celebrating the mystery and wonder of all life, including their own joyous sexuality.

But in the early phases of the final sex revolution, before these students, a decade later, become the new teachers, the federally funded courses on human sexuality will teach the history of human sexuality as a separate subject showing how "doing what comes naturally" became overshadowed with manmade taboos, sanctified by manmade gods, and became a weapon of male power, culminating in class structures that enslaved those without money and power and degraded the sexual act and life itself. The potential of human altruism and caring love for one another was vitiated. Man's multiple, sex-loving gods (paralleling each other in many different cultures), like men and women themselves, had multiple problems dealing with jealousy and too many lovers. The Jews stopped worshipping graven images and replaced the old gods with a stern and vindictive God. Jesus and Mohammed made God or Allah a bit more loving but, unlike their neighbors, the

Chinese and Hindus, of whom they knew little (there still is no global village), they insisted that the way to salvation, and a heaven where ecstasy is no longer sexual, is only possible through agape, the spiritual love of God, at the same time renouncing eros and human sexual desire.

In this last phase of the K-12 weekly seminar on human sexuality, once a month between seven and nine o'clock Friday nights, parents will be invited with their tenth-grade children to the school auditorium or for twenty-four two-hour sessions. Each group of tenth graders and their parents will be together once a month during the school years until graduation, when the students will be approximately seventeen and will celebrate their adult rite of passage birthdays. During these sessions a female and male teaching team will share with parents and their children a complete survey of human sexuality from 30,000 B.C. to the end of the twentieth century. These will be exciting, bonding evenings for parents and their children as they learn the long history of sexual celebration, devaluation, and denial, and compare it with the saner morality of today.

Well aware that, in this area, most teachers won't have adequate training to teach the multicultural aspects of human sexuality, the Future Families of America Commission and SIECUS will have had no problem in encouraging filmmakers to combine with historians and sexologists not only to produce SDH movies for general audiences with stories covering history in the new perspectives, but also to have one-hour teaching films narrated by experts that will provide the structure for these sessions and a prelude to later interactive discussion between teachers, parents, and students.

Parents and students will quickly learn that pornography—presumably the writing of prostitutes—is an eighteenth-century invention, and was unknown to early man, or even the Greeks and Romans who wrote and painted every aspect of their sexual lives with great aplomb and no shame or embarrassment. All students will have inexpensive paperback copies of Hans Licht's *Sexual Life in Ancient Greece* and Otto Kiefher's *Sexual Life in Ancient Rome,* which cover in depth many aspects of the average person's sex life in the world before Christ.

The first session will begin with films showing primitive men and women making love, and perhaps unable to evoke their deep emotions and feeling for each other, but later happily drawing vulvas and penises on the walls of caves in Europe. A 1980s film, *Quest for Fire,* will be recommended for home viewing. It shows that in the past filmmakers were fascinated but afraid of really dealing with the distant past. Later, during the Neolithic period (9000 B.C. to 7000 B.C.), after the Ice Age has passed, ancient people will be shown relaxing from hunting; playing with their children; women nursing, pushing overeager men away; and both sexes creating clay and stone figurines with protruding breasts and accessible vulvas as well as phallic charms.

Organized religion based on fertility worship was slowly evolving, and these carvings will eventually be refined into specific gods to be worshiped. During these years, with no sense of shame or sin, all over Europe and in the Middle East and Africa, primitive men and women were celebrating the mystery of their, and the earth's, fertility.

While these sessions will obviously be skimming the surface of human sexuality historically, they will be opening doors that were never opened before in most secondary education.Teachers will suggest many films old and new that can be watched at home to give young people and their parents insights into more recent past sexual history as well as their own lives.

Quoting from many sources that will be available in all school libraries for teachers, students, and parents, here's a fast survey of what these seminars will cover. As you read, keep in mind that there will be much verbal interaction, and some shock, as students, parents, and teachers interrelate the past with the new sexual morality.

Proceeding in the first sessions to early Egyptian civilization, a thousand years before Christ, the priests drawing on papyrus visualized the sexual activities of their gods. John Field, a contributor to Peter Webb's *Erotic Arts* (a book that will be widely available in low-cost editions), points out that in early Egyptian civilization drawings like that of Geb (the Earth god), with "his long phallus thrusting skyward in a vain attempt to unite with his beloved Easter wife," were common, but later, for some unknown reason, visual censorship came into existence, and sexual portrayals were barred by the establishment.

Worship of early gods who controlled the sun and rain and were responsible for the earth's fertility as well as their own will be dramatically shown on film, along with the rise of the medicine man, and tribal priests who preyed on man's early fear of the not-me, and the uncontrollable world of light and darkness, hurricanes, tornadoes, earthquakes, volcanoes, devastating snows and rains, and the seeming motion of the stars and planets, all of which became incorporated into myths and storytelling.

In these early societies fertility is soon related to the seeding provided by the phallus. Stone and clay reproductions of it are worshiped by males as well as females. Ideas of obscenity or pornography connected with sex do not exist. But gradually, as people gathered in larger tribes and males became responsible for the paternity of their children, the male sex drive, along with a fear of women— because of the male inability to resist the female's sexual attractions—was slowly built into the laws of various tribes and encoded on tablets that have survived in familiar Old Testament literature such as Deuteronomy and the Talmud. To give them force these laws became commandments of a fearful, often jealous, and vindictive God.

But from one culture to another sexual morality varied considerably and changed with the times. Teachers will explore many ancient taboos which the self-appointed avatars used to gain power over their particular people, and will reveal the almost complete male domination of women, along with the beliefs and powers of the gods with different names who often paralleled each other in their sexual activities. In the ancient Chinese, Indian, Egyptian, Greek, Roman, and Germanic civilizations many stories, which people believed and we now call myths, resurfaced in different forms in Gnostic and early Christian beliefs. Anything-goes sexual holidays were transformed into Easter and Christmas.

Inevitably, some Catholics and fundamentalists will object to the teaching of comparative creation myths, and other areas in which there is conflict with the creation of man and the Adam and Eve stories in Genesis, but keep in mind that the federally funded human sexuality seminars are optional, and a majority of Americans have agreed on the basic proposals of the Lovemore bill and the resulting NSME legislation.

A brilliant book, *Images of the Body* by Michael Gill, offers an excellent survey of the human body from ancient times to the present, as well as the Egyptian Isis and Osiris myth, which will intrigue many parents and students who have never read or heard about them. The story begins with the goddess Nut, lover of her twin brother Geb, the Earth god, whom she mounts (a modern version of the woman on top). By swallowing the sun each night and letting it pass through her body, she lays the groundwork for Christian resurrection. Nut also gives birth to Isis, who marries her brother, Osiris, whose image is a bag of seeds. Osiris is worshiped for his fertility, but is murdered by his brother, Set, who wants Isis for himself. Set dismembers Osiris and scatters his parts all over the world. Totally distraught, searching for him, Isis recovers every part of Osiris's body except his phallus, which was eaten by a fish after Set threw it in the Nile.

Multicultural teaching will reveal our common sexual heritages. In Mesopotamia, long before people were able to write, visual sexual art was widespread. As John Tierney, with a sly grin, writes in a lengthy *New York Times* article of January 9, 1994, "Porn [seems to be] the Low Slung Engine of Progress. Nearly 4000 years before *Playboy* or *Penthouse* ROM discs were making it possible for men to interact visually with their computer screens, and could tell women to take off their bras and go to bed with them vicariously, the Sumerians were writing smut."

But teachers will emphasize that Tierney, a fellow with the Freedom Forum Center at Columbia University, is wrong. Neither Sumerian nor Babylonian men were producing smut or pornography. They were fascinated and a bit frightened by their sexual compulsions, and their need for the female body. Long before Eve, they dreamed up Lilith. She was the first feminist who refused to acknowledge male supremacy. She is portrayed in stone "as a nocturnal succubus who causes erotic dreams," and who climbs naked on top of men while they are sleeping and rides their penises in wild abandon, thus providing an explanation for wet dreams.

Teenagers will laughingly applaud these stories and will contrast Lorena Bobbitt with Lilith and Isis, who restored her husband's manhood, and then, in a complete female-power role reversal, worshiped his resurrected penis by sitting on it. Continuing sessions will explore what is known as the Greek archaic period, when sex was humanized and immortalized on Greek drinking cups and vases, and later in the Hellenistic period on statuary and painting. Teachers will mention in passing that at the same time there were incessant wars between the Greek states and the Persians. These wars will be covered in detail in ancient history courses, revealing that in many areas the ordinary lives of the people were unaffected by the barbarian power grabbers. As Field notes in *Erotic Arts,* from the archaic period to the so-called Classical era, the daily lives of most Greeks revolved around "sex, religion, and magic, which were closely interwoven." Art objects including lamps, vases, paintings, and sculptures show explicit sexual activities in a completely open manner. "The close connection between sex and shame has yet to be invented." Or, as Otto Brendel, in his book *Studies in Erotic Art,* points out, "The artists of the time were simply portraying the erotic reality that was a customary part of banquets, symposia, and everyday life. Love was companionable."

Photographs of other drinking cups reveal men and women of all ages happily consorting together naked. Erect penises are being fondled by women and as Brendel points out, "Most of the participants busy themselves with railleries and preludes to love. Some chase each other, ready to catch and be caught." But teachers should raise the question: Although this was a society where there was presumably no shame attached to sex, do the cups, drawings, sculpture, and writings that have survived make it apparent that these were probably all created by men? That they are male sexual responses that didn't reflect the feelings and emotions of most women—all of whom were subservient? There was a subculture of *hetairae,* female courtesans who were presumably better educated than the women upper-class men married. They were available as mistresses. Brothels where whores serviced all comers for a few denarii, also flourished. A Greek cup now in the Louvre collection, showing a woman servicing four men by hand and in her mouth, vagina, and anus, makes it obvious that, like X-rated films in the 1990s, these were male creations. On the other hand students will be reminded that Socrates, who may have loved young boys but had a nagging wife, insisted in his *Symposium:* "Union between man and woman is a creative act and has something divine about it. . . . The object of love is a creative union with beauty on both spiritual and physical levels."

But in the Greek world sex was not degraded. Marriage was for life. People didn't live long lives and women did not expect sexual fidelity. In his study of

Greek art, Brendel offer three factors which he considered essential for the formation of erotic art on a quality level equal to the Greeks. First, "a closed social group of cultivated habits"—a society that enjoys both a secular and religious life and is not dominated by religious fears of their deities. Actually, as teachers will show students, the Greek gods were anthropomorphic. They enjoyed sex, were jealous, and had the same sex problems as average Greeks, but the gods could resolve them by turning enemies into animals or stone.

Secondly, Brendel believes, "A society must have a frankly appreciative and humanized attitude toward sex, and extroverted taste for the communication of sexual pleasure, and finally the social environment must be such that artists have a freedom to create an erotic art that demands a wide variety of expression." Both students and parents will discuss whether, with the new freedom to portray SN aspects of human life, filmmakers, and artists in general have been responding creatively according to Brendel's belief that "to make love is a part of a people's social life, and so the artists of that Greek time registered people's way of doing it with a keen perception of fact, and with a gusto that is most likely sympathetic." Students will find a quick survey of the sex lives of the Greek and comparable Roman gods in Roger Persall's book *Tell Me Pretty Maiden,* a study showing how Victorian and Edwardian painters used mythology as an excuse for painting popular pictures of naked ladies who presumably never existed.

The Hellenistic or Classical period of Greek art and literature persisted from 470 B.C. down to the first century before Christ. In later times Euripides, Sophocles, and Aeschylus, in their plays presented a more tragic picture of human sexuality; they also often put much bawdy sex in their dramas, so much so that Plato disapproved. And, of course, Aristophanes must have really shocked Plato with his play *Lysistrata*—was she the world's first feminist? "Let us wait at home," she advises the wives of their ever-warring husbands. "With our faces made up, advance to greet our husbands with nothing on but our little tunics. . . . Then, when they are panting with desire, if we slip away without yielding, they will soon conclude an armistice. . . . So no more legs in the air and no more playing the lioness at the cheese grater." Teachers will encourage a humorous discussion as to why this advice probably wouldn't work in the twenty-first century, with so many women pursuing military careers.

Moving on historically to Rome, teachers may read from John Field's essay, on "Sexual Themes in Ancient and Primitive Art": "The Romans inherited many of their ideas and customs from the Greeks, but the highly civilized attitude towards sexuality manifested by the Greeks in art and life did not find a parallel in Rome, where lustful brutality tended to become characteristic of sex relations as time passed." Nevertheless, before the gradual deterioration of Roman culture, the interlinking of sex and religion with phallic worship and fertility cults was widespread and produced both light-hearted, comic, and bawdy sexual literature such as *The Golden Ass* by Apulieus, *The Satyricon* by Petronius, Lucian's *Dialogues,* as well as Ovid's light-hearted sex manual *The Art of Love.* All of these books will be available for students and parents as outside reading.

As Field points out, the famous brothel paintings discovered in Pompeii in 1900, and long unseen by the general public, "are more concerned with love than wishy sex, and could be illustrations for Ovid's poetry." But the twenty-nine life-size paintings in the Villa of Mysteries in Pompeii, which will be shown with opaque projectors or on film, have a strange mixture of the sensuous and romantic along with sadistic approaches to sex, that may have been a part of the Dionysian rites, and although it may be shocking, teachers will show cuts of 1970–1980 orgy parties as shown on X-rated tapes, and will contrast the sexual devaluation that took root in Rome and continued almost nonstop for two thousand years, until the final sex revolution, engendered by the Lovemore Bill, created a saner sexual environment.

Was America in the mid-1990s approaching a similar decline and fall as the Roman civilization? Teachers will detail the American obsession in the mid-1990s with the sexual insanities of the rich and famous, as flagrantly displayed in the *National Enquirer* and told and retold in television dramas and in the novels of Harold Robbins, Judith Krantz, Sidney Sheldon, and many others. All this will be compared to Suetonius's stories about Tiberius, Caligula, Nero, and the twelve Caesars, where human sexuality among the ruling classes became totally sadistic and bestial and which were recreated, many centuries later, by Hancarville in three volumes of paintings illustrating Roman orgies, which he claimed were copies of Roman cameos produced in abundance at the time.

Before teachers move on to sex in other cultures, students will wonder with their parents whether, as Field points out, "The debauchery was merely symptomatic of the political and economic chaos of the times"—rather than being the cause of the fall of the Roman Empire. And they will wonder with their elders whether without the new moral direction, Americans in the mid-1990s might have drifted into a new repressive Christian era, where a combination of old-style Catholic theology and Protestant biblical fundamentalism, which reflects the religious beliefs of nearly half the population, might have ushered in a Middle-Ages-style morality, where nonmarital sex, human nudity, and the devil are almost synonymous. And they will compare the possibilities with Arabic countries dominated by Islamic fundamentalists who have created just such societies in the name of Allah.

The multicultural, once-a-week seminar on human sexuality now moving forward historically surveys human sexuality in ancient Incan and Mayan cultures, which had developed from 600 B.C. in South America until the Spaniards arrived and gradually supplanted the multiple gods of these societies with Catholic Christian beliefs. The Incan rulers evidently were opposed to sexual representation, but Peruvian pottery, well into the fifteenth century, portrayed heterosexual copulation and genital display. But, as Paul Gebhard points out in his *Studies in Erotic Art,* there is no visualization of masturbation, group sex, oral sex, or homosexuality in the artifacts of these cultures.

On Europe, discussing the same historical timeframe, Reay Tannahill's *Sex in History* will be an essential text for students. During the Middle Ages, as Tannahill points out, the Christian church fathers were blaming Adam, and particularly Eve, for the disgusting merger of their genitals. Arnobius called sexual intercourse filthy and degrading, Methodius called it unseemly, Jerome called it unclean, and Ambrose called it a defilement, but only a few thousand miles away, in India and China, people were being assured by their gods and priests that sex-making was not only a joy and pleasure, but could become a way of transcending oneself in an extended, ritualistic merger of male and female flesh. Lovers could, for a brief moment, glimpse nirvana, the godhead, and blend themselves with the ultimate.

Nevertheless, even though the yang and the yin, the lignam and yoni, the Shiva and Shakti became icons and symbols of the male/female balance in the world, Indian and Muslin countries, like the Christian world, were male-dominated. By the end of the eleventh century, in 1099, Jerusalem fell to the Christian crusaders in their first battle with the Muslims, who were polygamous. Christian men extolled their virgin Madonna, married their more earthly counterparts, but couldn't resist the tempting Eve seducers with their apples.

Teachers will explore why, in the nonwarring areas of life, in China and the Islamic countries there was practically no portrayal of naked females (or males) or of explicit sex action. The prohibition still exists today. The new, twenty-first-century American morality approving SN movies and television was, and still is, very shocking to Muslims. On the other hand Arab/Muslim believers never had a spiritual love affair with Mohammed (who had several wives) and would be horrified that many Christian monks and nuns were having spiritual love affairs with Jesus, who told his disciples to give up worldly pleasures, including sex, and, forsaking all others follow him, thus showing that some moral beliefs go beyond the golden rule.

Parents and students will become acquainted with the unexpurgated *Thousand and One Nights,* in the Richard Burton translation. By this time filmmakers will have rediscovered the stories told by Scheherazade and, unlike the Arabs, will be filming, often amusing, sexually natural stories along with later renditions by Boccaccio and Chaucer.

But Indian and Chinese approaches to human sexuality, in the same timeframe as early Christianity, will be far more intriguing. In China, while visual sex censorship prevailed, followers of Buddha were modifying his aesthetic teachings, which were not sex negative. A few hundred years later Confucius was telling his followers, "Male chastity shortens one's life." Reading from Jolan Chang's *The Tao of Sex,* parents and students will be amused to learn how some Chinese emperors pursued longevity

In China there were no visual portrayals of sexmaking until the fifteenth century, and Taoist theories of lovemaking depended on hand-copied manuscripts and remained the sexual secrets of the upper classes. One of the most famous instructional dialogues is that between the Yellow Emperor and the Plain Girl. It will give parents and students much laughter as Plain Girl divulges the secrets of the bedroom to her master, who has asked her to explain the benefits of not ejaculating. She (purposely?) ignores the advantages for the female who, the Emperor well knew, could reach orgasm after orgasm while he had only one shot at a time to impregnate her with his vital fluids. So, perhaps, Plain Girl by her answer was proposing a kind of birth control, which was practiced many centuries later by the Oneida Community and John Humphrey Noyes. "If the man performs the act once without releasing his semen, he will add to the vital flow. If he performs twice, his hearing and vision is sharpened. Three times and all illness vanishes. Four times his soul finds peace. Five times, the circulation of his blood improves. Six times his back is strengthened. Seven times his buttocks and thighs grow strong. Nine times he will be like the immortals." Presumably the Yellow Emperor who managed to have intercourse twelve hundred times without ejaculating, thus became immortal.

The Chinese were finally producing sex manuals with pretty drawings that not only taught the reader how to prolong sexmaking but how to make the act continuously interesting by trying hundreds of different positions such as the Unicorn's Horn, the Winding Dragon, the Fluttering Butterfly, the Reversed Flying Drakes, the Wailing Monkey, the Galloping Charger, and the Jumping Tiger, to mention a few.

The discovery that the Chinese artists finally were using drawings to teach the art of love was not revealed until 1951, when the amazing R. H. Van Gulik (famous, then, for his detective stories about Judge Dee), who had acquired many of the original drawings, published a collection, *Erotic Color Prints From the Ming Dynasty.* Van Gulik was a Chinese scholar, and, although he knew the prints were historically valuable, in those days he was embarrassed to show them and only fifty copies of this edition were made. Even later in 1963 and in 1970, when they appeared in English and in a Swiss edition called *Yun Yu,* they were considered, and at the end of the twentieth century were still considered, pornographic.

Like the Konarak sculptures in India, these prints exude a warm, loving ambiance, covering every kind of natural human sexuality except masturbation. There is no sadistic behavior illustrated. Heterosexual lovemaking was not only a religion but a part of life. Many of these prints and erotic art objects were common in the Ming dynasty but were driven underground by the Manchu conquerors and in the twenty-first century still have not reappeared in modern China. Mao, and later leaders, probably feared visualizing the natural sexual activities for a billion people, which despite government-forced birth control, might increase the birth rate. It is a moral position that NSME legislation will have resolved for twenty-first century Americans who, now with extensive birth control knowledge taught in the later secondary grades, are in wide agreement on the necessity for zero population growth—duplicating themselves with no more than two children.

Of course, teachers will be well aware that many of their young students, now approaching their seventeenth birthdays, have discovered the other sex, and while the majority have restrained themselves from actual sexual merger, many have enjoyed private, one-to-one foreplay leading to climaxing by mutual playing with each other's genitals. Now the female/male teaching team can discuss with their smiling, bemused males and happy females, and their parents, who are mostly in their late thirties, the Chinese and Hindu discoveries of how to prolong sexual intimacy based on "absorbing the female essence." This was the Tao, or Way, of sexual merger, and in India was practiced by Tantric tribes, to the horror of the British when they discovered it. Margo Ananda's book *The Art of Sexual Ecstasy*, which shows how the Eastern way of lovemaking can be enjoyed by Western people, will fascinate both parents and students. Not rushing to climax creates total involvement with a woman that young men can learn how to do as well as or better than they can hit home runs or throw forward passes.

The seminar will continue with an exploration of the first culture in the world where women achieved sexual equality with men, which was immortalized in stone sculptures. Filmmakers and narrators will take parents and students on a slow tour of the famous erotic sculptures of Meru, the home of the gods, in the temples at Kailasanath, Konarak, and Kuharjo located in southern Bengal. The sculptures were completed between A.D. 200 and 1200, a timeframe known as the Middle Ages in Europe. Narrators will read from the writings of Alan Watts, who describes the Sun Temple at Konarak as a vision or erotic spirituality. Watts asks his readers looking at the photographs (there are many portraying various acts of sexmaking) to imagine these figures as they were originally carved in stone, polished and given skin-color-like tints, and he says sadly, "Modern apologists for these images were doubtless right on one point: they are pornography in the eyes of people with dirty minds." But, as he points out, "We are not looking at some version of the stag film or girlie magazines, for the faces on these sculptures are innocent of the leer which always masks the shame and guilt of finding pleasure in filth. There is no attitude of secretiveness, or of intent to shock by doing openly what supposedly should only be done in the dark."

Since the insights of Eastern sexuality have never been taught in secondary schools, and coincide in many areas with the new sexual morality, parents, students, and teachers may decide for the next few months that the seminar should continue on a weekly basis.

Alan Watts's writings, coupled with new filmmaking, will provide guides. These statues suggest a state of reality-awareness ecstasy, or, as William Blake said, "Energy in eternal delight." As Watts suggests, most people living in the twentieth century have had little occasion for ecstacy in their lives apart from sex. "Ex-stasis means to stand outside—to be liberated from the bondage of oneself." Teachers will explain that in the twentieth century most Western people were conditioned by endless, how-to sex manuals that overemphasized technique to the detriment of mental rapport between lovers. Sexual devaluation was so prevalent that the ecstatic blending of one's genitals with a loved person was not a common experience. Sex in those days, for the majority of Americans, took approximately ten minutes and ended in an embarrassing convulsion.

Watt's essay on Konarak, with photographs, will be back in print and students will discover that the architecture of Konarak was conceived as an enormous chariot for Surya, the sun god. On his "diurnal joy-ride," he is accompanied by asaparas (courtesans) with full bosoms and curvaceous buttocks, and devas (angel gods) with erect penises. Most of the riders are engaged in some form of sexual play including kissing and enticing each other, enjoying erotic antics, along with oral sex, masturbation, and complete sensual merger. In essence what's happening is not reality but a kind of utopia heaven where among these angels "there is neither marrying nor giving in marriage."

Watts believed that sexual union could, given the proper instruction from youth which is now occurring as a result of NSME legislation, become an effective way of obtaining an undiluted awareness of reality. "But this will not be the wham-bang kind of intercourse that generally prevails throughout the world." By contrast, presaging the new morality, Watts offers the discipline of delights that is the essence of Taoist sexmaking. Tantric/Taoist sexmaking reflected in the Konarak sculptures is a ritual dance of joyous, laughing lovemaking. Love is the basis of religion, and it is not solemn, nor is it pompous. Making love is not work. It is play! Religion without sex, Watts reminds us, "is a rattling skeleton," and "sex without religion is a mass or mush. The whole human organism is an erotic zone."

Reay Tannahill calls the temples in India "the Kamasutra in the round," and while Vatsayana's *Kamasutra* and Pandit Kookoa's *Rati Rahasya*, subtitled *The Hindu Secrets of Love*, are not manuals for Tantric, extended sexual intercourse, they are amusing to read and will be available in school libraries along with Nik Douglas and Penny Slinger's *Sexual Secrets,* which offers a completely illustrated study of Tantric sexmaking

Watts concludes his essay on Konarak touching upon both Western Puritanism and Brahmin asceticism. "Which then is the most blasphemous sexual union, to see it as an image of the divine ground of the universe, or to see sex as mere fucking?"—as in the expression "Fuck you!"

Before teachers move on to Japanese sexual life in the late 1700s when it finally becomes visually portrayed, they will say goodbye to Chinese art with Peter Webb in his book *Erotic Arts,* who tells about the famous Shou Lou, the patron of longevity. An icon, he is portrayed as a very old man with a dragon staff in one hand and a peach in his other. The peach has a deep flesh color and a lovely, vulva-like cleft (more realistic than yang and yin symbols). "Shou Lou's portrait appears with horns (penises), and was reproduced on robes, porcelains, sculptures, and some drawings." He is usually in the company of dragons. "The celestial dragon, an imperial authority, represents heaven and is believed to have mated with earth (which is female), and is represented by a less ferocious dragon." Jade is so precious because it represents the dragon's semen (petrified). Students will be fascinated that these symbols clarify the many allusions to the female genitals, which were called the Gateway of the Jade, the Flute of the Jade, and the Jade Fountain—drinking at which, and bathing the male flute therein, assured a long healthy life.

The Japanese, like the Chinese, extolled human sexuality in their religions. Reproductions of phalluses were common in Shinto shrines, and "pillow books"—sex manuals—appeared in Japan in the eighth century. Only a few of their erotic scrolls have survived. Not until nearly a thousand years later, in the late 1700s, when Harnobu and other Japanese artists perfected the art of four-color wood block printing, had any large-scale method—in Japan, or elsewhere—been invented that would permit the visual celebration of human sexuality. By 1765, Japanese artists were creating drawings of "a floating world"—"ukiyo-e pictures." Known as *Shunga* drawings in their sexual aspects, or spring pictures, they portrayed every aspect of human sexuality. Students will discover Hanobu, Utarmaro, Shunch, Kiyonga, Eri, Maiko, and even Hokusai, Japanese artists who painted joyous, laughing sexmaking in their drawings.

In their book *Shunga, The Art of Love in Japan,* Tom and Mary Evans write, "The Japanese approach to sex (in those days) was conditioned by a moral system very different from our own. There was very little sense of personal sin, and the body was as important as the spirit. Sex, however, was not elevated to a mystical significance as it was in many Chinese and Indian systems. The sexual act was seen as a natural, intrinsically enjoyable event. There was no equivalent to the Western concept of pornography, and no connection was made between moral corruption and the representation of sex. The Shunga shows us the difference between erotic art and pornography. The Shunga, and under-the-counter sex magazines (in the twentieth century) of the modern, "civilized" West, are similar in the activities that they depict, but in their effect they are worlds apart. The Shunga represents sexual activity in many forms as the joyful and inspiring experience that it should be. The sex shop magazine is by comparison almost invariably sordid, meretricious and vulgar."

In essence, the human sexuality seminar will have revealed to students and parents that thus far in human history, in Eastern cultures, sexual devaluation, degradation, and decadence did not exist. But, up until the NSME legislation, western Christian morality has prevailed. When Americans "opened up" Japan to Western trade in 1853, the sexually explicit Shunga went underground. The Victorians had discovered pornography. Later, in the final roundup of the multicultural, sexual tour of the world, students and parents will contrast this history with present-day Japan, which censors SN filmmaking but offers many bondage and discipline and SD portrayals.

11

Teaching Pornography, A.D. 1500 to the Present

Twentieth-century readers of this book should keep in mind, as I have previously mentioned, that this phase of the value-laden human sexuality seminar is not so concentrated as it might seem in outline. The New Sexuality and Morality Education legislation will completely revamp high school curricula in liberal arts studies. Young people in the later ages—fifteen, sixteen, and seventeen—unlike students in the late 1990s, after a continuous one-hour weekly course in human sexuality from kindergarten through the ninth grade, plus the much broader education they will have experienced and will still be receiving, will be more sophisticated about the world in general than twentieth-century teenagers who have no depth of education. Two other things should also be kept in mind. Within ten years after NSME is fully functioning, the sexual devaluation comparisons with the past will be integrated into other liberal arts studies on a historical basis. During the first ten years, the two-hour parent-student session will also be invaluable for the large majority of parents who have no background in the history of human sexuality. Also, these parents, for the most part, will be in an age group, thirty-five to forty-five, that is sexually active, and will in the companionship of the sessions bond more closely with their teenagers. In passing, it should also be noted, as I will discuss in a later chapter, that the new sexual morality will be in conflict with orthodox Christian religious teachings; but Catholics and fundamentalists must make adjustments. There is nothing in the New Testament that can't be realigned with a new morality that sacramentalizes human sexuality as the basic element of a loving God.

The seminar now turns back to Europe, where the Catholic church's gradual suppression of sexual paganism along with worship of sexual gods throughout what is now known as continental Europe, England, and Ireland, continues.

114

Flagrantly sexual pagan holidays, times of sexual release in which to mourn or to celebrate the changing seasons with relevant gods and goddesses, were transformed into Christmas and Easter with only Mardi Gras remaining in a few areas today to celebrate the release of sexual inhibitions.

Students and parents will be shown how the church, with some tempering of male dominance, recreated the biblical Mary into the Holy Mother who gave birth to the son of God. Jesus' birth without sex offered an idealization of sexuality that didn't require the merger of "two sewer systems" (the way St. Augustine viewed sexmaking—"among stools and urine we are born"). For the first time, religion had established copulation as definitely dirty, but, unfortunately, a necessary adjunct of marriage to create human children. Virginity and celibacy were the only ways to escape to God pure in heart. No one dared to depict the Holy Mother naked, not really an irreligious idea. Some critics today are sure that Michelangelo, in *Pieta* sculpture, revealed the dying Jesus with an erection . . . a reflection of sexual ecstasy in reuniting with God.

Teachers will explore King Arthur's realm and the age of chivalry; love, presumably without sexual merger, will be examined as a byproduct of the more spiritual Christian approach to agape, as contrasted with the "anything goes" aspect of Eros. The surface hypocrisy was that knights of old clanked off to battle wearing the perfumed handkerchiefs of their female lovers, who were actually married to local barons. Before they departed to kill dragons and behead their enemies, they could sleep with their married lovers, kissing and sighing, but having no intercourse. High schoolers in their last year who have refrained from sex will agree that it is possible—but not forever!

By this time in the course teachers will be teaching students and their parents the fun of reading a few of Chaucer's *Canterbury Tales* in the original old English and learning that five hundred years ago, and centuries before, men and women rarely used a sexual word as a nasty, hateful verb spoken in anger, or as a putdown adjective, nor was there any false modesty about certain words that, up until thirty years ago, were kept out of most dictionaries or from being used in printed form in books, or in spoken form on radio or television. These sessions would reveal that our ancestors (and they are our ancestors no matter what our racial origins may be) enjoyed sex with laughter and double entendres, hence words like *acqueyntaunce,* derived from *queynte* meaning a woman's sexual parts, which eventually became *con,* then *conny,* and eventually the nastiest word of all, *cunt.* There are hundreds of other such words. *Chaucer's Bawdy* by Thomas Ross, an analysis of three hundred risque words used by Chaucer to delineate comic characters and make us laugh, will be a fun book to read.

Also teachers could recommend reading *Dirty Words* by Ariel Arango, M.D., who examines the dirty words of the past that have come into common usage, such as *piss, shit, ass, prick, asshole,* and why *fuck* is no longer such a forbidden word (because it doesn't convey the mental imagery of the act) while *cock, tit, cocksucker, motherfucker,* and *cunt* are still words that are mostly verboten in polite company because, for most people, they conjure up the physical reality that still embarrasses us, or makes us feel uneasy sexually. In the process, teachers will point out that the baby's need to suck his mother's titties remains imbedded in both the adult male and female's joy in sucking titties, cunties, and cockies (as the case may be, with diminutives supplied to give the verboten words a loving flavor).

Teachers could examine the long history of the word *fuck* and its equivalent in many languages, and construct an hour diversion into the thousands of words, similies, and metaphors that have been used in other languages, and in ours. Teenagers could be referred to books like *Slang* and *Euphemism,* by Richard Spears, and the three-volume *Historical Dictionary of Slang.* In the process, the human sexuality course would not only be exploring human communication via words but challenging teenagers to think of better words to express their anger than such boring (pun intended) phrases as "fuck you," or "asshole," or "shit head," etc., etc., to describe an unliked person. The dirty-word sessions of the human sexuality course would, like the entire seminar in the final high school years, be very popular and create a learning environment that would totally involve the student.

There always has been a high road to sex and loving in religion but it has never equated sex with joy or passion. According to the song, the low road gets you in Scotland first, but the message to young people in the human sexuality course will be that the sexual low road is a dead road.

The male/female teacher team will now move into the Christian Middle Ages. While India, China, and Japan were integrating human sexuality into their religions, in Europe any overt depiction of sexual action was being repressed. For more than a thousand years, in the fourth century, beginning with the triumph of Christianity and the disappearance of the Roman Empire, to the fifteenth century, the nude, with the exception of Christ on the cross, almost completely disappeared from Western art. In his book, *Erotic Art of the West,* Robert Melville offers the following reasons: "Iconoclasm, fear of pagan idols and a new condemnatory attitude toward the body and its pleasures," during which time the Christian fathers' interpretation of the Gospels was being grafted onto the pagan religion. "When the nude finally did appear in Christian art, the body had ceased to be, as it had for the Greeks, a mirror of divine perfection and had largely become an object of humiliation and shame."

Much of this feeling still dominates Christian cultures in Europe and America. It is even reflected in much erotica today, including sexvids. Eve's descendants were seducers of men who consorted with the devils and snakes. Their children today expose their genitals for male delectation in X-rated films.

Nevertheless, visual sex didn't go completely underground in the Middle Ages and, using the medium of woodcut engravings and painting and sculpture, many artists still managed to accentuate the erotic element in a society that condemned human sexuality. But, as Melville points out, "Not the vice itself; but the punishment." Depiction of toads eating female vulvas and female breasts, accompanied by snakes engaging in the feast, together with drawings of women copulating with goats (the goat was a symbol of the devil's virility) were common and they reappeared in the seventeenth century in Heironymous Bosch paintings, *Temptation of St. Anthony* and *Garden of Terrestrial Delights*. These paintings today reveal a sexual devaluation and a sad commentary on the underlying prurience (sexual itchings) of many religious leaders, who are still determined to restrict sexual pleasuring to monogamous marriage and the reproduction of children.

Films and slides will be used by teachers to show the first nudes in Western art, which finally appeared in the paintings of Lucas Cranach and Hans Baldung in the fifteenth century in northern Europe and approximately at the same time in Italy in Botticelli's *Birth of Venus*. To distinguish northern European paintings from the Italian paintings, which were not so erotic, Kenneth Clark has called the northern style of painting the "Alternate Convention." Cranach's and Baldung's paintings, among others, show Adam and Eve and other nude figures complete with pubic hair, penises, and slits in the vulva. But underlying the realistic portrayal of human nakedness is a negative feeling of lust. Orgasm and human sexuality are related to death and not to birth. It's a theme that still permeates much of the twentieth-century erotic paintings. Melville sums it up: "The sense of sin, essential to the Gothic nude and which adds an element of the perverse to its erotic appeal, is entirely absent from the classical nudes, which above all is an idealizing form, embodying a sane sensual eroticism."

Melville's appraisal underlines the new morality. For the first time in human history, millions of people are learning to celebrate the miracle of human sexuality and recognize that sexmaking is an ever-churning blend of idealization, lustfulness, playfulness, aggressiveness, and laughter, plus an overwhelming necessity to escape one's self by a complete merger with another person.

Influencing the idealization of the female portrayed by the Italian artists (and when reflected the romanticism of the age of chivalry) painters and sculptors created female nudes who seemed to be, at least on the surface, sexually innocent. But, nevertheless, Bottecelli's *Venus* is definitely enticing the male viewer. Of course, Italian art was influenced by Greek sculpture and painting and particularly Praxiteles, who was the first to sculpt totally naked goddesses. Prior to Praxiteles, early Greek artists, like the later Indian, Chinese, and Japanese artists, usually portrayed the female partially clothed and, even today, many men believe that wearing some clothing makes the female body much more erotic.

At this point, teachers will raise the question whether Fredericks of Hollywood and other companies selling female undergarments that eroticize the female breasts, pubic area, and buttocks, contribute to sexual devaluation, as many feminists claimed in the mid-1990s, or whether sexual tease isn't really a valid part of the human sexual experience.

Reflecting current morality, one art critic in the twentieth century insisted: "If the nude is so treated that it raises in the spectator ideas or desires appropriate to the material subject, it is false art and bad morals." This judgment so overlooks normal male reactions that Kenneth Clark in his book *The Nude in Art* responded: "It is necessary to labor the obvious," he said with some irritation, "and say that no nude in painting and sculpture, however abstract, should fail to arouse in the spectator some vestige of erotic feeling . . . even though it only be the faintest shadow . . . and if it does not do so, it is bad art and false morals."

Clark is careful not to specify whether the nude is male or female and in the twenty-first century, in addition to any erotic feelings from childhood, men and women will have been conditioned to enjoy other human beings in a totality that includes their hands and face as well as their entire bodies.

During the next three hundred years, naked goddesses and gods (deprived of realistic genitals, of course) cavorted over thousands of canvasses. Michelangelo set the pace in the 1500s by painting the ceiling of the Sistine Chapel with a naked Adam and other biblical characters in various stages of undress. Later, he sculpted David with a realistic penis nesting in his pubic hairs. But even though his subjects were religious, he was walking a razor's edge and defying Christian morality. Naked hasn't been nice since Adam first looked at Eve and got an erection.

Pietro Arentino, a total libertine himself, denounced the Michelangelo frescos in an open letter, and said, "They are fit for a brothel wall." Arentino insisted they should be destroyed or at the very least, Daniele da Volterra, "the trouser maker" as he was called, an artist employed by the Vatican, should paint out Adam's genitals and those of other biblical characters Michelangelo had painted nude. Fortunately, some kind of sanity prevailed, but not until Michelangelo's statue of David was adorned with a fig leaf. It wasn't removed until the twentieth century.

In 1549 Michelangelo's *Pieta* was attacked by Ninni Boscio Bigio when a marble copy was unveiled in the Florentine church of Santo Spirito. Bigio recognized something that has intrigued viewers ever since. Is the Pieta really an evocation of the dead Christ in his mother's arms, or is it really the sculpture of an excessively beautiful naked youth in the lap of a young girl who is obviously much younger than Mary would have been? In essence is this sculpture really the story of Venus and Adonis brought up to date? Not a Virgin Mother with her son but a passionate woman mourning her lover? Leo Steinberg explores the thought in a fascinating essay in *Studies in Erotic Art,* which is well worth reading.

Aside from Michelangelo, and far beyond him erotically, Guilio Romano, a pupil of Raphael, had created a series of totally explicit drawings that were later engraved by Raimondi to illustrate Argentino's bawdy sonnets on sexmaking. They created such a scandal that Raimondi fled to Mantua, where he painted one of the most erotic pictures to have survived from the sixteenth century, in which a nude Jupiter, with a big erection, is about to enter smiling Olympia. During the same period another artist whose name is not well known, Agostino Carraci, spent most of his adult life drawing and engraving detailed erotic pictures that have survived but are still interred in the restricted collection of the British Museum.

During the sixteenth century other painters such as Titian, Corregio, Clouet, Tintoretto, Caravaggio, Brueghel, Rubens, and Jordaeens (Melville lists more than twenty others chronologically) painted or sculptured erotic works, but it was not the main theme of their art, and they vacillated between the idealization of the female and her seductive potential and painted very few explicit acts of sexmaking.

Not until the eighteenth and nineteenth centuries did overt sexuality begin to appear regularly in works of art, but keep in mind that the spread of steel engravings, wood engravings, and stone lithography as artistic mediums was slow. Painters like François Boucher, who was one of the great erotic artists of his time, were subsidized by royal patrons such as Francis I and Henry IV. The greatest lover of women of all was Louis XV. Peter Webb points out, "French painting of the eighteenth century reflects the amoral, fun-loving atmosphere of the court life. The joys of lovemaking are celebrated with official approval." But painters like François Boucher didn't paint for the masses. Even today, only owners of expensive art books are aware of his nude painting of Mademoiselle O'Murphy, which Boucher painted in 1775 at Louis's request. The mademoiselle was one of his mistresses and the very erotic painting reveals a young woman lying on her stomach, legs spread, waiting for Louis. She is a total sex object.

At this point, teachers of the human sexuality seminar will point out that the major artists, for the most part, were no longer worried about sexual sinfulness, but were catering to the male's delight in the female body.

Linda Nochlin, professor of art history at Vassar, in a collection of essays *Women as Sex Objects,* fully reminds us, "The notion of erotic imagery (in nineteenth-century art) is created out of male needs and desires ... as far as one knows, there simply exists no art and certainly no high art in the nineteenth century based on women's erotic needs, wishes or fantasies. Whether the erotic object be breasts, buttocks, shoes or corsets ... the imagery of sexual delight or provocation has always been created about women for men's enjoyment, by men."

But finally, although other artists of the eighteenth century, such as

Fragonard, Watteau, Goya, and Fuseli, to mention a few, were still creating art for the elite, first in France during the Napoleonic wars and then in England, mass-produced sexual art for the man in the street (and his occasional bawdy mistresses) flooded the market. Cartoons satirizing political and military leaders show their heads filled with vulvas and penises. Drawings of lustful women holding engorged penises of generals and other officials with idiotic expressions on their faces were widely circulated. Drawings to illustrate the increasingly common written erotica, such as the Marquis de Sade's endless dealings with sick sex, portrayed for the average citizen everything in weird and kinky sex, from flagellation to shit eating, that was supposedly enjoyed by the upper classes.

In England, William Hogarth, followed by Thomas Rowlandson, was creating hundreds of erotic etchings reflecting with much humor the low-down sexual life of the common man and woman. In *Harlot's Progress* and *Rake's Progress,* and in Rowlandson's drawings, nothing was sacred. At the same time, explicit drawings of sexmaking, whipping, beating, orgies, and ejaculating penises were more available in sidewalk shops in London and Paris than sexvids are today.

But there was one difference. Hogarth and Rowlandson, and many of the anonymous artists, were able to stamp their creations with their own personalities and idiosyncrasies. The interaction between the medium and the message of the artist creates art. Humor predominated and it reflected the laughing bawdiness of the uneducated man in the streets.

During the schizophrenic, repressive Victorian era of the nineteenth century, a new morality crept into the world. Teachers of the seminar will point out that we are still living in the shadow of the sexual hypocrisy that motivated men like Thomas Bowdler, who, in 1818, insinuated his name into the language of Shakespeare by publishing expurgated ("Bowdlerized") versions of Shakespeare and Gibbons's *Decline and Fall of the Roman Empire* from which all dirty words and ideas were removed. By the end of the nineteenth century, Daniel Defoe's *Roxanna, The Fortunate Mistress,* John Cleland's *Fanny Hill,* and many other books had been declared obscene. Both visual and written sex disappeared as the Victorian guardians of human sexuality tried to legislate morality for the average man and woman. But, of course, the upper classes were not deprived. Written pornography was easy to obtain and visual sex for private art collections continued to be produced. Ingres, in his eighties, suddenly turned to erotica and produced many sensuous paintings, among them *Le Bain Turc,* with dreamily, lusciously naked young women lying around a harem bath obviously waiting for their master who, of course, the male viewer fantasized as himself. Gustave Courbet painted a female nude for Khalil Bey, the Turkish ambassador to St. Petersburg. With legs spread, it reveals genital detail that would have to wait another seventy-five years before *Hustler* magazine upstaged it. Many critics believed that Courbet was working with photographs (a new art form) when he created masterpieces like the *Sleepers,* a painting of two nude women locked in a loving embrace that was also painted for Bey. Corot and Diaz painted such subjects as *Women Masturbating before a Statue of Priapus* (1860) and *Women Embraced by a Goat* (1865). Painters like Honoré Daumier, or John Paul David (who charged admission to his studio, where he painted live women and then undressed them in paint later), and Charles Edward Beaumont were painting idyllic but not-too-explicit sexual paintings of sexmaking.

At approximately the same time that Renoir was busy painting buxom erotic ladies cavorting together without male companionship, Degas and Toulouse-Lautrec, fascinated with the sad underworld of sex, occasionally lived in whorehouses and painted prostitutes. While Rodin was idealizing human sexuality in stone, Gaugin and even John François Millet were painting much symbolic erotica. Later in the century, Achilles Deveria (reproductions of whose beautifully painted details of explicit human sexmaking are still not generally available) was finally topped by Aubrey Beardsley, Michel Von Zichy, and Constantine Guys, who came to earthly grips with penises and vulvas and finally ran smack into the law and censorship, probably because their drawings could be lithographed and thus be mass produced and were. Visual upper-class erotic art was no longer displayed with impunity. Edward Manet showed his *Breakfast on the Grass* in 1863. It was patterned after a subject that Girgione had painted three centuries before, in 1510. The art world of Paris was horrified, but relatively few people saw Manet's painting, or copies of it, with its intimations that after breakfast the naked woman in the painting picnicking with two fully dressed men would offer her sexual favors to both of them.

The last phase of this historical survey of human sexuality for tenth to twelfth graders and their parents can be covered on film and with opaque projectors in one or two sessions. With the invention of the daguerreotype process, the visual portrayal of human sexuality became more prevalent. In 1839, the *New York Tribune* estimated that three million daguerreotypes were being taken annually. Sixty-eight individuals were arrested for selling obscene photographs in that year alone. The obscene photographs, of course, were naked women. Nearly fifty years later, on April 23, 1896, using Thomas Edison's new gadget, the Vitascope, the first moving picture was projected in America on a large white sheet. Of course, the subjects were women and it wouldn't be long before young men were getting their sexual education from what became known as the "stag" film. But before that, even before World War I, Paris became known as the capital of the "filthy picture" industry. Still photography blossomed and erotic French postcards with real live naked women show breasts, behinds, and classical mons veneris, later called "pussies," without pubic hair.

For the first time, the average American boy was discovering that women, some women at least, were bubbling sexual creatures. The Victorian coverup was exposed. The French postcards gave the impression that if these women went to bed with you they wouldn't just lie there, or pray to God that the man would get it over with quickly. The viewer was given the feeling that these women enjoyed sex just as much as he did. But then, in the late 1920s, and for the next fifty years, stag movies became a sad, sleazy, sex-devaluing right of passage for millions of American men.

Teachers, using a book like *Nudes,* 1925, will reveal that the women in the French postcards, like the pinups that appeared later in World War II, were basically erotic sex tease pictures for men. They were not, by the standards of the new morality, sexually devaluing.

The unacknowledged author of the introduction to *Nudes* captures their mood: "The straightforwardness of these earlier 'daughters of joy' offers a pleasing contrast. Amplitude of breasts and buttocks seems a welcome alternative to today's extreme of near gaunt chic, reminding us of the pleasures that sculptors have always taken in richly curvilinear forms. Many of the subjects show attractiveness of personality, pensiveness, twinkling fun, poetic moodiness . . . these nudes were really never naked, there remains a personal reticence, a veil of aesthetic gracefulness and even in a coy, tantalizing look . . . there is an elegance . . . a restraint that keeps the sensuous enjoyment from shifting to overt sexuality."

But like stag films and X-rated films, French postcards in the late nineteenth century became an undercover sex revolution against superficial Victorian morality, setting the stage for a never-ending devaluation of human sexuality that became the keynote of twentieth-century art and literature. As William Oulette and Barbara Jones note in their book *Erotic Postcards,* "There were cards for tit men, bum men and flagelants. Many portrayed imaginary harems and white slavery and lesbians stroking each other." There were no naked men, nor any homosexual action, but in keeping with the male's sexual frustration and social conditionings many of the cards offered bawdy jokes with their drawings or photographs, such as two women wrapping a bottle of champagne in the shape of a phallus, or a man resting with a woman on a tree stump captioned, "When hiking, all girls like resting on a stump."

The first porno movies were produced in Paris by George Melies and Thomas Vaseltrap between 1893 and 1895. Based on the new sexual morality they'd be labeled Sexually Natural: "Now you are watching a young woman astride a horse. Her skirt is hiked above her well rounded thighs, which straddle a horse. A stable boy watches her pitching on the horse . . . now she's erotically enjoying her ride. The horse stops dead center in the frame. The boy helps her off the horse and her movements release her breasts. She embraces the boy and is kissing him passionately. They are soon tumbling in a pile of hay and she is caressing and kissing his swollen penis. She disappears in the hay as the boy mounts her."

In the last twenty years of the twentieth century practically all of the stag films produced between 1920 and 1960 were transferred to video and widely available to adult video stores. A few will be shown, along with the "tits and ass" movies that were shown both in major cities, like the Times Square area of New York City, as well as country towns where they passed censorship because they offered uplifting morals of what happened to bad girls who indulged in sex outside marriage, and because the Supreme Court had agreed in the *Sunshine* nudist magazine case (see chapter 2) that the human body was not obscene. Nudist magazines along with men magazines could print pictures of completely naked people, but not playing naked together or making love together in moving pictures so that children under eighteen could see them.

There are many books describing these movies and the changing sexual morality such as Al di Lauro and Gerald Rabin's *Dirty Movies, an Illustrated History of the Stag Film, 1915-1970,* Amos Vogel's *The Film as Subversive Art,* David Friedman's *A Youth in Babylon,* Friedman, and Kenneth Turin and Stephen Zito's *Sinema,* all of which detail the beginning of the X-rated porno industry. These will be available in the school libraries for parents and students who wish to explore the sexually sick and violent twentieth century where men, still in the driver's seat, instead of celebrating both the joys and wonders of male and female love and their fertility, wasted their lives in wars and self-made, often religiously inspired human catastrophes.

In twenty-first-century history classes, teachers will go beyond the surface facts of history and speculate on the sexual lives of the protagonists as conditioning factors. Along with their students, they can crawl into the brains of Julius Caesar, Marc Antony, Napoleon, Hitler, Henry VIII, Casanova, Don Juan, George III, George Washington, Abraham Lincoln, John Fitzgerald Kennedy, and thousands of others, revealing them as sexual human beings whose fame and deeds may well have been conditioned by sexual frustrations. Or, by contrast, the sex lives of men like Winston Churchill and Louis Mountbatten could be explored. How did they overcome jealousy and accept the fact that their wives had other lovers? Edwina Mountbatten shared her love with Jawaharal Nehru. Like Presidents Roosevelt, Eisenhower, and Kennedy, Churchill and Mountbatten were able to perform in their respective areas of command while they lived in a grown-up, future kind of pair bonding in which they and their wives could enjoy a sexual intimacy with another person without being troubled by "betrayal" of their primary partner or breaking a religious commandment.

As Isabelle de Courtivon, a professor of literature at M.I.T., asks in a review of a biography of Michael Foucault titled *The Passion,* "Should the revelations of guilt, revenge, contradictions, or misogyny, political incorrectness, and, most of all, human limitations lead one to rethink seriously a particular intellectual's contribution and to re-evaluate his or her work in the light of this personal information?"

The answer is yes. Foucault, who wrote a multivolume *History of Sex,* was gay. He was entranced with sadomasochism, had a preoccupation with death, and knowingly exposed himself to AIDS and may have spread it to others. Inevitably, his beliefs and attitudes toward human sexuality were reflected in his writings. The same applies, in retrospect, to Jean Paul Sartre. Simone de Beauvoir, famous as a feminist, finally revealed after she had given up much of her life to him that the intellectual Sartre, in his final years, was more interested in whiskey and young women than with the ramifications of his philosophy. And de Beauvoir herself, it is now apparent, was more intrigued in her youth with her lesbian companions than politics, all of which illuminates her famous book *The Second Sex.* In the twenty-first-century liberal arts' environment young people will learn very early in life how famous people have tried to transcend, or have been trapped by, their sex drive.

They will learn, as Kenneth Clark pointed out, "The desire to grasp and be united with another human body is a fundamental part of our nature."

In their literature courses, teachers will contrast Rabelaisian and Chaucerian humor with the sex-driven obsessions of Casanova, a few hundred years later, as he juggled politicians and bed companions. They will compare the happier sex drawings of Thomas Rowlandson with the sick sexual writings of the Marquis de Sade and the drawings of Aubrey Beardsley and the Marquis de Bayros. When they come to the surface repression of Victorian days they can peek behind the scenes and compare books like *My Secret Life* and *The Autobiography of Frank Harris,* and their author's attitude toward the female, with the dreamy evocations of Elizabeth Browning or Edward Fitzgerald's translations of Omar Khayyam. Skimming the history of men's feelings about their sex drives (women's feelings conditioned by male power have only begun to surface), these male writers vaccilitate between adoration and disgust of their need for women or a particular woman.

Now, the human sexuality teaching team, who may have been in their teens in the sexual explosion—not really a revolution—that began in the late 1950s, should keep in mind that their students weren't born yet and most of their parents were still playing in their sandboxes.

Thanks to Norman Mailer and James Jones (*The Naked and the Dead* and *From Here to Eternity*), the word "fuck" and other "dirty words" were finally permitted in print. For the rest of the twentieth century, fucking, with its overtones of hatred, became a commonplace word and beyond "having sex" or "making love," was the only word Americans had to describe human mating. As a nation, Americans were obsessed with the word and the act, not romantically or caringly, but mostly as an act of aggression in their novels, movies, television, and often in real life. Fucking made daily headlines. It was both nasty and titillating. During the 1960s and into the mid-1980s, when STDs and AIDS presumably cooled things a bit, sex exploitation was the medium and the message.

Students and parents will be amused by the report of the Commission Upon Obscenity and Pornography, released in 1971, which shocked hundreds of organizations like Morality in Media, who expected that the commission would give a report that would make it possible to criminalize visual sex portrayals in any form. Instead, the commission voted, in a twelve-to-six majority decision, "Federal, state, and local legislation prohibiting the sale of sexual material to consenting adults should be repealed!"

That did it! In the words of one of the dissenting members of the commission, the report was a "Magna Carta for pornographers." Within a few months, thousands of sleazily produced, fully illustrated books poured off the presses of New York and California publishers. They offered every aspect of human sexuality, in words and pictures, that most people had never seen before. Naked sex positions, oral sex, anal sex, sex orgies, threesomes, group sex, homo and lesbian sex, even animal sex. Most of the sex books published in the 1970s had a pseudo text appearance along with a publisher's blurb that they were scientifically or educationally oriented and thus within the law. They were sold by mail and in a new kind of bookstore for adults that also offered all kinds of presumably sex-enhancing gadgets from dildos to penis pumps.

Teachers will display these books and gadgets as a sad substitute for healthy loving and touching between two adults. And they will show that, from the late 1920s to the 1960s, certain areas of major cities (from early Puritan times) have always catered to male sexual frustration. In typical areas like lower 42nd Street in New York and, later, lower Washington Street in Boston, rundown theaters offered burlesque and police arrested young women who occasionally revealed their pussy hair. During the 1970s, these areas degenerated into even sleazier "combat zones" where prostitutes solicited and strippers could "show it all" as they danced naked behind bars.

Finally, the teachers will remind parents and students that rather than trying to legislate morality in the twenty-first century we have embraced human sexual sanity. We have come to grips with human reality; our joy in experiencing warm, loving human flesh; our human needs to touch, kiss, taste, and suck one another; our needs to join with the flesh of another human being, or to see photographic and living portrayals of other human beings experiencing each other. These needs are not filthy, evil, or criminal. What is evil and ultimately dangerous for society is to dehumanize these needs or devalue them either in the written word or pictorially.

Thanks to the New Sexual Morality and Education bill, young people no longer grow up in an environment that denigrates human sexual loving or gives it an aura of guilt, tainting it with a feeling that human sexuality is basically animalistic, cheap, vile, and depraved.

We have completed the final sexual revolution and created an entirely new environment where politicians, educators, and religious leaders can unite in the knowledge that the sex act should be warm, delicate, joyous, laughing, and an ecstatic blending and worship of life itself—sex as the basis for religion, a blending and rapport with whatever God we may prefer and with each of us loving ourselves and other selves and finding what the philosophers in India call "enlightenment."

12

Creating an Educated Person: Reading, History, Self-Disclosure, and Journal-Keeping

After reading the preceding chapters, you may think that sex is the primary subject in twenty-first-century K-12 education. Not so! The in-depth sex value education, running an hour a week, *plus* an extensive (ninth to twelfth grade), in-depth multicultural, historical education in all the arts and sciences from human origins to the present, are completely interwoven. On a person's seventeenth birthday—a celebratory rite of passage coinciding in most cases with graduation from high school—a student not only becomes a sexual adult but he or she will have acquired broad, upbeat historical, "Who am I, why am I here?" and "Where am I and where is the world going?" perspectives that intertwine her or his life with a fascinating past and a dynamic future.

Young adults will now go on and complete their four-year undergraduate, largely vocationally oriented education in the GLUE program. They will not only be able to quickly acquire a technical vocabulary in any subject, but read about it with complete comprehension. They will be able to express themselves in writing or orally with great ease, and will have been taught and learned the art of self-disclosure as the sine qua non of love and friendship.

In a social environment that guarantees all high school graduates four more years of undergraduate education leading to bachelor or arts or science or vocational degrees, all young people fourteen to seventeen years old can be given, and they will absorb, a general, liberal arts education, as good as if not better than a minority of undergraduate students ages seventeen to twenty-one today, who get this kind of education in dribs and drabs because they never had it in high school.

Once NSME has been functioning for a few years most high school graduates will be on a cultural and intellectual par with comparable college graduates in the twentieth century.

Looking back to the twentieth century, the problem of how to create educated men and women will be seen to have been a delayed product of a college or university education. In his book *Killing the Spirit,* Page Smith reviews the awakening fear, as far back as 1914, among college presidents and professors that undergraduates were too concentrated on their "majors" and not getting a broad general education. A few years after World War II, James Conant, president of Harvard University, published *Report on General Education in a Free Society.* It proposed a unifying purpose and idea from the study of Western civilization that must be conveyed to all students as a part of their education. President Truman's Commission on Higher Education reached the same conclusion. "A core of unity . . . a body of common experiences and common knowledge . . . and the transmission of a common cultural heritage toward a common citizenship."

By the mid-1990s it was obvious that common citizenship involved many cultures in addition to the Western European. In a full-page advertisement that appeared in many European newspapers in January 1994, Adelphi University President Peter Diamandopolus, in Garden City, New York, asked, "Does anybody need an education this good?" He went on to say that the twenty-first century presents a very different set of demands for ourselves and our children. Adelphia's answer is a liberal arts education with a core curriculum, continuing through all a student's undergraduate years, that "is an open-ended but coherent inquiry into the issues, origins, achievements and difficulties of the modern condition . . . We ask does everyone need an education this good?'" Diamandopolus responds, "We say no—everybody doesn't need an education this good or this radical—only your congressman, your doctor, your lawyer, your business partner, your accountant—your son and daughter." While Diamandopolus doesn't say it—of course it is assumed that the reader's son or daughter will become one of the upper-income, professional or business people that he enumerates.

The basic qualifications for an educated man or woman didn't change much in the twentieth century. In 1974 Dean Henry Rosovksky spelled them out: "1. An educated person must be able to think, and write clearly and effectively. 2. An educated person should have achieved some depth in some field of knowledge. 3. An educated person should have critical appreciation of the ways in which we gain and apply knowledge and understanding of the universe, of society, and themselves. 4. An educated person is expected to have some understanding and thinking about moral and ethical problems which enable him to make discriminating moral choices. 5. An educated American cannot be provincial in the sense of being ignorant of other cultures and other times."

For Rosovksky these were the minimal educational accomplishments of a Harvard graduate. This is not a premise of the NSME legislation. The twenty-first century concept is that *every* American will be given this kind of intensive liberal arts education beginning in kindergarten, with really educated young American men and women graduating from the twelfth grade. The only item missing from Rosovksky's description will be the second one. The twenty-first century high school graduate will acquire "depth in some field of knowledge" in the GLUE undergraduate program.

GLUE is also predicated on recreating a not-too-distant past educational history, similar to that of the seventeenth and eighteenth century, when the lifespan was ten to fifteen years less than it is now and leaders in every area of life from the arts to science to politics were completely educated men in their late teens and at the height of their creative abilities between twenty and thirty. For the most part women weren't expected or permitted to pursue education beyond grammar school, but could dabble in the arts or teach themselves.

But in the mid-twentieth-century, with parents and educators becoming so affluent that they could extend the joys of childhood, they inadvertently created a nasty byproduct. Between 1900 and 1950 very few people were aware that the so-called "generation gap" between the younger and older generation didn't really come into being until early 1950s with the "beatniks," flowering with the hippies in the 1960s, and for the remainder of the century becoming an accepted way of life. Prior to that there was the "Jazz Age." But short skirts, bobbed hair, sexier music, and drinking prohibited booze in speakeasies encompassed more of the past-thirty generation than it did teenagers. Ernest Hemingway, F. Scott Fitzgerald, and other "expatriates" were still very much the creatures of Victorian morals, and their rebellion for more freedom in the arts and personal freedoms was well documented.

The byword—"Don't trust anyone over thirty"—response of the 1960s teenagers continued into the 1990s with heavy rock and rap music, books, magazines and movies for the younger generation who were presumably much more sexually sophisticated, even if it didn't extend to birth control. During the last half of the twentieth-century the "generation gap" mentality was created, underwritten, motivated, and stimulated by the make-a-fast-buck mentality of many business leaders and trumpeted by the never-ceasing assault of television and the media. Very few people challenged the social disruption and moral questioning that occurred in creating separate teenage markets, for everything from music to dress styles, or the preferred cola—Coke or Pepsi.

It wasn't always so. Before and after the two world wars and throughout the 1950s, teenagers were carbon copies of their parents. There was no external mental conditioning force like television to show and tell them that their parents didn't really know the time of day. Neither the movies nor the magazines from 1900 to the 1950s, that young people read went all-out to create a pseudo-sophisticated, "live today, tomorrow we die" environment that thousands of gun-carrying teenagers in the mid-1990s identified with during their formative years. Until the 1950s, for better or worse, radio and movies aimed their fare at adults. Teenagers learned to empathize with movie heroines or heroes who even with all their fictional or real life trials and tribulations usually offered some kind of moral uplift that wasn't too far removed from church or parental teaching. Even the Shirley Temples and Jackie Coopers were adults in clothing, smaller size versions of the clothing mom and dad wore.

Along with teenage clothing, music, magazines, and movies, there were teenage books offered as "young adult fiction." Inspired by Judy Blume, who sold millions of copies of her books, the market was soon flooded by female writers (Norma Klein, Beverly Cleary, Paula Zanaiger, and Caryl Rivers to mention a few) who tried via their stories to resolve moral and sexual confusion of young women ten years old and up. Using the first person to make their stories sound more authentic, they explored such subjects as: "What if parents grow apart?" "What if big sister gets married?" "What if she can never find true love?" "Having a boyfriend isn't the answer", "How to deal with split-down-the-middle life styles" (divorce) or "Riding a bus between one's parents' home"—this one is titled *Divorce Express.*

The NSME legislation, without infringing on First Amendment rights, creates an entirely new sexually moral environment that very quickly will eliminate the generation gap and bond parents with their children with a common joy in their sexuality, and a lifetime goal of learning more about specific things, and anything, as a way of life. Concentrating entirely on K-12 liberal arts education makes possible many new approaches to public school education in all the grades. Comparisons between the new American approaches with the methods being tried in other countries become major news stories of the twenty-first century. As far back as December 2, 1991, *Newsweek* explored some of the ideas being used in what they called *The Ten Best Schools in the World.* Teaching reading ability in the primary grades in New Zealand, one half of the class day is spent reading and teaching reading. In the Diana School in northern Italy teaching art and drawing is combined with science and math. At the Greydamus School in the Netherlands, realistic math is taught to ten-to-fifteen-year-old students who become totally intrigued with practical math by reinventing mathematical concepts.

In Japan, whose ministry of education directs national educational goals, Shigeki Kadoya, the ministry's specialist for elementary sciences, was moving the secondary school curriculum away from pure science. "We are not here to produce more effective economic producers. The new concept is to create a real human being—and a human who creates!" In Dutch schools young people of necessity learn to speak three or four different languages. Unlike the overall GLUE plan, the Germans go all-out for vocational education through grade ten.

Those who plan to go college, if their grades are high enough, attend the gymnasia for a more liberal arts preparation. Young Germans completing grade ten who don't go on to the universities are hired as apprentices to particular industries, where they continue their vocational training. The German concept is close to the American experience before NSME. Ultimately, the German program will continue to produce a divided working class structure. By contrast, American students with a complete liberal arts education who pursue undergraduate vocational degrees in the GLUE programs will be much better educated in several specific vocations, and will, in addition, have general abilities and perspectives on life and living that a strictly job education can never provide.

There will be many new approaches to K-12 education. Theodore Sizer's fascinating book *Horace's Compromise—The Dilemma of the American High School,* published in 1984, quickly evolved into a nationwide Coalition of Essential Schools. In 1995 its basic theories are still being explored and experimented with in more than eight-hundred public and private schools. Sizer wrote in his widely acclaimed book, "What is especially troubling is the low level of high school student reasoning skill. While students seem to be improving in rote level, concrete learnings—vocabulary recognition and in mathematics and simple addition, for example—their ability to think resourcefully is lamentably weak and is continuing to weaken. Sizer offers many solutions to the problem.

In their big complex book, *The Bell Curve,* published in September 1994, Charles Murray (who unfortunately died just after the book was published) and his coauthor Richard Herrstein uncorked the old IQ race issue, which William Schockley and Arthur Jensen had done previously in 1969, claiming that the black-white IQ gap is overwhelming and unsolvable, and is the reason that so many blacks, with this intellectual disadvantage, are doomed to remain in poverty. Murray and Herrstein are totally pessimistic about improving black IQ rate. I disagree with this aspect of the Bell Curve completely, and I'm sure that when GLUE becomes the main thrust of American politics—giving us all a long, lasting sense of national purpose, and making us fully aware that the IQ problem, black or white, is nurture not nature—in a very few years the lower black IQ discrepancy will vanish forever.

But before he died Murray did put his finger on the basic problem. Asked whether the *Bell Curve* was related in any way to the pessimistic, surly mood of America in 1994, he replied. "If you're asking the broader question this book addresses—an underlying sense that that this country is becoming unhinged?—I sure do agree!" There isn't any question that he was right. We need the Lovemore legislation passed before we are all flapping hopelessly into cyberspace—wondering where in hell we are going and why. These are questions that Laurence Shames tried to resolve in his 1989 book *The Hunger for More—Searching for*

Values in an Age of Greed. Shames pin-points the shuck values—middle-class Americans being brainwashed and transformed into a nation of shoppers by the media, and trying to find happiness in material possessions, but like Murray and Herrstein he has no answers. Guaranteed Loving Undergraduate Education (GLUE) does! It's within your power to make it an American way of life!

The basic underpinnings of reading, writing, and arithmetic-merging-into-mathematics can be taught by parents to their pre-schoolers, but for the first ten to fifteen years, until the many of the first GLUE graduates are filtering back into the teaching system, K-12 teachers will teach all subjects, except computer abilities, via printed books and reading.

Showing children how the printed words of any author can be more exciting than anything they may watch on computer monitors, reading to each other and learning to read rapidly with in-depth comprehension, gives young people a new sense of power, especially when the reading is praised by other listeners. By the time they are in the third grade nine-year-olds should be able to read silently and so fluently that the words in the book come alive, almost as if the author is talking directly to them, so much so that in later grades, as they learn to read with a pen or pencil in hand, they can bracket an author's thought—check it to come back to—and even learn to argue with the author in their own words in the margin of the book. Long before they graduate from high school they will not only have learned how to be "interactive" with anything they read, but they'll discover that almost any author writing fiction, biography, autobiography, poetry or scientific subjects not only sounds in the reader's brain as if he's talking directly to them, but the author can expand the reader's imagination and creativity far beyond any comparable visual attempt on film or television. Young readers and an author can ruminate together—a subjective chewing of the cud that not only produces educated men and women but provides endless sharing of ideas with others.

Inevitably, all schools and millions of homes will have complete reference libraries available on computer disc, and young students will be able to call up any subject instantly on their computer monitor. The subject may be illustrated and even be read aloud to them. There will be book-size read-only-memory trade books and fiction produced on small discs. The pages can be turned with light finger pressure on the machine. These discs will eliminate most text books, which in the past had to be printed in huge volumes and updated annually to keep abreast. Textbooks on large computers will now have print-out abilities to capture underlined material that must be learned. These machines will make many old-style printed books obsolete, but they won't accelerate the learning process. Over and above pictures, learning requires an ability to read words and transform them into brain knowledge. Assimilating the kind of twenty-first-century knowledge that will create a person who cannot only get one or more specific, well-paying jobs, but enjoy a self-fulfilling life as a complete, knowledgeable American citizen requires sixteen years of education. Reading ability, along with the ability to transform reading words and numbers into retained knowledge, is the prime objective of K-12 education. In the process, this twenty-first century approach will expand the unused potential of the human brain.

In late 1994, Harold Bloom in his book *The Western Canon* wrote, "I have very little confidence that literary education will survive its current malaise." Essentially Bloom meant book reading and learning from our heritage extending back from ancient antiquity to the present, which he believes is essential to human understanding. He lists thirty-six pages of these books in the appendix.

Sven Bijerts, in his 1994 book, *The Gutenberg Chronicles,* is even more depressed than Bloom. He imagines his daughter in a post-book world inhabited by college freshmen who are so enmeshed in electronic information, so tuned in not just to television but to pervasive, interactive multi-media, so besotted by on-line data services, and so attuned to the rapid rhythms of MTV that they have grown up barely able to understand the printed book and are totally deaf to the inner voices of print.

Amusingly, in the February 27, 1995 issue of *Newsweek,* which is almost totally dedicated to the future wonders of the technoworld and cyberspace, Clifford Stoll, author of a 1995 book, *Silicon Snake Oil—Second Thoughts on the Information Highway,* challenges the twenty-first-century-media, hyped-up dreamland. He writes,

> Visionaries see a future of telecommuting workers, interactive libraries, and multimedia classrooms. Commerce will shift from offices and malls to networks and modems. . . . Baloney! Do our computer pundits lack all common sense? The truth is that no on-line data base will take the place of competent teachers. What is missing from the electronic wonderland? Human contact! Discount the fawning techno-burble about virtual communities. Computer networks isolate us from one another. A network chat line is a limp substitute for meeting friends over coffee. No interactive multimedia display comes to the excitement of a live concert. And who'd prefer cyber sex to the real thing?

In a parallel *Time* magazine, Spring 1995 issue, Welcome to Cyberspace, Robert Hughes joins Stoll in a two-page article titled "Take this Revolution . . ." ("and shove it" isn't part of the title). Among other things Hughes gives his "Bah" to Internet which,

> it seems speaks to America's unappeasable terror of loneliness; a fear that overflows into a mistrust of one of life's most precious assets—optional solitude. Americans, it is said, already watch seven to eight hours of TV a day. Not all that

many at present, but their numbers are growing, spend 25 hours [a week] on the NET, goggling at another kind of screen and calling it community empowerment. To them one is tempted to say: Get a life!

During the early years of the NSME legislation, the media, including television, can help create a new generation of avid readers by offering prizes for reading comprehension and ability. In place of largely moronic spelling contests, children at different grade levels can compete in programs that reward their ability to read, and prove they understood what they were reading with a quick verbal test, thus combining learning with play. Even closer parental involvement will be achieved by asking parents to contribute the dollar they might spend on the local lottery for monthly prizes given to young people in the first six grades who demonstrate their reading and comprehension abilities in school auditoriums or gyms on a monthly basis.

History and literature teachers will praise and use public television series like those that were offered in the mid-1990s covering the Civil War, Columbus, and the Age of Discovery. They can even pause in whatever historical era their students may be studying, and in the classroom broaden the television series with in-depth explorations of the entire fifteenth- or nineteenth-century world depicted in these programs.

A good example of this approach was provided by the National Gallery of Art in 1992 with an exhibition titled "Circa 1492: Art in the Age of Exploration." Contemporary with Columbus were the artists Albrecht Dürer, Leonardo da Vinci, Michelangelo, Hieronymous Bosch, Donatello, Botticelli, and Piero della Franseca. Some of their works were shown in the European section. While Columbus never got to the Orient, in Japan, Sesshu Toyo was creating magnificent landscape scrolls, and in Ming China, Shen Zhou was painting in metaphorical styles that would have surprised the Europeans. In the African gallery were masterpieces of Benin sculpture, and in the American section was a life-sized god, Xoxchiplli, an Aztec masterpiece. This is only a small portion of the artists exhibited, but assuming that films were made, they could be available on cassettes for teachers.

Despite the multicultural approach, students will be reminded, as art critic Jack Flam pointed out, quoting philosopher Lesek Kolakowski: "In these times, unlike the rest of the world, European culture had developed a self-critical faculty that is generally lacking in other societies, and it is this self-critical faculty that impels us to take a sympathetic interest in the culture of others."

In the ninth and tenth grades, and even earlier, young people are capable of learning how to use a quadrant and why Columbus was sure that the world was round because of his dead reckoning, as well as his ability to place himself on primitive maps with an early knowledge of latitude and longitude. Math, history, geography, politics, and the discovery of how to put words—handwritten and spoken—into print, can be made totally fascinating when teachers turn historical learning into multicultural drama with thousands of people in Eastern and Western cultures searching for answers to every aspect of life and living.

Young people who have shallow family roots, and even those who can trace their ancestry back many generations can adopt an ancestor—learn everything possible about some person who may not have been very important historically and learn all about him or her. This can become a fascinating, fun way of resurrecting the dead and bringing them back to life. Speculating on how they might respond to the twenty-first-century world will create enthusiastic young people involved with past lives. Using books like *The Age of the French Revolution,* Claude Manceron's five-volume panorama revealing the emotions, words, and actions of people long forgotten, in their own words, can also provide many ancestors waiting to be adopted and live again. Every young person, or his family, should have a copy of James Trager's *The People's Chronology—A Year by Year Record of Human Events from Prehistory to Present.* Using Trager's book is a fun way to involve young and old and let them discover what was happening in the world on their birthdays—twenty-five, fifty, a hundred and a thousand years before they were born—thus establishing human continuity both for themselves, their parents and their friends and not only give them a gold mine of ancestors they can adopt but heroes and heroines of the past they can emulate.

Underlying all the K-12 teaching is the continuing need to create a long-term sense of national purpose for new generations. All high school graduates will not only have broad historical perspectives but common beliefs that the history of man and woman is not circular, but upward and forward. In the twenty-first century teachers will not only plumb the mysteries of life and the universe, but will help create new generations who are learning that one of the real joys of life is not the "I gotta be me" discovery, but rather "I've got to dare to be you!"—both past and present.

To accomplish this teachers will have carte blanche to explore with students the entire history of man and woman on this planet and teach sciences, the social sciences, literature, drama, poetry, sculpture, music, and architecture as a reflection of not just human abilities during particular times but human values and morality as well. A study of slavery, for example, will reveal that it was a way of life in Roman times. A thousand years later Columbus's plan to enslave the Caribs and Arawks and make them Christians was approved by the pope, just as Francis Drake's expedition to enslave blacks in Africa and bring them back to the West Indies was approved by Queen Elizabeth. And, in this multicultural approach, Africans selling their captured enemies to American slave traders will also be noted.

All young Americans participating in the GLUE educational plan will acquire a wide historical background in all areas of human endeavor, along with the slowly changing moralities and values as humans struggled for freedom from the money and power-hungry people who controlled their lives. Knowing where we've been, how far we've come, lights the way into the future and how far we still have to go.

Young people will not only learn how the Soviet Communist leaders rewrote history to justify their regimes, but will discover in their high school courses how American history has been slanted. They will learn the complex motivations behind the scenes that led to the American Revolution, our Civil War, World War I, and World War II, and the emergence of United States in the twenty-first century as a world policeman. And they will discover the pros and cons of why most leaders of Western nations in the twenty-first century, along with our leaders, refuse to create a world federalist government and to give armed sovereignty to the United Nations to create one international army, navy, and air force that could rapidly move in on aggressors of any kind who refuse to resolve their problems by discussion and majority rule.

Twenty-first-century students will learn that despite the end of Communism in the Soviet Union the new Russian regime couldn't make the transition to laissez faire capitalism, and they will discover that many economists and world leaders do not believe in a completely laissez faire market system. In the twenty-first century, with broad perspectives on the past, they will learn that all the nations of the world, including the United States, are still learning how to merge economic freedom with communitarian/socialistic, democratic structures. Teachers may even raise the question whether after the demise of the Soviet Union, Americas should have lifted the embargo against Cuba, and helped Fidel Castro experiment with a socialistic economy, thus learning answers for good or bad to our own economic problems.

From the ninth grade on, young people will discover that every aspect of former lives, and our lives today, are reflections of the same fundamental urges—love, fear, anger, self-enhancement, acquisitiveness, curiosity, creativeness, gregariousness, hunger—that motivates all of us. They will learn that the writers of other eras and civilizations have offered insights into how these urges affected them and other people. But whether it be Greek philosophers, religious prophets, or in later centuries storytelling playwrights, poets, and novelists, neither the solutions offered by Plato, Jesus, or Mohammad, or the problems dramatized by Sophocles, Shakespeare, Moliere, or Ibsen, to name a few playwrights, can resolve most twenty-first-century problems. Oedipus, Hamlet, Ophelia, Lear, Tartuffe, and Nora in her doll's house can all be enjoyed in historical performances on video tapes, and students can follow them in annotated editions, approving or disapproving, with their teachers, of editing and cuts. Momentarily, they can adopt these ancestors and sympathize with their man-made tragedies. But the emphasis will be on man-made and man-created tragedies. Students may gain some insight into how far humans have progressed from the tragic (or comic) events that affected past generations, but in the twenty-first century there will be diminishing sympathy with man-made tragedies emanating from religious and political differences and personal hatreds ending in wars that dominate human history, and more for real human tragedies that were and still are beyond human knowledge to prevent.

In essence, in this new liberal arts environment, teachers will teach history and literature as reflections of the emotional and moral values as well as the economic conditions of particular times. What was happening in the world when Shakespeare wrote a particular play? In 1606, while he was complaining via Macbeth that "Tomorrow and tomorrow creeps into this petty pace from day to day,"—evoking another time, there was a gun-powder plot to blow up the House of Commons, Puritans were being persecuted by Archbishop Laud because they refused to follow the Church of England ritual, and Queen Elizabeth, daughter of Henry VIII and Anne Boleyn, died in 1603—still a virgin, presumably. Everywhere in high places there were sex scandals. Why wasn't Shakespeare interested in contemporary events? Maybe he was, but only dared to confront them with allusions from the past.

Learning this dramatic kind of real-life history, young people will discover that during the previous hundred years the invention of moveable type and printing on paper was making the Holy Bible everyone's property. Catholics weren't supposed to read the Old Testament, but thousands of dissenting Protestants were cooking up their own Christian religions and proselytizing for their own routes to eternal salvation. And young people will learn that most of them became seeding grounds for the "poisoning of eros" that ultimately led to the final sex revolution.

Two other aspects of the twenty-first-century K-12 liberal arts training that are interwoven with other courses and will accelerate reading and thinking abilities is teaching young people the art of self-disclosure and journal keeping. In passing it should be noted that in addition to continued reading and math ability, testing scoring on Scholastic Aptitude Tests will continue. Scores of 600 or above, in the mid-1990s, had dropped from 11 percent of the students to 7 percent. All students will be aware that their scores will determine whether they have the option of pursuing a career in vocations that require graduate study, or taking the vocational route during undergraduate years. In any event (see chapter 14), all students in the GLUE programs will be required to take a unifying undergraduate course called Human Values that will continue to broaden their liberal arts training.

In the mid-1990s it was standard practice for teachers in the early grades to have their young students, several times a week, write a few paragraphs on what they did on vacation, or over the weekend, or write how they felt about their pets, or characters in a book that they have learned to read, and have the young people read what they had written to each other. Realizing that all young people should develop the ability to express their thoughts in writing, and this is by no means as easy as verbal expression, in the seventh grade young people will be encouraged to keep a daily journal of their activities, and put in writing not only what is happening in their lives, but to try and reveal in their own words, without too much worry about grammar or literary construction, their innermost feelings—how they are reacting to school, their parents, their teachers, their friends, and the world in general. To do this effectively will require an honesty and a willingness to record one's true feelings at particular times, and discover later that they may change rapidly. While the book wasn't written for young people, teachers will try to convey the idea expressed by J. H. van den Berg in his book *The Changing Nature of Man,* which devotes more than half the study to adults versus children, and the confusing, multivalent society children experience as they try to find roots and meaning in constantly shifting social and home environments.

In the twentieth century, twelve- to seventeen-year-olds, becoming aware of their burgeoning sexuality and that their loving needs carried an aura of sin and shame, had few people, if anyone, to whom they would dare to reveal their real problems and feelings. Teacher will encourage older students that keeping a day-by-day journal in spiral-bound school notebooks with lined paper—one notebook for each month and writing in it a half hour a day, perhaps before—can be an adventure in self-discovery, and help them develop the ability to self-disclose their most intimate feelings and frustrations.

Teachers will explain that in the nineteenth century almost everyone who could write wrote long letters, and letter writing became a high art for many. In the twentieth century if you wanted to tell someone something, no matter where they were in the world, the telephone—telecommunications did it faster, and a person could get his thoughts across with a limited vocabulary. Some people might have been able to tell another person their intimate fears and worries, hopes and despairs, but, as Ira Progroff, who wrote a basic text on journal keeping as a form of long-term therapy, points out, keeping a journal is a way to let people discover their own inner processes of development and "look behind their own minds." Reading ones own words at a later date not only gives a person perspective on him or herself, but lets them monitor their own growth.

Journal keeping would not be compulsory but could be integrated into English courses. Students will become familiar with journals kept by many famous people. A collection of diaries, *Heart Songs,* kept by ten young ladies, including Selma Lagerlof and Anaïs Nin, will interest both boys and girls. In these intimate diaries young female adolescents describe their sexual awakenings, philosophical searchings, and cultural transitions in their own words. As Laurel Holliday, the editor, points out, "This is the one book I was looking for when, as a lonely and somewhat lost teenager, I tried to find other girls on library shelves who would help me with what I was going through. Needless to say, I never found the documents I was looking for in the local library."

Teachers will explain that keeping a journal in the twenty-first century should be a person's private space to vent himself, to write what he or she really thinks about their own sexual feelings, as well as moral and religious beliefs or the lack of them. Young journal keepers, learning about the past history of sexual devaluation and degradation, can decide whether they fully agree with the new twenty-first-century sexual honesty and restraining their own sexual drives until they are seventeen, or not. They can contrast the past, when boys thought they had to maintain a macho image with their male friends and never reveal any deep emotions that might betray a "female" outlook on life or cowardice, and young girls were conditioned never to reveal intimate feelings to anyone except their best girlfriend. As teachers will show, in the mid-1990s it was acceptable for people to spill their guts on afternoon talk shows but anyone, especially teenagers, who kept journals were "ranked" by their friends as "nerds."

In this twenty-first century environment teachers can create journal-keeping excitement with a monthly journal lottery. All those in particular classes can agree in advance that the girls draw the names of participating guys from a hat, and they will exchange journals. Not only can a guy read a young woman's intimate thoughts, but she can read his. Before they recover their journals each can write a note to the reader with his or her reactions. Young people experiencing the flow of their hormones, and a driving interest in the other sex—in a wait-until-you-are-seventeen social environment—will find this voyeuristic game of journal exchange an exciting experience. And, from the standpoint of learning to write well, knowing that they will be judged by one of their peers, they will go all-out to try to express themselves coherently.

In the area of journal keeping, teachers will explore the social environment of the twentieth century, where children, parents, friends, husbands, and wives were often unable, or afraid, to reveal the kind of people they really were. In a collection of essays, *Environments for Man, The Next 50 Years,* Christopher Alexander discussing the city as a mechanism for maintaining human contact wrote:

> Modern urban society has more contact and communication in it than any other society in human history. . . . But as the individual world expands, and the num-

ber of his contacts increase, the quality of the contact goes down. A person only has twenty-four hours a day. . . . As his contacts increase his contacts with any one person become shorter, less frequent, less deep. In the end from the human point of view they become almost trivial. . . . People who live in cities may think that they have lots of friends, but the word friend has changed its meaning. Compared with friendships of the past, most of these friendships are trivial. *Intimate contact in the deepest sense is rare. Intimate contact is that close contact between two individuals in which they reveal themselves in all their weaknesses without fear,* in which barriers that normally surround the self are down. It is the relationship which characterizes the best marriages and all true friendships. We often call it love. . . . We can make it reasonably concrete by naming two essential preconditions. These conditions are: 1. The people concerned must see each other very often, almost every day, though not necessarily for a very long time. 2. They must see each other under informal conditions without any special overlay of role or situation which they usually wear in public. . . . It may help to keep in mind an even more concrete criterion of intimacy. If two people are in intimate contact, then we can be sure that they talk about ultimate meanings of their lives. . . . If they do not talk about these things then they are not really reaching each other and their contact is superficial. By this definition it is clear that most "friendly" contacts are not intimate.

Alexander continues these thoughts vis-à-vis the family and I will pick them up in a later chapter. But the basis for building a healthy personality, according to Sidney Jourard (and many psychiatrists) is the ability to self-disclose.

In their first few years of life, children reveal their feelings and needs completely, but then parental repression sets in as they soon learn what is bad and what is good to put in their mouths or diapers. "As children," Jourard wrote in his book *The Transparent Self* (which should be used in the later years of the human sexuality course)

we are, we act our real selves. We say what we think, we scream what we want, we tell what we did. These spontaneous disclosures meet variable consequences—some disclosures are ignored, some rewarded, some punished. Doubtless, in accordance with the laws of reinforcement, we learn early to withhold certain disclosures because of the painful consequences to which they lead. We are punished in our society, not only for what we actually do, but also what we think, feel or want. Very soon, then, the child learns to display a highly expurgated version of his self to others.

Jourard points out that it takes "courage to be" and as a result of early conditioning many people would rather die than become known. "When I say that someone achieves personality health, I mean something like the following. . . . It is not until I am my real self, and I act my real self that I am in a position to grow. . . . People's selves stop growing when they repress them." In his book Jourard covers the many aspects of self-disclosure in marriage; the lethal male role in which many men soon lose the ability to reveal their real selves; and the psychiatrist's and nurse's role in aiding self-disclosure. "Through my self-disclosure," Jourard writes, "I let others know my soul." The word soul may be too ephemeral. Jourard really means what makes us tick as human beings. "I'm beginning to suspect," he continues, "that I can't even know my own soul except as I disclosed it. I will know myself for real at the exact moment that I have succeeded in making it known to another person."

In the next chapter, we follow the new liberal-arts-educated high school graduate into a very different, four-year undergraduate environment with a Roommate of the Other Sex Option, but readers may be interested in my following, personal experience in twenty-first-century journal keeping, *Jennifer's World,* and an excerpt from my novel, *The Oublion Project* (both as yet unpublished), revealing a new breed of twenty-first-century young people in action. If you question the validity of this kind of nine-year-old mentality in the Oublion excerpt, read the biographies of Descartes, Pascal, Goethe, and Mozart to mention a few brilliant children, all or whom were created by their familial environment.

"Jennifer's World"

In the mid-1990s, a few years after I had lectured to an audience of teenagers at Thayer Academy, a nearby private school, a young woman who I had never met phoned me. "I've done it!" she told me triumphantly over the phone. "Done what?" I asked warily. "I've followed your advice. Like the kids in your novels *The Harrad Experiment* and *The Premar Experiments,* I've kept a journal for one full year. You said that if anyone listening to you would actually do it that you probably could get it published. Do you want to read it?"

Of course I did. But waiting a few days until she delivered it, I couldn't help thinking, "Oh brother—now you've done it. Some unknown teenager is going to bring you a boring catalogue of the daily events in her life with little or no attempt to correlate them in a way that would reveal the kind of person she really is."

Then Jennifer, a pretty, vivacious, blue-eyed young lady just past her fifteenth birthday, arrived carrying a knapsack. When she opened it—to use a teenage expression popular at the time—"It was awesome." She handed me six spiral-bound notebooks, 730 pages, written on both sides averaging 125 to 150 words per page. It was an unbelievable 250,000 words or more. As I pointed out to her later, it would make a book larger than a Stephen King novel.

For the next few days, via her journal, I really got to know Jennifer. Going on sixteen, she was (and still is) a fearless young lady who dared to ask questions about herself and everyone and everything she came in contact with. I was privileged to go inside a teenage mind and read her journals before her parents did. They were in the process of divorce, and I doubt if, even today, they could cope with Jennifer's cool appraisal of their problem—she loved them both, but was living with her upper-income yuppie mother since her high-income daddy had moved out and was living with his new friend. Interestingly, she was a woman about the same age as Jennifer's mother, indicating that her daddy was not in search of a youth, but rather a woman who was perhaps not so career-oriented as her mother.

Jennifer is now a graduate of Columbia University. During the year that she kept the journal she hoped to become an actress or a writer, or even to go into politics. Unlike Michael Apted, who made a career of keeping track of a group of British young people and filmed and recorded their thoughts and aspirations in remarkable films every seven years of their lives—the latest at age thirty-five—I haven't heard from Jennifer for several years. But I made her promise to keep a typewritten copy that I helped her prepare to the five-hundred-page manuscript. Her written words give you insights into the life and thoughts of a twentieth-century young woman that no flat visual portrayal on film ever could. Jennifer reveals herself totally, including what she laughingly refers to as the "juicy parts"—and her transition from a virgin to an almost virgin who would give oral sex to her boyfriend and let him explore her pussy with his tongue but no sexual merger. Finally, well into her seventeenth year, thus presaging the new twenty-first-century sexual morality, and after months of self-discovery of herself as a woman who enjoys sex, she tries to envision the kind of man she needed to confirm herself and him in their lifetime pursuits.

"The Oublion Project"

That night after dinner, and after the loving, still starry-eyed, holding Kara's hand, Raini listened while Kara told Tenzin and Persephone: "Each generation can climb a stage closer to a better world, not on the backs but on the brains of our ancestors. Unfortunately, the best minds of our generation are usually outnumbered by those who have just evolved beyond an eye for an eye, and a tooth for a tooth mentality."

He opened a bottle of French Bordeaux, explaining to Raini that on special occasions, Arkheans Tenzin and Persephone, who were nine and ten years old, could mellow their brains with a glass of wine at dinner. He toasted them all: "In the words of that old song 'The world is waiting for the sunrise.' It's up to us to make sure it does."

To Raini's surprise, by their tenth year, all Group Fivers had pretty much absorbed algebra and Euclidean geometry. At the same time they were exploring the development of natural-language thinking versus artificial intelligence, or computer language—all of which, Raini had to admit, was a mystery to her.

Sipping her wine, Persephone told them that their preceptors traced the search for ultimate truth back to Aristotle and his development of syllogisms whose premise, if true, could be developed into truthful conclusions.

"A thousand years after Aristotle," Tenzin added, "a Muslim mathematician, Al-Khowarazmi—they named algorithms after him—wrote a book called *Kitab Aljabr, w'almgabala,* which is where algebra came from."

"Al-Khowarazmi had a new idea," Persephone interjected. "He figured out how to solve propositions by substituting letters for the unknown. He probably never heard of Aristotle but, like him, he was searching for new ways to find true answers to everything."

"A few hundred years later, in the eleventh century, a Spaniard named Raymond Lully invented a logic machine," Kara told them. Like a wheel of fortune, it had letters and words that could be combined to help discover the basic equations in any philosophical problem."

"Maybe he could have found the answer for Arkheans," Raini suggested a little sarcastically. "For example, does the end justify the means? And is the Arkhean end—or plan for the world—just a pipe dream?"

"That takes us back Euclid," Kara smiled. "What do you think Perse? Did Euclid have the right approach?"

"Maybe," Persephone said very seriously. "That's what we've been studying. First you develop a proposition and then prove it by other propositions and axioms that you know to be true." She stared at Raini thoughtfully. "Here's a proposition. If humans breed a race of superior men and women who can be educated to use all their powers to improve the lives and environments of every person on this planet—and not take advantage of any person—is that good or bad, and does the end justify the means?"

"That's a mouthful." Kara grinned at her. "What true proposition can anyone offer to sustain that one?"

"We know that man has bred superior animals of many kinds," Tenzin said. "We know that man can breed a new race of superior men and women. We're doing it here on Arkhea."

"We know that human beings would like to stop all wars," Persephone said, correcting herself. "Well, most human beings anyway. But most people believe that their leaders might be right. If they're not ready to fight back, then people in another country might conquer them."

"That could lead to an axiom," Kara said. "What if nations all over the world had new leaders who dared to tell them the truth? Without guns, war ships, attack airplanes, submarines, bombs, missiles—in this modern world no nation could conquer another with just sticks and stones, swords and bows and arrows."

"Quod erat demonstrandum," Tenzins and Persephone chorused. "We need new leaders."

"That's silly" Raini said. She was enjoying the discussion but decided to punch a hole in it. "Read your history—the Romans, the Crusaders, only had swords and bows and arrows. They tried to conquer the world. How do you know that your new leaders won't become the future Genghis Khans and Adolph Hitlers and go into business for themselves?"

"They obviously might," Kara said. "But if they invaded a modern city with sticks, stones, swords, and bows and arrows—even on horseback—they'd soon be wiped out by people in automobiles running them over. Anyway, the new leaders won't be interested in conquest of others. Brought up like Tenzin and Persephone—as philosopher-kings and queens, they will have a new mission to make as many people as possible philosopher kings and queens so that they won't be lonesome."

Before they finished the dinner of grouper that Kara had scooped out of the nearby fish hatchery, and which Tenzin and Persephone had cleaned, broiled, and served with tomatoes and rice—all the while discussing the problem of whether what was happening on the island of Arkhea was good or evil—Kara and Tenzin had meandered into a discussion of Descartes, Leibniz, George Boole and Boolean algebra, Newton's axiom of the laws of motion, and Nicholas Lobachevski's proof that Euclidean theories weren't the only ones that could be derived from his proposition—Raini was totally bewildered couldn't believe that Persephone knew as much or more than Tenzin.

"Women weren't supposed to be so good, or give a damn about such things," she said.

"Arkhean women and men are now a part of an exciting historical continuity of people searching for answers," Kara told her. "In the twenty-first century we can no longer afford to leave it to chance, or to let superior minds be exterminated by barbarians whose brains haven't evolved beyond the primitive stage."

13

GLUE and the
Roommate of the Other Sex Option

The Clinton Goals 2000 educational bill daydream is that by the year 2000 the high school graduation rate would be at least 90 percent—and American students would be first in the world in mathematics and science.

In the mid-1990s, according to Paul Barton of the Educational Testing Service, the difference between student proficiency in the public schools of various states could be explained by five factors: number of days absent from school, number of hours spent watching television, number of pages read for homework, quantity and quality of reading material in the home, and the presence of two parents in the home. In 1993 the estimated graduation rate from high school was 77.1 percent. In 1991, American thirteen-year-olds ranked thirteenth among fourteen nations surveyed in math, and twelfth in science.

George Will, in a 1994 article, "Goals 2000," was convinced, "The government can do next to nothing quickly about the quality of families." He tackled The National Education Association for having a vested interest in preventing "parents from being active shoppers for their children's education and using school choice programs."

Will and others who fear governmental leadership are wrong. The NSME legislation and the GLUE programs will create a new kind of sexual and educational environment that not only sets the stage for a 90 percent high school graduation rate but will ensure that liberal-arts-educated teenagers will excel over students in every nation of the world.

Looking back to the twentieth century and remembering the futurists and those with solutions to the problems of human sexuality and disintegrating family values will be an important prelude to understanding why GLUE is the answer and why the ROSP alternative, which in the initial years may only attract 15 per-

145

cent to 20 percent of the A13ers, will ultimately become an educational way of life—not only to give every man and woman a complete education but in the process educate them for each other.

During the 1990s many of the problems enumerated in chapter 1 were spelled out, for the second time in 1994, in a book called *The Index of Cultural Indicators,* a volume of tables and graphs assembled by William Bennett, formerly secretary of education, and examined more fully in *Values and Public Policy,* a collection of essays published by the Brookings Institute. Rutgers professor David Popenoe declares that, "As families go, so goes the nation. . . . Every society must be wary of the unattached male, for he is universally the cause of numerous social ills. The good society is heavily dependent on men being attached to a strong moral order centered on families, both to discipline their sexual behavior and to reduce their competitive aggression. . . . Almost a quarter of all men between twenty-five and thirty-four live in non-family households. . . . The proportion of the American adult's life spent with spouse and children has declined from 62 percent in 1960 to 43 percent in 1994 . . . this trend alone probably helps to account for the rising crime rates over the past thirty years."

Contrast his feelings with the reaction of Alan Berkowitz, who directs a course, "Men and Masculinity," at Hobart and William Smith Colleges: "This is a very confusing time for heterosexual males," he writes in 1991. "Young men are caught between the traditional macho ideal and the alternative of being open and pro-feminist. But they fear if they go too far in that direction, they may be labeled 'fag' . . . so they are on the defensive. Many feel if a woman has second thoughts after sex, she can always say it was rape, and get the guy in trouble unfairly."

Feature articles like Lance Morrow's "Are Men Really That Bad?" in *Time* (February 1994) and Warren Farrell's book *The Myth of Male Power,* exonerating men and blaming women for the lack of rapport between males and females, were the subject of billions of words written by pop psychologists in the 1990s—all providing no answers at the educational level.

The World Future Society, "An Association for the Study of Alternate Futures," devoted issue after issue of its monthly magazine, *The Futurist,* as well as many books, to every conceivable aspect of the future from world economies to space travel, and current buzzwords like telecommunications. But futurists, for the most part men, rarely offered any alternatives in the areas of marriage, the family, or human sexuality that dovetailed with the education of the younger generation or that proposed that educationally a mental as well as physical merger of the male and the female was possible.

An amusing prognostication from the 1970s was given by William Simon and John Gagnon. They were senior research sociologists in those years at the

Institute for Sex Research (no longer operating). In an article, "Prospects for Change in American Sexual Patterns," they wrote:

> The yeasayers and the naysayers both make forecasts of the future. The yeasayers focus on a glorious sexual re-evaluation that will release human energy to produce Utopian social fulfillment. The naysayers forecast social and moral collapse and point to the pseudo parallel of Rome. The naysayers are those for whom any sexual change is seen as the inexorable decline in the moral condition of society. Opposing them are the yeasayers who feel if only sexual problems could be straightened out, then every one would able to live a happy productive life, that sexual freedom will somehow reduce sexual tensions, improve the lot of the poor, educate the illiterate, and put an end to causes of war. Both of these groups suffer from the same delusion (as perhaps do all of us) that sexuality is the prime moving force in human experience, and if it were regulated either by suppression, on the one hand, or total freedom on the other, the problem would be resolved.

Simon and Gagnon's further conviction was that,

> The future drift of society will be to a situation where sex will diminish in importance in terms of being a source of major guilt or passion. . . . Sex will move out of the center of the stage as a source of passion and return as a form of play—as a parallel to gourmet cooking. There will be no Romeo and Juliets because no one will be able to develop a level of passion sufficient to die for sex. The likely outcome for modern society will not be the sudden release of sexual passion, but sexuality played out in a new key, less important, less central, less over determined.

The New Sexual Morality and Education legislation gets to the root of the problems and provides sane goals and a sense of purpose by embracing human sexuality and putting it back on the church altar not for worship but for human joy and wonder. At the same time, during their school years, the new sexual morality lays the groundwork for mutual male/female commitment to sexual restraint followed by a coming-of-age reward at seventeen that includes four more years of education during which cohabitation is a structured way of life in the optional phase two of the GLUE/ ROSP program, or is left to more random choice in phase one of GLUE. But in each area the guarantee continues and is based on no marriage and no children until graduation—approximately at age twenty-one. Obviously, those who are sexually oriented toward their own sex won't have these problems. Gay and lesbian students, representing about 5 percent of the population, will be accepted in phase one of the GLUE programs, and similar to the accommodation made by the military services, will not have to reveal their sexual preferences. They will, however, be discouraged from rooming together. Getting involved in flagrant, unstructured, multiple sexual contacts (either hetero or homo) will be cause for expulsion. In the late twentieth century Gay Talese in his book *Thy Neighbor's Wife* and Stevie Chappie and David Talbot in their book *Burning Desires* sum up the hit-and-run mentality and sexual frustrations of the thirty years between 1960 and 1990. These books will be required reading in human values undergraduate seminars to give young people background on past sexual searching and devaluation, along with the writings of Betty Friedan and Germaine Greer and later, more belligerent women who changed the original thrust of female liberation to an all-out, never-ending war between the sexes.

During the anything-goes sexual freedom era of the 1960s the message to young women (aided by the birth control pill and as yet no fear of AIDS) was that the male/female merger was basically a merger of genitals for a moment of pleasure and not a merger of minds. It could be summed up by the male adage, "He who fucks and runs away lives to fuck another day." Any merger of minds on undergraduate coed campuses was not accelerated by feminists like Andrea Dworkin. In one book after another, she insisted, "The penis must embody the violence of the male in order for him to be male. The male is his penis, violence is the penis or the sperm ejaculated from it. . . . Men love death. In everything they make, they hollow out a central place for death. They like its rancid smell that contaminates every dimension of whatever still survives."

Paving the way for the jury that acquitted Lorena Bobbitt, Dworkin and many feminists, countered and abetted by male chauvinists all screaming their downbeat sexual devaluations, will be explored in human values sessions throughout the entire four-year work/study undergraduate years. I have shown how the seminars may function in my novels *The Harrad Experiment* and *The Premar Experiments*.

In the twenty-first century, whether a student is enrolled in the regular Phase One, GLUE program or in the phase two, ROSP program (which I will detail below), all student roommates will meet in prearranged groups of not more than forty-eight students, equally divided between men and women. Informal meetings take place once a week for one hour after dinner on Friday evenings, during both work and study months. One male and one female graduate student will chair the meetings and guide the discussions each week. All students are assigned one book each week (fifty-two a year), which will be a partial focus for the HV meetings. Graduate students who are known as "Compars," communal parents, function like older brother and sister siblings to the students.

During the first six months assigned books in the human values seminar will be oriented around the sexual lives of the students—active or not—as well as their work and study problems. Obviously the HV seminars for students enrolled in the ROSP program (see ahead) who will have roommates of the other sex will be on a different level than students in the regular GLUE program. Young people with roommates of the same sex will have many of the same problems of twentieth-century undergraduates. They must find loving companions of the other sex on their own and contend with AIDS or sexually transmitted diseases. The weekly HV seminars, equally divided male and female, will have approximately 20 to 25 percent of the students of other races or ethnic cultures. In many sessions a kind of group therapy will occur that not only provides answers to learning and work problems, but will create a safe environment for dating and ultimately sexual relationships with other students.

In Europe, before universities developed into degree-granting institutions, the idea of attending a university (males only) was to learn from teacher/scholar interaction. The search for knowledge and the attempt to unify human thinking was a search for roots (the basic definition of the word radical will apply). The two-way interaction in these weekly seminars with two graduate students presiding, and directing traffic, provides a learning atmosphere that was lacking in undergraduate life in the twentieth century. In a very real sense as the HV seminars continue into the last two undergraduate years they become a deconditioning process. Each student gradually creates a moral and value structure for him or herself. Over and above their particular courses of study, vocational or bachelor degree oriented, they are, in essence, teaching each other.

Obviously, in addition to their regular courses, HV students will not be able to read completely every book that is assigned on a weekly basis. But roommates, regardless of what other courses they may be taking, will be absorbing ideas from the same book. They will learn the art of skim reading, plus the joy of sharing particular authors' ideas, which are being explored at the same time with their peer group. In the process, they will reexamine the values acquired from their parents, teachers, and religious leaders. There will be no attempt by Compars to indoctrinate or teach "this is better than that," but rather to engender an exploration of all human values in all societies. Helping each student shape his or her own values, morals, and ethics, and opening strange doors for many students, lays the foundations for a lifetime of creative searching for answers as the key to a self-fulfilling life.

As they did in their K-12 human sexuality course, college students in their HV seminars will continue to compare past with present and ask why, as a nation, we finally agreed to legislate our way to the final sex revolution. They will discover that during the 1980s male/female sexual devaluation became a way of life. Andrea Dworkin was joined by Erica Jong, who after extolling the zipless fuck for women, joined aging Germaine Greer, Nancy Friday, and Shere Hite. All abandoned sexual liberation. They were in general agreement with Susan Forward, who wrote a book, *Men Who Hate Women,* which sold millions of copies and created an avalanche of similar books. The concept was basically that men only wanted women they could control—female empowerment could never happen. One proof of male reality was that men reveled in X-rated films, renting or buying five hundred million annually so they could watch women on their knees adoring and sucking the male penis.

During the Human Values survey of twentieth-century sexual confusion that may not have been covered in their K-12 courses, first-year undergraduates will be amused to discover that many of these new-style feminists jumped on Jerry Falwell's Morality in Media, anti-porn bandwagon. An evangelist, preacher, and president of Liberty College, Falwell, backed by millions of dollars pledged by Southern Baptists, made it clear to Ronald Reagan and later George Bush that the sure way to get the southern vote and get elected was to join the battle against abortion and pornography—especially X-rated movies and videos. Meanwhile Catherine MacKinnon, a lawyer, and Andrea Dworkin, working together, almost persuaded the Minneapolis City Council to pass a law that would give a woman who might have been sexually harassed or raped by a man who had been incited to such action by watching a porno movie to sue the producer of such a video or film. The law, which was never passed, was a current feminist attempt to put an end to porno movies, but not erotic ones. Alas, none of the ladies could agree on what was erotic and what was not.

The HV seminars are organized around a continuing search and creation of human values and sexual morality that will work for society as a whole as well as create an environment for individual happiness. During a reexamination of the sexual furor of the late 1990s, the question will be raised why, then and now, do the Christian conservatives refuse to accept or feel uneasy about the new sexual morality and educational environment, since the basis of Christian belief is that the Word is God, and God is Love.

Despite the K-12 human sexuality conditioning, the question of rape on campus as a possibility, especially in the ROSP program (see ahead) continued in the early years to be a topic of discussion in the HV seminars. In the late 1980s, statistics provided by the National Institute of Mental Health revealed that one in four college women were the victims of rape, or attempted rape, and 84 percent of the victims knew their assailants. Studies in previous years had shown that 30 to 40 percent of college men might force a woman to have sex against her will, if they were sure they wouldn't be caught or punished.

Fraternity Gang Rape, subtitled *Sex, Brotherhood and Privilege on Campus,* written by Peggy Reeves Sanday, professor of anthropology at the University of Pennsylvania (in the words of the publisher), reconstructs daily life in the fraternity, showing the role played by pornography. Most fraternities have a collection of porno videos—male bonding, degrading jokes, and ritual dances all shaping the fraternity's attitude toward women and toward sexuality. Sanday's documentation is compelling—gang rape occurs widely on college campuses. It is a common pattern for the brothers to seek out a "party girl," a vulnerable young woman, one who is seeking acceptance, or is high on alcohol. They take her to a room where she may or may not agree to have sex with one man, but generally passes out and a "train" of men have sex with her.

During the early HV seminars, Compars will contrast the twentieth century with the twenty-first-century sexual moral environment that has recognized age seventeen as a rite of passage into sexual adulthood, and encouraged one-to-one, premarital sex between sexually caring men and women who are completely trained in birth control and are well aware of their joyous sexual drives, as well as the ameliorating effect of Sexual Stress Relief Clinics (see ahead) for older men and women who cannot find sexual companionship on their own.

In the *Village Voice* (April 1991) Sarah Ferguson calls sex on campus "the Vietnam of the 1990s." She covers the Dartmouth Affair, during which Dartmouth "womyn" (a spelling to disassociate themselves from men) joined together to warn others to beware of Kevin Acker, a student who presumably raped Christine Hwang, a first-year student. Acker was finally suspended although Hwang admitted that she hadn't physically or verbally rejected Acker's advances. Meanwhile, on college and university campuses throughout the nation "Take Back the Night" marches, instigated by young women to protest sexism, date rape, and homophobia, were given full media coverage.

At Brown University women scrawled names of men on bathroom walls who they claimed had harassed or assaulted them. They discovered that the brothers in one Brown fraternity had a collection of homemade porno tapes—shot with video cameras with unsuspecting women having sex with various brothers. At Rutgers University, a feminist coalition posted signs along fraternity rows that read "Caution: Rape Zone," and at Duke University, a female task force roamed the campus slapping "Gotcha" stickers on lone men walking home at night. Syracuse University organized five hundred or more women into a group called SCARED (Students Concerned About Rape Education). Their concern was to change male attitudes reflected in words such as: "I got some. I jumped her bones."

As Sarah Ferguson pointed out in her article, "45 percent of the people in their twenties are children of divorce. So many feel a bit jaded to equate a good fuck with true love, and a bit wary to pursue sex for the sheer pleasure of it."

In the late twentieth century, because of AIDS, many college students associated sex with dying. Deb Silverton, director of student health services at the University of Maryland in Baltimore was convinced that "virginity was making a comeback—21 percent of UMB undergraduates had never been sexually active. Jay Segal, professor of sexuality at Temple University, who wrote *The Sex Lives of College Students,* said after comparing 5,400 "sexual autobiographies" written by students in 1982 that the frequency of sex reported by men dropped from 2.6 times per month in 1982 to 1.8 times in 1989—while women's sexual activity dropped from 1.9 per month to 0.8 times per month. According to Segal "The main problem is anxiety. students not only don't engage in sex, they don't want to start relationships." The message was, "It's not in vogue any more to be sexually active. You know that you could get AIDS even if you have sex with a condom, and you really don't want to get involved with a person who has been sleeping around."

In the last years of the twentieth century this downbeat attitude toward sex was rampant. Until the passage of NSME education the civil war environment between men and women was growing in intensity. Marriage, divorce, and trying again in a second marriage became a way of life. There was no attempt to educate young men and women for each other mentally or sexually. And no one raised the question, "How do young men and women students, age seventeen to twenty-one, studying for undergraduate degrees, at the height of their sexual drives, sublimate their need for human loving and caring sexual merger? And if they manage to do so—say no to sex, with little premarital sexual experience, or brain merger with the other sex during these years—how do they find a lasting marriage partner they can love and grow with for a lifetime?"

The twenty-first-century answer is ROSP—phase two—the optional Roommate of the Other Sex, GLUE program that is available to all unmarried and childless high school graduates with C or better average who are enrolled in the GLUE programs.

A13ers, as they are generally known, who select the ROSP program are also known as Premars—premaritals (see my novel *The Premar Experiments*—published in 1975, it covers some of the interpersonal aspects of the Premar experience). During their entire junior and senior years in high school all young men and women who wish to take the ROSP option must provide ELISA credentials that they have been AIDS-free during these two years. They will not only have had their blood tested every six months during this preliminary period, but they would agree to blood testing every six months throughout their entire four-year undergraduate work/study education.

In addition, before arriving on campus they will have passed physical exams making sure that they aren't carrying any sexually transmitted diseases and that they are drug-free and in good health. The large majority of Premars will have been raised in an environment where they heeded the emphasis to delay sexual merger until their seventeenth birthday. Thus, most Premars may still be virgins in the technical sense of never having had penile/vaginal intercourse. Many will have experienced little love affairs with their peers, kissing and body touching, and they will be fully aware via movies and films they have watched and their K-12 sex educations of the coming joy of sexual merger.

ROSP students will have agreed in signed documents that during the ROSP work/study years they will have four roommates of the other sex, and at least one person from a different racial or ethnic background—in essence a new roommate every six months during their first two years in the ROSP undergraduate living program. They will also agree that regardless of previous at-home romantic attachments to another person, they will now be rooming with a person of the other sex *not of their own choosing,* and every six months that the roommate exchange will occur with a person who they already know in their forty-eight-member HV seminar group, and, also despite attraction to a previous roommate, they will accept the roommate shift for the first two years.

During these two years if a Premar cannot adjust to a particular roommate, he/she will have the option of rooming alone for one six-month period, or can completely withdraw to phase one of the GLUE program, where roommates are of the same sex. This will be a carefully considered option since once they have left ROSP they cannot rejoin at a later date. Students who have chosen phase one cannot later transfer to ROSP, or phase two.

In addition to agreeing, in writing, to confine all sexual intimacies to other ROSP students in their forty-eight-student HV groupings, Premars also agree to be "monogamous" with each roommate in turn with whom they are paired. Thanks to strict, ongoing surveillance and blood testing, combined with the fact that all female students will be using birth control pills, or a Norplant injection, the use of condoms by students will be a matter of roommate choice.

All Premars understand that ROSP is not a wild sexual environment, and continuation in the program is based on maintaining good grades in their studies, and performing to the best of their abilities in work assignments during the thir-teen-week work cycles. Work cycles will be arranged so that roommates are on work or study cycles at the same time. Matched couples will see each other naked in their rooms, and all students will use coed showers and washrooms, but keep in mind that Premars in their social and K-12 training have been conditioned since childhood that this is quite normal. Now they are adults, and based on mutu-al agreement, which may not, at the beginning of the first semester, occur for a few weeks, they can experiment with caring foreplay and sexmaking. During the first two years, they will gradually discover with their alternate roommates are the kind of sexual person they are. There will be no sexual forcing. The twenti-eth-century rape environment they will have discussed in their HV meetings will be recognized as a time of total sexual decadence.

If a particular young woman prefers to "go slow" with her first or subsequent roommates, or not to have sex with a particular roommate, these feelings will be quickly aired in the HV meetings, and an open forum of sexual discussion will develop during which all Premars and Compars try to resolve particular problems between roommates and wonder and laugh about their own sexual and interpersonal needs. In this environment "date rape," even between roommates, would be an unlikely occurrence, since an overly aggressive male would be quickly pinpointed by his peers.

All students will make an initial agreement that should a pregnancy occur, the morning after pill, RU486, would be used, or if not possible, the woman could have an abortion, or, the male and female students involved, if they were in love, could get married. But, in any of these cases, neither student could continue in the GLUE Program. There will be no married students in either phase one or phase two of the GLUE program. All students in either phase will be very knowledgeable about birth control, and the use of any addictive drugs, including the excessive use of alcohol, is cause for expulsion.

During their junior and senior years, students enrolled in the ROSP program can choose their own roommates, and may shift as often as they think desirable. But they must continue in their HV seminar, where jealousies and many other interpersonal problems may emerge, and be resolved. By this time Premars who have survived "mental incompatibility" between roommates, and learned the fun of adjustment to a young man or woman from entirely different backgrounds, or literary-style females, may discover the fun of rooming with a "jock" roommate who prefers sports to her academic pursuits, or roommates who are too fat or too thin, too homely, or too messy, or want too much sex—all these will have been the focus of many HV sessions.

In their last two years following Future Family of America guidelines for HV courses, they will continue to explore past sexual values as espoused by Alex Comfort's *New Joy of Sex, A Gourmet Guide to Lovemaking,* with its updated advice on AIDS. They may question Comfort's consistent overemphasis on the mechanics of sex, which becomes a kind of sexual devaluing since the great satisfactions, according to Comfort's kind of teaching, is in performance, and varieties of places and positions to avoid boredom, rather than brain awareness and appreciation of the other person as a complete, amazing vulnerable person, daring, because of her or his love and confidence in the other person, to experience a complete surrender of his or her self.

Compars and students will contrast Comfort's approach with Margo Anand's in her book *The Art of Sexual Ecstasy,* subtitled *The Path of Sacred Sexuality for Western Lovers.* Comfort tells his readers, "A woman who has the divine gift for lechery and loves her partner will masturbate him well, and a woman who knows how to masturbate a man—subtly, unhurriedly, and mercilessly—will always make a superlative partner." Comfort also details the joys of "sexual sauces" and the use of sex toys—dildos, knobby condoms, vibrators, penis rings as well as porno videos—to heighten sexmaking and the ultimate orgasm. Premars will be amused that Comfort never wonders if after the loving there is a brain merger and overtone of wonder.

And while Premars will gradually discover that it is possible to love, in both a mental and sexual merger, more than one person of the other sex, they will have learned that Comfort was wrong about performance sex, and in his belief "there's no reason why stable couples could not make love in each other's company," or that "this could be a liberating experience or disruptive . . . but there is something to be said for anything which breaks down the equally numbing convention of sexual privacy."

Comfort's beliefs, published in books that were read by millions in the late twentieth century, contributed to the total sexual degradation and devaluing of sex in life and in the arts that led to the final sex revolution. The twenty-first-century moral emphasis is that while it is possible for those who have had the ROSP experience to learn how to become mentally and sexually attuned to one or two other people in a long lifetime, there must be time for each relationship and the sexual time is private time. Group sex is simply a form of gymnastics that devalues the wonder and communication possible in a one-to-one merger of two minds and bodies.

Margo Anand, however, pointed the way for twenty-first century lovers in various chapters of her book such as "High Sex and the Tantric Vision," "Awakening Your Inner Lover," "Opening to Trust," "Honoring the Body Ecstatic," and a total approach that sacralizes human sexuality and is compatible with twenty-first-century religions that encourage a transcendental awareness of life and the human need to merge, even momentarily, in the Ultimate—the Cosmic, or, as Abraham Mallow puts it to enjoy a "peak human experience."

In all probability, after two years most Premars will have discovered a person within their own forty-eight HV group, or other ROSP human value groupings on campus with whom they prefer to room during the last two years. Ultimately, after four years of the ROSP undergraduate, work/study program, most Premars will be more compatible with ROSP graduates than any others and Premars will probably marry Premars. They will also be the kind of people most interested, most able to live in, and most amenable to new-style family groupings that Future Families of America will be exploring.

Not only will these new families will be far more cosmopolitan, but the GLUE work/study program in either phase one, phase two/ROSP, or both of which eliminate campus enclaves and require a complete racial and ethnic mixture of roommates by the mid- twenty-first-century will have created a racial and environmental intermixture of all Americans. In the last of the "American Civilization" series run by the *Wall Street Journal* (December 2, 1992), Dennis

Farney asked, "Can Americans Live Together?" As an antidote to the race riots in Los Angeles in April 1992, and the abandonment of many areas in major American cities to blacks, Hispanics, and Asians with the "whites" fleeing to sur-burbias, Farney extolled Occidental College, only fifteen miles away from down-town Los Angeles, which, in 1987, aggressively recruited minority students until 40 percent of the students were from minority racial and ethnic groups.

"The goal is a community in which students may in some small measure experience a world that could be," said President John Slaughter, who is black. Professor of anthropology May Weismantel called it "a laboratory for the future." As Farney points out, in Los Angeles County there are were at the time 3.4 million Hispanics, 900,000 Asians, and 935,000 blacks. Together, prefiguring America by the middle of the twenty-first century, they comprise 59 percent of the population.

But Occidental College was/is too small an effort, and the "great realign-ment" didn't occur in the twentieth century. By contrast, in the fall of 1992 the University of Massachusetts at Amherst, with 23,000 students, was plagued by race riots to a point where a United States Department of Justice mediation team was brought in to heal the campus. Chancellor Richard O'Brien pointed out that the university's attempt to create multicultural diversity had the paradoxical effect of magnifying intolerance.

Heather MacDonald, a lawyer, in an a article in the *Wall Street Journal* September 29, 1992, called "Welcome Freshman," pinpoints the problem. "In one college after another two themes predominate at freshman orientation pro-grams—oppression and difference—foreshadowing the leitmotif of the coming years. Orientation presents a college picture in which bias lurks around every corner. This year, for example, the University of California at Berkeley changed the focus of its freshman orientation from "stereotyping" to "racism, homopho-bia, status-ism, sex-ism, and age-ism."

Unlike the twentieth-century campuses, in the twenty-first century multicul-turalism begins with a total intermingling of human beings at the undergraduate level racially, ethnically, in courses of study, and in the work they are assigned to earn their education. Thus work/study students pursuing bachelor of arts or sci-ence degrees may be rooming on a day-to-day to basis with students of other races and colors who may be working for vocational degrees. But, in any case, because of a prior K-12 liberal arts education which they've all had in common, they will be able to communicate easily with each other, and despite their differ-ent undergraduate educational goals leading to thousands of different careers, a new kind of loving, caring unification will continue in their weekly human val-ues sessions.

14

Twenty-First-Century Solutions to Prostitution and Drug Problems

In the late 1990s, according to Frieda Klein, a management consultant, as the result of the Clarence Thomas "trials" on television, 90 percent of *Fortune* top companies began to offer special training courses on sexual harassment—voluntary, one-day sessions, in many cases covering work environments that women considered "hostile" and where some men not only posted pornographic pin-up pictures of naked ladies, but in hundreds of other ways harassed or tried to "make out" with them.

In 1991 Sen. Joseph Biden introduced a "Violence Against Women Act" that created new penalties for sex crimes, encouraged women to prosecute their attackers, authorized $300 million for related law enforcement and $25 million to create safer parks and public transit, created a National Commission on Violent Crimes against women; protected women from abusive spouses with a variety of additional penalties, and authorized $25 million to develop special spouse abuse court units, triple present funding for battered women shelters, and create a program designed to stop family violence.

Sen. Biden's concern was not only male sexual harassment. The FBI reported that in 1991 four million women in United States were kicked, smothered, knifed, or shot to death by their male partners. In Massachusetts alone, one woman died every sixteen days because of domestic violence.

A few years before, in 1986, President Reagan and Attorney General Edwin Meese tried to legislate morality, and disprove the 1970 report of the Commission on Obscenity organized by President Johnson that concluded pornography was not a significant cause of sexual crime and recommended better sex education. The 1986 commission report insisted that the 1970 report was "starkly obsolete," and that sexually violent pornography lead to greater acceptance of the "rape

157

myth"—that women enjoy being coerced into sexual activity, and that they are basically enjoy being physically hurt during the sex act.

Edward Donnerstein, a well-known psychologist, reported to the committee: "If you take out the sex and leave the violence, you get increased violent behavior. . . . If you take out the violence and leave the sex nothing happens." Barry Lyndon, a lawyer employed by the American Civil Liberties Union, summed it up: "The report masqueraded behind social science jargon. . . . The commission are quintessential censors. . . . They truly want to regulate every one's sex life. . . . If they had their way they would truly crawl into your bedroom and tell you what is appropriate."

In his book *Liberty and Sexuality,* subtitled "The Right to Privacy and the Meaning of Roe vs. Wade," a nearly thousand-page study published in 1994, David Garrow reveals how rapidly the old sexual order has crumbled. While sexual harassment went under cover, violence of men and women against each other continued unabated, and X-rated movies were more or less absolved of being pornography; in other areas with no alternatives, the old order continued to crumble.

Within the lifetime of a person born after World War I, as late as the early 1950s, getting a divorce could jeopardize a high level job, a divorced man could not be elected president, premarital sex was frowned upon by a large majority, teenage pregnancy was a family disaster, visual sex shown in print or on film was a quick road to jail, abortion was a seedy and criminal business, adultery ended in heartbreak or suicide, as did homosexuality, if it was discovered, and the nuclear family seemed to be the backbone of America.

Forty years later, all these moral and sexual underpinnings had collapsed or were trembling in continual sexual seismic shock. But by the end of the twentieth century the final sexual revolution was in the making. All it needed was leadership that dared to contest outmoded religious values and accept human sexual realities. The overarching reality is that some time in their lives, early or late, the vast majority of men and women discover that sex and loving another person offers a momentarily joyous escape from oneself and a world that is too often with us. So do alcohol and drugs.

At relatively small cost, by changing the focus of human nakedness and caring human sex, and creating a new kind of guaranteed education for all men and women from kindergarten until they are twenty-one, a vast majority of Americans will find other persons with whom they can enjoy sexual and mental merger during a long lifetime, and occasionally, not as solitary drinkers, but in company, sex and a "tickling" of alcohol combined.

But for those who, for one reason or another, are unable to find surcease from sorrow with another person, Future Families of America proposed a twenty-first century approach for the legalization of prostitution and all drugs, with moral blessings in the one case and moral concern in the other. Thus will the final sex revolution will be completed.

Let's look at prostitution first. In the nineteenth-century, brothels and the madams running them in red light districts were an accepted way of life. They provided a man who couldn't find a woman a moment of escape with a female who might not be a dream girl, but who for a relatively small amount of money could be a momentary friend and help him escape himself. In upper-income levels, ladies of the night were tolerated by more virginal women who had married for reasons other than sex. By the turn of the century, police-protected brothels and whorehouses had been eliminated by the same people who believed that virtuous people who loved God didn't need a rose garden in which to escape. Every man and woman should trust in God, and pray to God for salvation from their sinful need to find solace in wine, women, and song. The eighteenth Amendment to the Constitution outlawing the sale of alcohol became law January 16, 1919. Prohibition wasn't repealed until December 5, 1933, when Franklin Roosevelt dared to confront reality. As Ronald Siegel points out in his book *Intoxication* (required reading in HV courses),

> Over the centuries people have sought—and drugs have offered—a wide variety of effects including: pleasure, relief from pain, mystical revelations, stimulation, relaxation, joy, ecstasy, self-understanding, altered states of consciousness and escape. The motivation to use drugs to achieve these effects is not innate but acquired. . . . The pursuit of intoxication is no more abnormal than the pursuit of lower, social attachments, thrills, power or any number of acquired motives.

Siegel didn't include sexual build-up, foreplay, and orgasmic release as a drug-free form of intoxication, but it is, and its repression in the Freudian sense raises all kinds of devils that can be tamed in a sexually sane society.

Sexual release, including the joy of sexual intoxication with "the real thing," a loving female, and her vagina, was so difficult to obtain on a regular basis in the twentieth century, or was fraught with disease danger outside marriage or a marriage commitment, that millions of males, depending on their financial resources, got their momentary escape from reality with masturbation and the aid of men's skin magazines (or with prettied-up young ladies in *Playboy* or *Penthouse*), X-rated videos, 900 numbers with seductive female voices adoring cocks at a safe distance, women advertising as escorts, street prostitutes, and, for the upper-income high-class prostitutes. All were, separately and together, creating sexual devaluation, degradation, as well as a disease-transmitting and potential crime environment.

While no national figures are available, hundreds of thousands of women were arrested every year for prostitution, but within a few days were back on the streets again. In November 1993 the San Francisco vice squad logged 2,324 arrests for prostitution, including young boys offering their services. A task force was created to explore the legalization of prostitution with city-run brothels along German lines that would create "love hotels" to rent rooms to prostitutes. The National Organization for Women and the American Civil Liberties Union argued unsuccessfully for the decrimalization of prostitution.

The twenty-first-century answer is Sexual Stress Relief Clinics available in all cities with a population of 50,000 or more people. Self-supporting, they are licensed by the state but must follow standards and methods and offer similar environments nationwide that have been set up by the Future Families of America Commission. Clinics are run by one male and one female registered nurse who supervise and hire Sexual Companions, or SCs, as they are known. Female or male SCs must be age twenty-one or over. Stress Relief Clinics run explicitly for male homosexual men hire only male homosexuals. Heterosexual clinics offer males of varying ages for widows, and unmarried women seeking male companionship. To obtain employment they must be HIV negative for the past six months and take blood tests and physical exams once a month. All sexual services they provide are by hourly appointment at a fixed, national, hourly rate equivalent to the national average in service industries. (Twenty-first-century rates average $15 an hour). The client pays $30, with the additional $15 being for room fee, clinic nonsexual payroll, and maintenance.

SCs can only offer their services at state-run clinics designed with attractive bedrooms, which in many larger cities are former small hotels or motels. The rooms are equipped with television, radio, and audiotape music, and a refrigerator with snacks and soft drinks. No alcohol is allowed, and no clients who have been drinking will be served. All clients must establish their identity with friendly documentation. Appointments may be made from one hour up to eight hours, thus a client wishing to spend an evening with an SC may do so if he or she can afford it. All SCs will have taken training courses in interpersonal relationships, and are able to give body massage with the masseuse seeking, in the process, to establish a friendly relationship with the client by masturbating him or her digitally, if they wish. SCs may offer oral sex or vaginal sex to clients who have kept up regular HIV blood tests, and can do this on their own as a separate transaction, but no client can demand it. An SC's primary job is to offer an hour or more of friendly companionship, and caring, not in a hurry, and manual orgasm in a specific encounter. Clients may try to get appointments with the same SC, and some SCs may agree with a particular client to reduce his or her hourly rate for a regular clients. If an SC refuses a repeat appointment he or she must explain in writing to the clinic managers her or his reasons. Once Sexual Stress Relief Clinics are easily available women arrested for street soliciting or private prostitution will be given the opportunities to work at clinic. A second arrest will mean a jail sentence.

During the twentieth century there was some pro and con discussion about the legalization of drugs. But in 1993, when Surgeon General Joycelyn Elders suggested that the possibility should be explored, she unleashed a storm of negative protest. In January 1994 President Clinton asked Congress for a record $13.2 billion to combat drugs—with $448 million going to community-based education and prevention programs. Drug treatment would increase by $360 million with the remainder going to criminal justice—meaning as under President Bush, a confusing war on drugs costing billions of dollars annually. "If we want to reduce crime and cut health care cost," Clinton said, "If we want to rebuild our families and communities, all these things require serious effort."

Thinking more realistically, in Columbia the novelist Gabriel Garcia Marquez and Prosector General Gustav de Greiff, who was planning to run for president, proposed that Columbia give up the fight against drug traffickers and legalize drugs, specifically cocaine, of which Columbia is the world's largest producer. Statistics showed that after five years of the drug wars set in motion by President Bush, police had seized only 5 percent of the hundreds of tons of cocaine that flow annually from Columbia. As de Grieff and Marquez pointed out, "You can't shoot down the law of supply and demand with bullets. In Columbia a kilo of cocaine costs $50. It's sold in consuming countries for $5,000 to $10,000. There will always be someone who will run the risk for that kind of money."

In the twenty-first century reality finally intervened. Drugs have not become like alcohol. There is no free capitalistic market where marijuana cigarette producers compete for business as they still do for tobacco cigarettes. Following a carefully worked out plan, a new law was proposed to establish Federal Drug Store Clinics, and make them easily available in all towns and cities with a population of 50,000 or more people. Marijuana, cocaine, and heroin, and even synthetic laboratory-created varieties, are available. A purchaser, anyone twenty-one years of age or older, can buy a predetermined, one-week's supply at a time. A week's supply of the preferred drug is sold at a price of $5. No one is permitted to buy more than a one-week supply.

To qualify as a purchaser, all the drug user has to do is sign a form that appraises him or her of the dangers of the particular drug they are using. In addition the form spells out severe penalties, including a possible death sentence, for resale of the drug to anyone else, or if the user commits any criminal act whether under the influence of the drug or not.

All purchasers signing the purchasing agreement understand that they will not be forced into any drug treatment programs. The agreement will establish whether the purchaser is a first-time user. If so, the clinic manager, who is a licensed pharmacist, will ask the purchaser to spend a few minutes in private with him and discuss his or her reasons for wanting to try the drug. The discussion is friendly, with no recriminations. It is recorded on audiotape. A copy of the tape and literature describing use and dangers of the drug is given to the prospective buyer with the suggestion that he or she think it over for a week. If the purchaser wishes, she or he may apply for free counseling by established medics for problems that make "intoxication" a seeming way out.

After a week, if the purchaser still rejects these options, with no questions asked, he or she is not denied the right to purchase a particular drug, which like marijuana, might be a palliative for people stricken with cancer or AIDS, or people who need help from the pain of chemotherapy.

In addition to the signed application form, the purchaser will also be warned verbally that reselling his or her weekly purchase is a criminal offense. First-time purchasers are given a plastic card similar to a credit card that is used to record their weekly purchase. The purchaser will understand that the purchase is being recorded in a central computer system, and that he or she cannot purchase another supply for seven days in any clinic.

Using this procedure, for the first time the federal government became totally aware of practically everyone over twenty-one in the United States using these drugs. Because of the very low price the illegal market for cocaine and hard drugs rapidly disappeared. Purchasers quickly became aware that the federal drug clinics were not only selling higher-quality drugs than street versions, but that the drug clinics would also supply free needles or whatever paraphernalia that an addict might need to use a particular drug. Pharmacists also counsel cocaine users not to convert their weekly allotment into crack, which the drug clinics do not supply, but try to adjust their needs to a less dangerous quality cocaine. Purchasers who use their weekly supply before the week has elapsed, and can't wait for a new supply, will be referred to a rehabilitation treatment center.

All federal drug clinics are networked with local hospitals. Posters and literature in the clinic constantly advise addicts and junkies that medical help and counseling is available at no cost, if they wish. There are no recriminations and users wishing to kick the habit can make their own decision on a voluntary basis.

During the twentieth century several million children were born to and became the victims of drug users. Most of these children have congenital brain damage caused by the mother's drug use, and millions of them became twenty-first-century problems in public schools because of acute learning disabilities. Federal drug clinic pharmacists are on the alert for pregnant drug users and they are quickly assigned to drug treatment centers. All female drug users are warned to use birth control pills, which are supplied at very small or no cost if necessary.

Federal drug clinics recover some of their costs from the sale of drugs. The difference is made up by the federal government, leaving billions of dollars of savings in the federal budget over the former war on drugs. The savings are added to the GLUE subsidy, which along with billions of dollars saved by disappearing teenage pregnancies, and additional billions made possible by a vast reduction in unemployment rates, have made the federally guaranteed work/study undergraduate subsidy self-sustaining.

Two other drug-related problems, alcohol abuse and an increase in marijuana smoking, became major problems among teenagers in the late 1990s. Many attempts were made to legalize the sale and growing of marijuana, and alcohol presumably couldn't be purchased until the consumer was twenty-one.

In 1990, 33 percent of all high school seniors admitted that they had tried at least one illicit drug—down from a peak in of 54 percent in 1979. Twenty-seven percent of seniors had smoked marihuana, down from 49 percent in 1980. In 1991 Surgeon General Antonia Novello reported that drinking among minors was out of control. Her office reported that 8 million of the 20.7 million youths in grades seven through twelve drank alcoholic beverages at least once a week. In undergraduate areas according to study made at George Mason University and Westchester University, 41 percent of all academic problems and 28 percent of college dropouts were caused by alcohol abuse. The federal Office of Substance Abuse Prevention reported that undergraduates spend $4.2 billion a year on booze.

Andrew McQuire, head of the Trauma Foundation in San Francisco, California, was certain that, "Alcohol was the number one health problem in the United States," and it was probably the leading cause of death among teenagers, with 3,539 deaths due to drunken driving in the fifteen to twenty age group reported in 1989.

Time magazine of December 16, 1991, asked, "Why are so many kids drinking themselves into a stupor? Boredom, peer pressure, escape from psychological pain and wanting to feel good are the usual answers." But David Anderson, a research professor at George Mason University, came closer to the answer: "Kids delude themselves into thinking they have found their identity with alcohol. These kids are in search of community—and they have a quest for intimacy—who can I be at one with."

At the annual meeting of the American Council on Education in February 1994, more than a thousand educators worried about the college dropout rate and the current estimate that 40 percent of all students who enroll for a four-year undergraduate work suffered "academic difficulties, financial pressures, home sickness, and isolation." None of them mentioned that the alcohol escape route was symptomatic of all these problems. Educators who tried to predict twenty-first century higher education had no solutions except elimination of vacations and three years to get an undergraduate degree, less tenure and more emphasis on student-directed learning. President Clinton addressed the gathering calling for innovations, and offered a typical, hot-air, seven-point agenda that would ensure that every child was healthy and ready to learn, setting standards and achieving world class standards, opening college to every qualified American, expanding opportunities for community service, easing the school-to-work transition, retraining the unemployed and promoting life learning. How? Not a new sexual morality and education legislation. This would have to wait for the twenty-first century, and legislators not afraid to light bonfires.

The missing link were leaders who dared to question twentieth- century moralities, and create a new moral environment where teachers, educators and religious leaders flowed with the tide of caring human sexuality and understood the ever-present human need to experience transcendence and a new meaning of intoxication—the need to wake up each day with a personal sense of purpose. To discover and rediscover daily, with the help and enthusiasm of an older generation, that lasting ecstasy, rapture, and joy can be achieved without alcohol or drugs, and that it is good to have more than one mission in life, sharing at least one other person's mission, living creatively, or determined to find just one answer to one of the billions of questions human can ask.

Areas of inquiry include: studying chaos with the new physicists who are trying to answer questions neither Newton nor Einstein ever dreamed about; finding the answers to why humans propagate sexually, when thousands of asexual, mostly female creatures and plants, toss their pollen to the wind, or simply divide and clone themselves, doing the job more efficiently; drawing or painting a picture; learning to play a musical instrument; going for the gold in sports; playing in rock or chamber groups with others; singing in a choir; assembling a computer; growing perfect roses or tomatoes; or, like Fabre, discovering the world of ants and bees in one's own backyard. Learning to live and love creatively is intoxicating.

The key to finding the person with whom you can share each other's mission is a new sexual morality and education through the age of twenty-one, during which men and women learn how to blend intimacy, joy, and the pleasure of sex, and even enhance it with a glass of wine or one drink because occasionally two people need to escape themselves together. As Barbra Streisand once sang, "People who need people are the luckiest people in the world."

While it may seem a far call from a new approach to sexual morality and education, a twenty-first century thinker, Leon Wieseltier, literary editor of the *New Republic,* summed it up in an interview with the *Boston Phoenix*: "I think Woodrow Wilson once said that a man goes to college to become as much like his father as possible. A Jewish man or woman should not go to college to become Jewish. An African/American, man or woman, should not go to college to become African/American. . . . College is the only time in a person's life when he or she is encouraged to experience the Other, to fantasize about the Other, to try to become the Other. But now people go to college to become what they already are. I think that is not just a terrific cultural mistake, but a terrific personal mistake."

It's the kind of mistake that twenty-first century leaders will resolve with GLUE and a new sexual morality.

15

The Twenty-First-Century Merger of Church and State

Is the New Sexual Morality and Education legislation a pipe dream? If you are an *ardent* Catholic, *fundamentalist* Southern Baptist, *orthodox* Jew or Muslim, you may think so. But note the emphasized adjectives. You are a minority, not only in your own Christian, Jewish, or Muslim beliefs, but in the total number of Americans.

In 1989 the Yearbook of American and Canadian Churches revealed that there were 147.6 million Americans who were listed as members of religious organizations. The U.S. population in 1990 was 248 million. Most religious groups list children as young as thirteen as members. And there is general agreement that in the mid-1990s there were about 60 million Americans of voting age who may believe in God but are not affiliated with any religious organization or indoctrinated with particular religious beliefs.

There were 58 million Catholics, 57 million Protestants (split over many different denominations), 4 million Jews, and about 6 million Muslims. But how many are ardent, fundamentalist, or orthodox, and wholly committed to the beliefs of their particular religious leaders?

In June 1992 a synod of Catholic bishops completed the first revision in the Roman Catholic catechism in four centuries. Approved by John Paul II, it was published in French, and in 1993 in English. The five-hundred-page document has ten pages covering sexual morality. The Vatican and Pope John Paul II were still united against abortion, euthanasia, masturbation, premarital sex, birth control, adultery, pornography, prostitution, and homosexuality. With the exception of birth control, most fundamentalist Protestants were in total agreement. But most Catholics weren't *ardent* about birth control. In their book *The Contraceptive Revolution* Westoff and Ryder insist that nearly 70 percent of all Catholic women

166

practice birth control. A National Opinion Research poll revealed that Catholics were also very liberal about premarital sex, with 84 percent of Catholics agreeing that premarital sex was not a sin versus 69 percent of all Protestants.

In the mid-1990s there was a growing American Catholic resistance to the sexual morality being preached by Pope John Paul II. The Catholic Theological Society, American based, declared that "no single question will suffice to determine the morality of any sexual behavior," and suggested "that there were instances where pre-marital sex, and unwed sex, along with homosexuality were moral." During the 1991 National Conference of Bishops, they renewed their "Statement on Political Responsibility." Abortion is not a legitimate method of family planning," they said, but they faced the reality that "the fundamental dignity of the human person includes the right not to procreate," and the necessity to teach all young people how to prevent birth (not with birth control devices) and stay free of STDs, and not to depend on "safe-sex abstinence." Archbishop Daniel Pilarczyk of Cincinnati, who advocated "postponing sex" until marriage, was following the Vatican encyclical.

Many Catholics will have no difficulty in adjusting to the very practical GLUE approach, which offers the carrot incentive but also accepts age seventeen as a rite of passage opening the door to caring, responsible premarital sex. Keep in mind that with the exception of the voluntary rating system on the arts, the rest of the NSME legislation is optional. Any parent who decided that K-12 sexual/value education was teaching moral values that they believed was their responsibility, or the church's responsibility, could reject the twelve-year seminars for their children.

Phase two of the GLUE (ROSP) program is also optional—as is phase one, which most medium-income parents will enthusiastically approve. Seeing people who wish to be naked where it is convenient to be naked does no one any moral harm, and viewing sexually natural one-to-one, caring sexmaking between a man and woman can be avoided by television control boxes sex chips, as well as violence chips, which automatically cut off offending sequences.

The naysayers may be horrified by some aspects of NSME legislation. But, on the positive side, they must agree that tying federally guaranteed undergraduate education to the condition that there will be no children until participants have completed their additional four years at approximately age twenty-one, and giving all young people a thorough education in birth control, and at the same time counteracting sexual devaluation and exalting caring human sexuality, it will eliminate the abortion problem, as well as the problem of teenage mothers on welfare with no husbands. Abortions will no longer be an alternate form of birth control for teenagers and married adults who wait longer to marry, and have children who will be far better adjusted to family life.

Fundamentalist Protestant Randall Terry, executive director of Operation Rescue, proclaimed, "I don't think Christians should use birth control. You consummate your marriage as often as you like—and if you have babies, you have babies." Judie Brown of America Life League insisted, "We are opposed to abortion under any circumstance. We are opposed to abortifacient drugs like the pill, the IUD—and all forms of birth control with the exception of natural family planning." Joseph Scheidler, executive director of the Pro Life League, said, "For those who say I can't impose my moralities on others, I say just watch me!" All of these, and thousands more, were a leftover fringe with no positive approaches who must, eventually, embrace the final sex revolution.

At their annual convention in June 1992 the Southern Baptists, without offering any solutions, were pointing the way. They assailed the "moral breakdown" in our society, and condemned suicide, assisted suicide, abortion, and abortion-related research, and the distribution of condoms in schools. Representing 15.2 million Baptists they also encouraged the Boy Scouts of America to ban homosexuals from leadership, and condemned television as a corrupting influence by offering themes, plots, images and advertisements that promoted and glorified sexual promiscuity, violence, and other forms of immorality.

Leaving aside their negative beliefs about euthanasia and homosexuals, all the Christian Coalition and the American Center for Law and Justice (activist arms of the religious right, headed up by Pat Robertson and Ralph Reed, with a million or more contributing members in the mid-1990s) had to do was accept human nudity, agree that young people should grow up seeing one-to-one caring sexmaking in the arts as normal aspects of human life, and that premarital sex, delayed by common consent to age seventeen so that young people could qualify for GLUE and four more years of education, was morally sound; if they agreed they would not only resolve most of their problems about the moral breakdown of American society but they could help merge church and state with a common sense of national purpose, as well as have common cause with Norman Lear's People for the American Way.

Timidly leading the way in the mid-1990s were President Bill Clinton and Vice President Al Gore, both Baptists. Gore, with a divinity degree, dared to write not only a history of religion in his book *Earth in Balance,* but in the chapter "Environmentalism of the Spirit" revealed a twenty-first-century approach as he chastised religious leaders, regardless of their beliefs of who or what God is or may or may not be—for not listening to James Lovelock and his Gaia hypothesis "that the entire complex earth system behaves in a self-regulating manner characteristic of something alive," as well as Lovelock's insistence that "while this relationship between life and non-living elements does not require a spiritual explanation, even so, it evokes a spiritual response in those who hear it."

Verging on twenty-first-century approaches to morality, Gore deplores the separation of religion from science, and he castigates conservative clergy who are "deeply suspicious of any effort to focus their moral attention on a physical crisis in the natural world that might require, as a part of its remedy, a new exercise of something resembling moral authority by the state." Gore continues, "All discussions of morality and ethics in science are practically pointless as long as the world of the intellect is assumed to be separate from the physical world." Summing up, Gore quotes Teilhard de Chardin: "'The fate of mankind as well as religions depend on the emergence of a new faith in the future.'"

The key element of the NSME legislation that unites church and state is a new faith and a common belief arrived at long before Christianity. Heraclitus defined the *Logos* (the Word) as the rational principle of the Universe that is at once the moving and regulating principle in all things. In later Greek philosophy, the Logos became the principle between the ultimate and living reality and the mind of man. John, writing in the fourth gospel agreed, and simplified. The Logos and the Word are synonymous. The Word is God. Above all the New Testament God is no longer a vindictive God. He is a loving God. First and foremost God is Love. Thus the NSME legislation, summed up in the new creed, "In love we trust," unites man's need for religious transcendence with lifetime exaltation of caring mental and sexual merger.

Can the major religions find common ground by sacramentalizing both the erotic and spiritual aspects of human sexuality? Catholic theologians can show the way. In his book, *These Are the Sacraments,* Bishop Fulton Sheen described the symbolism of the seven Catholic sacraments, the Sacrament of Baptism, the Sacrament of Confirmation, the Sacrament of the Eucharist, the Sacrament of Penance, the Sacrament of Anointing the Sick, the Sacrament of the Holy Orders, and the Sacrament of Marriage.

"No one can understand the sacraments," he writes, "unless he has what might be called a divine sense of humor. . . . Our lord has a divine sense of humor because he revealed that the universe is sacramental. . . . A sacrament in a very broad sense combines two elements; one visible, the other invisible—spiritual. One that can be seen, or tasted, or touched or heard; the other unseen to the eye. . . . Thus a handshake is a kind of sacrament; a kiss a kind of sacrament." Bishop Sheen points out that sacrament means mystery.

Pope John Paul II's adamant stand, at the September 1994 International Conference on Population and Development in Cairo, during which he condemned both contraception and abortion as evil and unacceptable for inclusion in the final United Nations document, may give the impression that Catholics are irrevocably committed to his views. To top it off, in 1995 he issued a 190-page encyclical, *Evangelium Vitae* (Gospel of Life), in which he excoriated techniques of artificial reproduction, the moral corruption of the medical profession, the temptation of eugenics euthanasia, and contraception as "illegitimate means of population control." But if Catholicism is to survive as an American religion with the passage of NSME legislation, and a federal government finally committed to sexual sanity now, a new pope will eventually have to climb on the bandwagon and face the reality that the Western democracies cannot support a doubling or tripling Third World population, let alone problems like our welfare mess. As Robert Samuelson points out in a March 27, 1995, *Newsweek* essay, "Welfare Can't be Reformed," without a dramatic decline in single parenthood, and a strong family safety net, there are no solutions. Foes of teenage contraception and abortion have no alternative except to really educate coming generations about how to enjoy sex, before marriage, without having children.

If you read Pope John Paul's best-selling book *Crossing the Threshold* of Hope—after publication of which in late 1994 he was forced to apologize for his hasty, ill-considered characterization of the Buddhist faith as being "negative" compared with the "positive" attitude of Christianity, and stating that in Islam "all the richness of God's self-revelation has been definitely set aside"—you may look forward to a new day when a new pope will gradually issue new encyclicals modifying John Paul II's diatribes against chemical contraception and opening the door for the Vatican to add an eighth sacrament, the "Sacrament of Caring Sexual Merger." This would occur during a church service on a person's seventeenth birthday. Thus the church underwrites the same moral environment as the state. This sacrament, confirming that a young man or woman of seventeen is an adult and can enjoy responsible premarital sex, coincides with the GLUE subsidy. In the process, sexual abstinence, until one is seventeen, becomes a moral way of life.

At the same time the sacrament of marriage can be modified to adjust to twenty-first century realities, and could agree that adultery is not a sin if caring, responsible sexual merger occurs with other persons during a long lifetime, and all concerned are determined not to destroy the original pair bonding but preserve and enhance it in carefully structured group relationships (see ahead, chapters 16 and 21).

Along with this new approach to sacramentalizing the act of love, the church can resolve the problem of celibacy that emerged as a disrupting force in the mid-1990s, proving, in sad reality, that even priests cannot forswear their sexual drives. According to Gordon Thomas, in his sympathetic study *Desire and Denial,* subtitled "Celibacy and the Church," at the beginning of the twenty-first century there be will only 21,000 diocesan and 13,000 other priests—a decline of 45 percent from 1985 figures. Lack of interest in the priesthood is directly related to the twentieth-century reality, priest or not, male or female, that most human beings cannot, and don't wish to, repress their sexual drives. Male or female priests who will receive the revised sacrament of marriage are completing the essential merger with the God of Love.

In the mid-1990s Catholics were not alone. Liberal Protestants, in many denominations, were trying to get their leaders to face modern sexual realities with new religious moralities. In June 1991, the Rev. John Carey and the Special Task Force on Human Sexuality that he had mustered, presented a two-hundred-page report to the General Assembly of Presbyterians in Baltimore. No major Christian denomination, up to this time, even the Unitarian/Universalists, who could boast only about 200,000 members, has dared to consider how traditional Christian ethics could be brought up to date, and, as the report suggested, "conform to the changing mores of our society."

In a chapter of the report, "A Reaffirmation of Christian Ethics," the question is asked,

> What does the coming of age about sexuality in the church require?—At the very least, moral maturity requires an acceptance—and a celebration of diversity of sexual relations which have integrity and moral substance. . . . As James Nelson [a Presbyterian leader] notes, "One of the basic challenges of the church, and the synagogue is to change the sexual hegemony of the family, and the resulting tendency to police the sexuality of everyone who does not fit the mold. . . . We have enforced a sexual model on the nuclear family which excludes countless persons."

Offering a concept the writers called "Justice Love," the report committee proposed that Presbyterians should adopt a Christian ethic that

> will operate with one moral standard . . . a Christian ethic that honors, but does restrict, sexual activity to marriage alone, nor blesses all sexual activity within marriage as morally acceptable (sexual violence and coercion within marriage is obviously unacceptable). . . . We ought to respect Calvin's insight that God's intention for us as sexual persons lies not only in procreation, but even more fundamentally in loving companionship. Indebted to that tradition, we may develop theologies of sexuality to encourage sexual expression which genuinely deepens human intimacy and love.

The report goes on to insist that sexual gratification is a human need, and the right ought not to be limited to heterosexual response (thus putting the report's blessing on homosexual relations within the parameters of "Justice Love." Not only was the committee asking Presbyterians to condone masturbation and premarital sex, but it proposed that the church not pass moral judgement on sexual relations between "responsible" teenage lovers. It noted that a third of

Presbyterians were single women and men, and the report warned that the unmarried might leave the church unless the clergy cease their "painful" assumption that single people should remain celibate. "It is wrong to condemn non-marital sexual activity as unacceptable simply because it falls outside a particular, formal institutional arrangement. It's time for the Presbyterian Church to offer a creative alternative."

The twenty-first-century vision of this report blew the top off of conservative Presbyterians, who insisted, with no realistic alternate proposals in full-page advertisements in local newspapers, that, "Sex would split the church by advocating sex outside of marriage, abandonment of traditional family values, and would end up with homosexuals in the pulpit." A majority of 2 million Presbyterians rejected it, but the straw was blowing in the wind.

The Episcopalians also held a general convention in July 1991 in Phoenix, Arizona. Despite the fact that membership had dropped more a million, from 3.6 million to 2.4 million in the previous twenty-five years, the convention did little to resolve "simmering issues of sexuality" that revolved around the ordination of women, homosexual priests, and gay and lesbian marriages. Two homosexuals had already been ordained as priests. Bishop William Frey threw fat on the fire when he proposed a canon law forcing the clergy to abstain from sexual relationships outside of marriage. It was defeated.

But in the grassroots there were far more interesting twenty-first-century realities simmering. In 1987, the 113th annual convention of the diocese of Newark, New Jersey, offered a visionary report that stated:

> A major change is occurring in religious thinking regarding sexuality and the body. . . . Whereas the ancient Greeks regarded the mind or spirit as able to reach its triumph only by freeing itself from the corrupting captivity of the physical body (and this teaching was incorporated into Christian thinking), the Hebrews knew no such separation in Hebraic thought. One does not have a body . . . one is a body. What we refer to as body, mind, spirit, were in Hebraic thought dimensions of an indivisible unity. The contemporary, more Hebraic understanding of persons runs counter to the traditional dualistic teachings of the Church. . . . The contemporary attitude views sexuality as more than genital sex, having as its purpose procreation, physical pleasure, and release of tension. Sexuality includes sex, but is a more comprehensive concept.

This Episcopalian report also suggests in addition to accepting responsible premarital sex and gay/lesbian relationships, that

> given the Church's traditional view of the exclusive primacy of marriage and the nuclear family, the Church must learn how to continue to affirm the conven-

tional without denigrating the alternative sexual and family relationships and their potential for developing responsible persons in the Realm of God. The Church must affirm persons as they faithfully and responsibly choose to live out other modes of relationships.

During the mid-1990s the Evangelical Lutheran churches offered a fifty-thousand-word study on human sexuality, as did the United Church of Christ, and it was increasingly apparent that Americans were searching for a national consensus on sexual morality that is finally provided by the NSME legislation.

But the way the moral compass was pointing is reflected in the teachings of many minority religions such as the Jews, Quakers, Unitarian/Universalists, and humanist groups. Leading the way in 1970, the Friends Service Committee in London issued a booklet that reflected much Quaker thinking. In retrospect, the following quotation is the basis of many of the Future Families of America approaches (see ahead):

> Nothing that has come to light in the course of our studies has altered the conviction that came to us when we began to examine the actual experiences of people, the conviction that love can be confined to a pattern. But the waywardness of love is part of its nature and this is both its glory and its tragedy. If love did not leap every barrier, if it could be easily tamed, it would not be the tremendous creative power that we know it to be, and want it to be. We recognize that while most examples of the "eternal triangle" are produced by boredom and primitive misconduct, others may arise from the fact that the very experience of loving one person, with depth and perception, may sensitize a person to the loveable qualities in others. We think it is our duty not to stand on the peak of perfectionism, but to recognize in compassion the complications and bewilderment that love creates, and ask how we can discover a constructive way in the immense variety of particular experiences. It is not by checking the impulse to love that we can keep love sweet. The man or woman who swallows the word "I love you" when he meets another woman or man, may in that moment, for that reason, begin to resent his spouse's existence. But it is also true that love may be creative, if honestly acknowledged though not openly confessed. We need to know much more about ourselves, and what we do in our inner life when we follow codes or ideals that do not come from the heart.

While the Quakers admit in this statement that they do not have the answer, they dare to face the questions that will be raised but not answered in the K-12, federally financed human sexuality seminars, and will be faced squarely in the optional ROSP program, where young unmarrieds explore their sexuality in an upbeat way with four roommates of the other sex, and possibly a few others, before they complete GLUE. Later, many of theses pioneers may join experimental, new-style families being run by Future Families of America.

Despite Orthodox Judaism, and many conservative Jews, who in aggregate will become fewer in the twenty-first century, millions of Jews, unlike Christians, have been conditioned by their religion that love of God and love in the sexual merger are one and the same. During the mid-1990s, 52 percent of all Jewish marriages have been with people of other faiths, creating, in many cases, more of the millions of Americans without any church or synagogue affiliation.

While the kibbutz environment was slowly disappearing in the mid-1990s, it provided a much saner approach to some aspects of human sexuality that prevailed in the twentieth century, where young girls and boys were segregated in their play and sports activities, as well as their bedrooms. As M. E. Spiro points out in his book *Children of the Kibbutz,*

> Girls and boys age one to five sleep in the same room. They shower together and go to the toilet in co-ed facilities. They often run around naked together before getting dressed in the morning, or at night, before going to bed. It is not surprising that in this positive setting, some spontaneous age concordant, gender different, sexuoerotic sex play occurs with children embracing, stroking, caressing, kissing and even touching each other's genitals.

As Robert Francoeur comments, "It is hard to see this approach to child rearing being supported by either Protestant or Catholic doctrine." Francoeur, who was a tenured professor of embryology at Fairleigh Dickinson University, was originally a Roman Catholic priest. When he married a woman, Anna, he believed that the Vatican might accept his marriage and make the first break with church doctrine requiring priestly celibacy. It didn't happen. Francoeur has written many books on twenty-first-century approaches to human sexuality. In an essay that appears in the *Handbook of Sexology,* volume 7 (1991), he gives a broad background on current religious doctrines, and contrasts the sexual moralities in Judaic, Christian, humanist, Latino/Hispanic, Islamic, Hindu, Buddhist, and Confucian/Taoist faiths with their theologic beliefs.

"The advent of sexuoerotic drives and interest at puberty, and the postponement of adult status, leaves the adolescent in a state of limbo," he writes.

> Religious doctrines, and their adherents, can be divided by the weltanschauung which underlies their religious beliefs. If one believes that purposes of sexuality and human nature were established in the beginning (Genesis) then one finds it congenial to believe that evil results from some original sin, a primeval fall of the first human from a state of grace. If on the other hand one believes in an evolving human nature, physical and moral evils are viewed as inevitable, nat-

ural growth pains that come as humans struggle toward the fullness of their creation.

Francoeur analyzes the moral and ethical systems of all the major religions and points out that the anti-sex ethic of Catholic sexual morality is based on the beliefs of Jerome, Augustine, Aquinas, and hundreds of other self-appointed guardians who dominate Protestant moral thinking. In his book *Innocent Ecstasy,* subtitled "How Christianity Gave America an Ethic of Sexual Pleasure," P. Gardella believes that contemporary sexual ethics, without reference to God or theology, is part of the Protestant/ Catholic struggle to overcome original sin and without guilt find the innocent ecstasy of sexual merger.

Pointing the way to the twenty-first century were the Unitarian/Universalists and the humanists, who were offering new approaches to sexual morality that helped pave the way for the NSME legislation. But, unfortunately, a combination of avowed humanists—not more than fifty thousand (many of them are Unitarian/Universalists [U/Us] although they foreswear an active, interested God), and many U/Us who believe in God (but not necessarily a Christian one, with a son offering salvation)—in aggregate about two hundred thousand, during the last decade of the twentieth century could not consolidate their resources and present a united, sexually moral stand against the religious right, who denounced them all as "secular humanists."

In the East, Unitarian/Universalists were the first to accept homosexuals and lesbians as their ministers, and U/U churches in New York City, and areas like Provincetown, Massachusetts, with large gay memberships, flourished, but they were all much closer to their seventeenth-century Congregational roots than the U/Us in California, where many U/Us were experimenting and still are deeply involved in alternate lifestyles in the mid-1990s. They had, long ago, shrugged at the famous article in *Time* magazine (April 1984), which declared "The Sex Revolution is Over." According to *Time,* intimacy and relationships, the buzzwords of the time, were in vogue. Because of the fear of herpes, STDS, and AIDS, *Time* was convinced, "The national obsession with sex is subsiding . . . veterans of the revolution, some wounded, some merely bored, are reinventing courtship and discovering that often they need not sleep together on the first or second night. Many individuals are even rediscovering the traditional values of fidelity, obligation and marriage."

Eight years before that, in 1976, before *Time*'s futuristic probe that soon proved to be on a wrong trajectory, Lester Kirkendall, who will be remembered by millions as one of the first writers of textbooks on human sexuality, put together for humanists a *New Bill of Sexual Rights and Responsibilities,* which was published in a booklet, with twenty-first-century photographs showing a naked man and woman embracing, as well as a naked dad piggybacking his naked son and daughter (about five or six years old), a naked mother playing with her naked baby, three naked children taking a shower together, and a naked mother nursing her child.

The New Bill of Sexual Rights includes a brief discussion about the boundaries of human sexuality needing to be legislated; developing a sense of equity between the sexes as an essential feature of sexual morality; eliminating repressive taboos with a more balanced and objective human view; every person's right and obligation to be fully informed about civic and community aspects of human sexuality; and the right and responsibility of planned parenthood. But along with insisting that physical pleasure has a moral value, and in all sexual encounters humane and humanistic motives should prevail, Kirkendall missed the essential element.

"Sexual morality," he wrote, "should come from a sense of caring and respect for others. It cannot be legislated." The reality, of course, recognized by the benign sexual environmental legislation of the NSME legislation, is that without creating the environment for the final sex revolution, Americans would have sunk deeper into sexual sleaziness and dehumanization, which probably would have been terminated by the religious right with the enthusiastic approval of millions Americans who had been convinced that sexual repression is better than sexual expression with no boundaries.

While the Unitarian/Universalists offered no single twenty-first-century sexual perspective such as sacramentalizing human sexuality (see the addenda and the sermon from the *Immoral Reverend* that infuriated many U/U leaders), they were the only organized religion that dared to offer a twenty-first-century approach, similar in many aspects to the optional, federally funded K-12, human sexuality seminars (see ahead, chapter 18).

Recognizing that they had to compete with other kinds of entertainment if they were going to attract the younger generation, and the importance of having a gathering place for young people who had to escape their often very small home environments and meet a wider variety of potential mates, many Baptist churches in the 1990s tried to put the Christian sexual morality into a new environment of fun and games. The Second Baptist Church in Houston had a Sunday morning turnout of six thousand people on 32 acres of land, and membership of twelve hundred thousand who "worship" in a million-square-foot complex that offered not just a place to pray—but a place to play. Within the church, a member could lift weights, shoot pool, eat lunch, or even see a Broadway style musical show with a religious message.

Writing in the *Wall Street Journal*, May 13, 1991, R. Gustav Neihbur approvingly called Second Baptist, "A megachurch—the hottest thing in Protestantism.

The Christianity they serve up is mostly conservative and to the point, stripped of the old hymns, liturgy, and denominational dogma that tend to bore the video generation." One of the teaching staff, the Rev. Charles L. Martin III, calls it "The Fellowship of Excitement," and he was sure that in the late twentieth century the word "Baptist" would be the same. In the Shepherd Hills Baptist Church in Los Angeles, the Lutheran Church of Joy in Glendale, Arizona, and many other Protestant churches, the music of Bach, Beethoven, and Buxteheude is being replaced by "sacred pop music."

In a feature article, "In Search of the Sacred," *Newsweek,* November 28, 1994, contends that in one way or another millions of Americans are on a quest for spiritual meaning that coincides with current realities. As Harvey Cox reveals in his 1995 book *Fire from Heaven,* Pentecostal-based religions are the fastest-growing religions in America and in the world, with more than 500 million people who take the story of the Pentecost (occurring fifty days after Passover, or Easter, if you prefer) seriously. Described in the biblical Acts of of the Apostles, believers take the words literally: "Suddenly, a sound came from heaven like the rush of a mighty word and it filled the house [where the disciples were sitting] and it appeared to them in tongues, distributed and resting on each of them." Today, speaking in tongues in Pentecostal churches like the Assembly of God, as well as singing, shouting, trembling, falling down in ecstasy as each individual in his or her own way personally experiences God, is a way of life for many people.

Ralph Reed, who heads up the Christian Coalition, in his 1995 book *Politically Incorrect,* takes a new, low-key approach to creating a sound Christian America, and he plays down the fundamentalist belief in the inerrancy of the Bible. But he admits that Pentecostals and charismatics make up at least 20 percent of the Coalition. And while he doesn't cite the Willow Creek Community Church in Barrington, Illinois, founded in 1985 by David Hybell, the Coalition obviously approves of Hybell's approaches, which are described in detail in the Willow Creek Association's Church Manager Handbook. It's a book which should be read by all clergy, whether sympathetic or not, for insights into the American mind today. The Willow Creek Community Church not only has more than a thousand churches affiliated with their new approaches to bringing "Unchurched Harrys back to church," but it proves every Sunday, and through the week, that its methods work. It offers three Sunday services in its huge sanctuary/auditorium. All 4500 seats are fully occupied in each service. It is totally fundamentalist—the Bible is the word of God—and the big attraction is a spectacular Sunday theatre, which in music, sermons, and specially created dramas presumably modernizes Jesus' message. With no pressure the church is giving hundreds of thousands of baby boomers and Generation X'ers the opportunity to discover Christianity for the first time.

According to *Newsweek,* it is now even chic to use the "s words"—soul, sacred, spiritual, and sin. Spiritual novels like the *Celestine Prophecy* by James Redfield, and soul music with chants on CDs by Benedictine monks, along with the Beastie Boys doing Buddhist rap, have all become million-copy best sellers.

To top it off modern physicists, in search of the final nature of things, are merging quantum mechanics and thermodynamics with probes into religion. Frank Tipler's 1994 book, *The Physics of Immortality,* and a 1994 compilation of the views of ten physicists and biologists, called *Evidence of Purpose—Scientists Discover the Creator,* in various essays discuss whether the intricate harmonies of the cosmos testify to the workings of a divine hand. Along with *The Faith of Physicist: Reflections of a Bottom Up Thinker,* by John Polkinghorn, who is a particle physicist and a priest in the Church of England, and many other books, these writers point the way for a religious merger with NSME legislation.

For the record in my just completed novel, *Dreamer of Dreams,* I have offered a new religion, Wondering—with Wonderers believing in a Wondering God who, following the thinking of Alfred North Whitehead and Charles Hartshorne, is not an unchangeable "being" God, but is a God who together with humans is in the process of becoming.

The final sex revolution in the form of the NSME legislation gives both church and state a common objective in revaluing human sexuality by restoring sex worship and, in modern terms, equating caring, loving one-to-one human mating as merger with God or the underlying principle of the universe. Religious leaders discovered, once again, how to make the church, the mosque, and the synagogue a focus of human activity—and that none of us "live by bread alone."

In passing, it is interesting to remember the fears about separation of church and state. *Newsweek* in 1984 pointed out, "the sermonizing over religion and politics had become a code word symbolizing serious divisions in American society. In the 1984 political campaign, Walter Mondale accused Ronald Reagan of trying to transform policy debates into theological disputes." And Reagan responded, "Politics and morality are inseparable, and as morality is the foundation of religion, so religion and politics are necessarily related." Much of the issue revolved around "school prayer." In the twenty-first century this became an obsolete worry, since prayer in all young people's minds is now merged with the Word, and the Word is simultaneously God and Love, realized in icons of caring human sexual merger. When Mondale was contesting Reagan, Mario Cuomo wisely pointed out that (at the time), "Most people don't know the difference between values and morality, and the church and religion. They are all different terms being used interchangeably." In the twenty-first century one overriding value, caring human sexual love as God, superseded the endless debates over "born again" Christians, or whether Catholics, Jews, Protestants, males or females, of any race, religion, or ethnic group could be elected and function as president.

In September 1960, speaking before Protestant clergy, John F. Kennedy summed up the twentieth-century religious environment that caused so many problems that no longer exist in the twenty-first century. "In America the separation of church and state is an absolute. No Catholic prelate would tell the president (should he be Catholic) how to act, and no Protestant minister would tell his parishioners for whom to vote." Justice Hugo Black reaffirmed the First Amendment and said bluntly, "Neither federal nor state governments can pass laws which aid one religion, aid all religions, or prefer on religion over another."

The NSME legislation has done that by creating a church/state consensus on the nature of God. Individual religions still will diverge in rituals and have many theological differences, but they all have one common belief—God is Love, or, in some religious theology, "the Light within us." Even atheists who refuse to trust in God, can learn to trust in Love. Equating God with Love in a very human sense, the problems of prayer in schools and at public assemblies disappeared. Extolling human sexuality is tolling a bell we can all hear, or learn to hear. The bell tolls not for death but for life. In the twenty-first century Christians, Jews, and Muslims are praying to a God of Love who is encapsulated and expressed in a laughing, joyous, sexual merger with another human being.

16

Marriage and the Family in the Twenty-First Century

Ultimately, in the twenty-first century, since the Future Families of America Commission will be catalyzing policy and action in many crucial areas. The FFAC Secretary will have a cabinet position. Children of the twentieth century, so-called baby boomers, will be in charge, and they will be well aware that although a sound family structure is the sine qua non of a stable nation, the family structure in the United States didn't emerge as a problem for them that must be solved until the late 1960s when, largely for economic reasons, as Alexander Cockburn pointed out in an article in the *New Republic,* slavery was reintroduced into the United States. It now took two wage earners, a husband and wife, to achieve the same middle-class lifestyle that one could provide in 1965.

Coupled with this partial return to primitive times, when women were expected to work in the field, was the discovery that many women no longer needed men to support them, and thanks to the birth control pill women could enjoy sex without getting pregnant. Within the last forty years of the twentieth century women were liberated from male domination. But the trade-off would have shocked their mothers and grandmothers. Seventy percent of married women *had* to work if they wanted to live with anywhere near the affluence their parents had. Some militant feminists tried to sell the joys of being a career woman, but most of the serious ladies soon gave up marriage. They couldn't juggle work, career, and children unless they could afford nannies. For Mrs. Average American the nuclear family—husband and wife earning just enough money to babysit two kids when they were young and barely saving enough so they could go to college when they completed high school—became a joyless existence.

By the 1970s the divorce rate became 50 percent of the marriage rate, and a worried President Jimmy Carter, instigated by a Carnegie Council on Children report, "The American Family Under Pressure," proposed a White House Conference on Families. By June 1981 a 745-page document had been prepared and Secretary of Health, Education and Welfare Joseph Califano, Jr., had solicited more than four hundred politicians, writers, academicians, religious leaders and members of professional and special interest groups to participate in state level conferences. More than three thousand volunteered, but Hale Champion, undersecretary of HEW, was still seeking conference leaders, and the federal or White House phase was postponed. When Carter's White House Conference on the Family was finally held, Ronald Reagan was president. So many groups championed their particular views that no solutions to any problems emerged, and it was a total fiasco.

Neither Carter, Reagan, Bush, or Clinton dared to face the twenty-first-century reality. If the American family was going to prosper and survive, we had to go all out to control our population growth globally as well as at home. A capitalistic system that corrects itself in economic cycles, in the short term, destroys millions of low- and middle-income family structures and breeds crime waves. The twenty-first-century reality is that with a one hundred million increase in population, the percentage of the unemployed may remain the same but the absolute number of people and children involved grows enormously. On top of that we have greater longevity.

What we needed in the late twentieth century were leaders who endorsed planned parenthood, birth control, and zero population growth—leaders who dared to defy a religious minority who had been indoctrinated with theological moralities and values that no longer worked.

It didn't happen. When Reagan became President in 1980, Congress slowly began to undercut family planning services and the Population Research Act of 1970 (referred to as Title X funding), which had supported a nationwide network of birth control clinics. Reagan not only didn't approve of the Supreme Court *Roe v. Wade* decision, which legalized abortion, but he wasn't about to advocate birth control knowledge, which would have solved some of the abortion problems before they began. In 1991, the population crisis committee estimated that spending on contraceptives and voluntary planning services must rise to $10 billion annually by the year 2000. By the mid-1990s the United States was contributing very little to assist in worldwide population control. Both Reagan and Bush refused to get involved in birth control solutions that might offend Catholics and fundamentalist Protestants.

The Clinton Administration took a broader view and Clinton requested $585 million in his 1995 budget for spending on population programs. Timothy Wirth, undersecretary of state for global affairs, talked of raising $1.2 billion by the year 2000, based on the premise that the 5.5 billion population of the world would double in forty years and reach between 13 billion and 15 billion by 2050.

"Everything we would think of doing to further our goals of increasing stability and living standards around the world," Wirth stated, "can be compromised by unchecked population growth."

But Wirth and Clinton, like their predecessors, ignored the at- home problem of population increases within the United States. There was an euphoric feeling that the United States could easily absorb another hundred million people. That was America's strength, and how we grew from many people into one nation. But our forebears didn't arrive here seeking entitlement or dependency on government handouts. Freedom from government was their goal and they were willing to work hard for that freedom. People haven't changed—but the American environment has drastically. There's no land or gold waiting for the taking, and there isn't much freedom without jobs that pay better than minimum wages and poverty-level income.

But twentieth-century zealots preached the sanctity of human life in the womb, and the pope excoriated birth control. The basic philosophy was that increasing populations were God's will. In God we trust. But not in Love. Millions of children must have their God-given right to live, but not to have a more basic right—to be loved. And everyone ignored the reality that a million of them were in jail, and millions more lived lives of desperation that were not always quiet.

In May 1991 the Supreme Court, in the case of *Rust* v. *Sullivan,* endorsed what became known as the "gag rule." Family planning clinics could not receive government funds if they *even discussed* abortion with pregnant women, or told a woman where she could get information about abortion—even if a woman specifically asked for information.

Meanwhile, Reagan condemned China's "coercive abortion policy" to enforce a population control plan of "one child per family." China's leaders were well aware that with one billion people the country was walking a razor's edge. It was bad enough that the Chinese were rapidly acquiring material goods and demanding more, or that the doubling of such a huge population in a land mass smaller than United States could, in the case of crop failures, mean mass starvation. In any event there was simply not enough human space in which to live.

At the same time, in what became known as the Mexico City policy, the United States eliminated all U.S. funding to any international organizations that offered abortion information as part of their programs. Within the United States, the major problems of crime and unemployment were rarely linked with family instability.

In 1992, in a typical twentieth-century failure to get to the roots of the problem, David Blankenhorn, president of the Institute for American Values, believed that by focusing on women, the plight of children, day care, and whether Johnny could read, we missed the real problem, which is male responsibility.

Championing him, Louis Sullivan, secretary of the Department of Health and Human Services, detailed the economic, social, and health problems that children suffer when raised in fatherless families. The *Boston Globe* reported, "Sullivan's comments reflected a consensus across the political spectrum that increasing divorce rates have weakened family relationships. A bipartisan National Commission on Children suggested that children are best in families formed by marriage." Louis Sullivan told the Council on Families, "The greatest issue of our era is fatherlessness. . . . I'm here to put the issue of fatherless families front and center on our national agenda, and to call for national action on what is surely the most important family challenge of the 1990s."

Sociologist Sara McLanahan disagreed with Sullivan. "I think the most important problem is poverty, and it's not just poverty in single-parent families. More than half the children are living in two-parent families. The costs of poverty are even greater than the family structure itself."

No one in the twentieth century ever mentioned education, or a belief in the future and a sense of national purpose as the basic long-term solution to the problem of both old-style and potential new-style family stability. The extensive twenty-first-century, K-12 liberal arts and sexual education that all young people will receive does something for the first time in the history of education. Young men and women are being educated with common historical perspectives on every aspect of the world and human life. Whether they have taken the ROSP option or not, men and women have learned how to love one another, and have much more in common than most married couples in the twentieth century.

FFAC will continue to explore the problems that led to the high divorce rates and family breakups in the twentieth century. A new generation with wide background in the liberal arts and more than one vocational aptitude will be aware that over and above having children, which hopefully gives a married couple at least one common goal and focus for their lives, common interests are the only solid foundation for long-term relationships and stable families in twenty-first-century America.

In a society where the majority of husbands and wives must work to support a family, each with different jobs, the odds are that neither spouse is very much interested in the other's job. But if they're both happy, or even totally involved, in their work, they must learn to share each other's commitment. If both are working, not because they want to but because they have to, then the necessity for other common, shared interests is even more critical.

In the twentieth century millions of spouses discovered that they not only didn't enjoy the other person's hobbies, but they didn't like each other's friends. Early in marriage, many wives discover that her husband has a few male friends, like him, who have common interests in sports, or computers, camping out, owning guns, or even playing cards—things that don't interest most women. Or men find themselves married to women who enjoy the arts, music, literature, or just "shopping." In upper-income marriages, stories of which the middle-class enjoying watching, the spouses have affairs and find other lovers. In many marriages the spouses are often more intimate, "down to earth," with friends of the same sex than they are with each other.

Dining out, exploring different restaurants—anything to get out the house—was a national hobby that millions of husbands and wives in the late twentieth century shared. Understandably, working wives were not in the mood to prepare gourmet dining, and what was there to do in a small home or apartment, anyway, except look at television or go to bed?

But there was little intimacy or exciting exchange of ideas. James Ramey points out in his book *Intimate Friendships,* that the average American couple engages in about 27.5 minutes of conversation per week. People in traditional marriages cut down verbal input and depend on nonverbal communication. Not talking, because they had little to communicate, watching other noncommunicative couples "dining out," became a lifestyle for millions of married couples in the twentieth century.

Before NSME and GLUE in the twentieth century most couples, after a few years of marriage, lost the art of receiving self-disclosure from another person, noncritically. They avoided areas in which they were totally in disagreement. In the sexual aspects of their lives, they didn't dare to discuss, with some sense of laughter things they enjoyed doing or not doing with each other. Each carefully censored his or her thoughts because they might lead to arguments or because they were embarrassing. "As spouses come to know each other better," as Ramey points out, "the safe areas of conversations are 'talked out' and eventually they have little to say to each other or discuss." With insufficient secondary education, they never learned how to input their lives with hundreds of exciting ideas that could give their lives new directions or enliven the old ones.

Future Families of America, exploring old-style twentieth-century relationships that might be teetering on divorce or boredom, will be experimenting with new-style extended family relationships that expand the one-to-one mental and sexual intimacy of monogamous marriages (see part two for excerpts from my novels that offer many different approaches). FFAC will also have funding to explore adult sexual behavior as well as study the sexual patterns that govern choice of sexual partners among adults and teenagers—an $18 million program of this kind was shelved by the National Institute for Mental Health in the mid-1990s. The survey was blocked by Louis Sullivan for fear of political opposition from President Bush and Congress, and perhaps because of what might have been revealed.

People working for Future Families of America and those who will be funded to explore the problems that can occur in ménage à trois, corporate marriages of two couples, and other styles of extended families, will be well aware that in the late 1960s and 1970s many college professors teaching in the areas of psychology and sociology believed that some of what they called alternative lifestyles would become a way of life in the twenty-first century.

Robert Libby and Robert Whitehurst, both college professors with doctorates offered two books, *Renovating Marriage* and *Marriage and Its Alternatives* (Consensus Publishers, 1973 and 1977), which had essays by well-known marriage counselors and college professors such Jesse Bernard, Gordon Clanton, Joan and Larry Constantine, Anna and Bob Francoeur, Vera Mace, Ron Mazur, Pepper Schwartz, Rustum and Della Roy, and many others.

Group Marriage, a detailed study written by the Constantines, explored the problems of mental and sexual sharing when a group of adults and children move into a single house and try to share spouses and their monetary resources. During these years practically all colleges and universities offered courses in marriage and the family, which, at the sophomore and junior college level, were taken largely by women students. Relatively few men took the courses, which were backed up by thousand page textbooks covering every aspect of human sexuality as well as marital problems. By contrast, textbooks such as Robert Francoeur's *Becoming A Sexual Person* (MacMillan, 1992) are now used in the federally funded human sexuality courses from grades nine through twelve.

In these weekly seminars high school students also become familiar with Gordon Clanton's study, *Jealousy* (Prentice Hall, 1977), in which leading sociologists explore the dynamics of jealousy and how to overcome it, as well as the best selling book of its era *Open Marriage,* by George and Nena O'Neill (Evans 1972). The book asked and answered the question raised by Rustum and Della Roy in their essay "Is Monogamy Outdated?" They all believed that it was, but a few years later, revealing the sexual confusion and rebellions without focus of the last thirty years of the twentieth century, Nena O'Neill, after George's death, wrote another book excoriating what had proved to be an an unworkable concept—a lasting prime marriage where the original pair bonds could date other persons and go to bed with them, if they were so inclined.

From the 1970s to the end of the century the baby boomers whether they were still striving to maintain an original nuclear family, or were divorced and remarried, or were divorced and still hoping for a lasting marriage, all were searching for some kind of marital (and sexual) stability in a world where it seemed to be vanishing forever.

Irving Kristol, one of them, and a conservative grandpa, in an article called "Reflections on Love and Family" (*Wall Street Journal,* January 7, 1992) was daydreaming.

> The nuclear family is once again respectable, even popular. Unfortunately, this popularity is promoted by pop psychologists and their Hollywood screenwriters,

who haven't the foggiest idea of what real family life is about but are determined to counsel us as to its virtues. Parents are supposed to go around telling their children "I love you," and children are supposed to respond in kind. The other night I saw on a television sit-com, a ten-year-old boy come down to breakfast and kiss his mother and father before sitting down to eat. Surely, not even in Hollywood do ten-year-old-boys behave that way. Had I ever tried it my mother would have promptly taken my temperature. Families are not about "love" but about sensed affection plus, above all, absolute commitment. Children do not yearn for "love," they desire and need security that comes from such absolute commitment, spiced with occasional demonstrations of affection. In real life, we do not honor our father and mother because of the kind of persons they are, but because they are our father and mother. We do not recognize their authority because they, in any sense, deserve it. We do it, and are pleased to do it, out of a natural sense of piety toward the authors of our being.

Kristol's concept of family worked well for the nineteenth century—and mid-twentieth-century Jewish families. In the twenty-first century much of that old-time flavor of commitment not only to children but to "landsmen" and the older generation will be integrated into new-style extended families where millions of people rediscover, in a lifetime learning environment, that the joys of community in larger "created" family groupings can resolve many of the man-made tragedies of the twentieth century.

On October 25, Herbert Stein, a fellow of the American Research Institute, in a *Wall Street Journal* article titled, "The Show is Over," proclaimed, "Whether or not there is poverty in our private lives there is poverty in our public life." The reason for this state of affairs, according to Stein, is similar to the thesis of this book: "We have no sense of national purpose." Stein calls for a goal that would inspire and energize the American people. "The goal would be to improve the quality of life of the least advantaged among us, and reduce hostility and fear among races."

Alas, like most of our leaders, Stein is spouting soap-bubble solutions—fairy talk. Sounds great but adds up to nothing. There's only one way to improve the quality of life—politicians, leaders, and a president who makes no bones about it. We must extend the education of all Americans now in high schools and give them all the assurance of a Guaranteed Loving Undergraduate Education. Neither Clinton nor the new Republican Congress, nor any of the candidates for a Republican presidency thus far in 1995, have offered any specific national purpose. Instead of blowing soap bubbles and letting democracy continue to drift to disaster, NSME legislation is the only hope.

17

Love Me Tomorrow

Before the K-12 human sexuality and GLUE human values seminars became a way of life in the total educational environment, in the mid-1990s, Kate Roiphe wrote the book *The Morning After,* subtitled, "Sex, Fear and Feminism on Campus." With a twenty-first-century perspective, the author questioned the feminist movement and its "obsession with date rape and sexual harassment." Perhaps the hysteria had something in common with the Salem witch trials.

Meanwhile, female students at Antioch College, once the 1960 undergraduate bastion of sexual freedom, in 1994, with an enrollment of 650 students, 70 percent of whom were female, published a nine-page "Sexual Offense Policy" advising their male peers what was fair play and that obtaining sexual consent was an ongoing verbal process in any sexual interaction. The media immediately pronounced it "a Byzantine consent code" and a menace to spontaneous sex. But the reality, as Allan Guskin, president of Antioch pointed out, was, "The nineties are a time for searching for new norms of behavior. How do we relate? What is the nature of relationships?"

Women at Antioch (unlike the young women who take the ROSP option, during their continuing education) were trying to find their way in a hit-or-miss sexual environment. Along with the dating code were their "steam orgies" where young men and women showered together in their dormitories. With many young women daring to say to a male fellow student, "I'd like to fuck you," they were trying to find a balance for male/female sexual responses that made sense. In essence they were laying some tentative foundations for the final sexual revolution.

By contrast here is a "Love Me Tomorrow" message for the twenty-first century, and the basis of K-16 education, and twenty-one years of learning to love.

1. You must learn how to be you—and simultaneously, a less involved you,

187

watching you. You may even discover how to be a third you watching the other two. Soren Swedenborg summed it up: "You must learn how to be subjective toward others and objective toward yourself." If you learn this, you'll never be afraid to make the opening move and deflect hatreds, cynicism, and verbal nastiness by a simple: "I know how you feel, *but,* I wonder if . . ." thus opening other possibilities.

2. You must learn, and dare to reveal to at least one or two intimate friends, all the conflicting aspects of the different "yous"—the grim you, who thinks you want money and power and fame, versus the laughing you, who is very well aware that your fifteen minutes of public adoration, if you ever achieve it, can't compare with the bliss, and long-term happiness of a man and woman, alone, daring to self-disclose and become transparent selves before and after a sexual merger. This is a great deal more than role playing. You must be unafraid to accept the responses you may evoke when you reveal some of your conflicting emotions and ambitions to an intimate friend or spouse. He or she may not have learned how to interact with you on the same basis. He or she may stand in judgment on you and pronounce you a weirdo, a kook, or a person who is trying to swim upstream and downstream at the same time.

The twenty-first-century life-style is "daring to be defenseless with another person." Initially, if you are male, many of your male friends may come to the conclusion that you are pretty naive, or are ingenuous. But often you'll discover that instead of endangering your masculinity, verbal intimacy breeds verbal intimacy. Most women have been conditioned by the male game of never revealing fears or weaknesses. But, fortunately with people they love many women dare to abandon their mental defensiveness much more quickly than the average male. But, sadly, after they were married, most twentieth-century men and women never learned how to "let go" and achieve the kind of mental intimacy with a spouse or lover that lays the foundation for great sex.

3. In the twenty-first-century liberal arts program in secondary school, young people will be taught not only how to self-disclose, but to accept self-disclosure from a friend or lover, noncritically, and never become judgmental or play God. In addition they will learn how to resist the temptation to believe that another person's openness with them is casting some reflection on their own ego identification. If either person doesn't affirm or confirm the other's ego problems, petty or not, they will laugh, even call each other "assholes," but still love each other.

4. Underlying all continuous K-16 teaching and the foundation of a new national morality and ethics, is to teach a new generation how to learn from the past, and live in the present, guided by the American Indian wisdom, "You can not understand me, or my life, until you have walked a few miles in my moccasins," and another: "I cried because I had no shoes, until I met a man who had no feet."

5. All young people should be taught in schools as well as in churches and

temples, an underlying awareness that they are mortal and time is precious. You are going to die, but you have a good chance of living four score and ten years. In the meantime, right now in your K-16 schooling, you are becoming the kind of person that you will be for the rest of your life. The essence of you—the energy that is you—will live forever, and who knows, you may live again in some other form, *but you won't live long enough to hate or to be jealous or envious of any other person.* Disappearing from earth this time around is nothing to be afraid of, but some of the joy of living is trying to achieve a limited immortality, first in the memories of your friends or lovers, and second as someone who contributed a bit of knowledge or happiness and a sense of wonder that may spark the lives of others.

6. The role of all teachers in the twenty-first century and during the final phase of the sex revolution will be to continuously project for their students a sense of awe and sheer amazement at life and human intelligence. Parents, knowing that their children will receive a complete education K-12 through GLUE, as well as teachers and religious leaders, should reinforce the lasting joys of curiosity, and should combine to create lifestyles for their children where asking why, and finding answers—or no answers—is the essence of life. This kind of curiosity is built into the genes of young children, but in the twentieth century was put down. You grew up and didn't ask so many questions, or you were even derided by too-easily-bored young people. In the twenty-first century, curiosity will become a happy, infectious disease, creating the kind of dis-ease that makes life endlessly exciting. Once it takes hold there is no surcease from it—the more answers you find, the more questions you raise. Laughingly, aware that no one can ever know it all, young people will discover, early in life, that they are happiest when they are fulfilling their destiny in man's never-ending search for answers both to specifics and to "What's it all about?"

7. Finally, young people who have had a complete education from kindergarten through one GLUE work/study program or the other will have learned that in all interpersonal relationships, monogamous, triadic, two-couple pairings, or experimenters in other family styles that are being funded by Future Families of America, another real joy in life is to learn to function like a chameleon. If you dare to take on the coloring of another person, you can still hang onto your own identity as a laughing, contingent human being. In the process, you will not only find yourself by escaping yourself, but you will discover the essence of sexual merger. *I am you!*

Freedom of expression was the byword of the twentieth century. Beyond anything else, this was a First Amendment right and prerogative. But gradually people became aware that freedom of negative expression had created a "put down" society. Millions of people were compensating for human drives and motives that they didn't understand, were afraid of, or uneasy with—especially in the sexual area—by using derogatory words. Other than making love, or having sex, screwing and fucking were the basic words to describe the joy of mating—and neither of the last two are joyous words.

The "D" words seemed to verbalize reality. Deface, degrade, defile, denigrate, deprave, derange, denounce, deplore, destroy, disgust and a late-twentieth-century addition, "dissed." The nation was "de profundis," out of its depth and without a sense of purpose; millions of people were playing a minor key in a continuous downbeat.

Way back in 1986, the Reagan/Meese-instigated Commission on Pornography offered one sensible statement: "We all agree that some degree of individual choice is necessary in any free society, and we all agree that a society with no shared moral values is no society at all . . . and although there are many members of this society who can make affirmative cases for uncommitted sexuality, none of us believe it to be a good thing."

Eight years later, in 1994, Sheldon Hackney, former president of the University of Pennsylvania and currently president of the National Endowment for the Humanities, was calling for an "American Conversation," and a search for values during which Americans at all levels could find agreement on "What it means to be an American, and define a clear sense of where we're going and what we want to be." In the late twentieth century thousands of Americans were looking for national goals, but few seemed to realize that it could only come with an entirely new approach to education, and a moral compass that NSME legislation would provide.

In my novel, *The Harrad Experiment,* Beth Hillyer, after watching the opera *Lucia* and its mind-blowing "mad" scene, asks a twenty-first-century question: "In our future Utopian world with no conflict, with every one in full accord finally, with no wars, no murders, no hate, no jealousy, what in heaven's name will be the subject matter of the arts?"

And many years ago, long before NSME legislation, Harry Schacht responds,

There's a thousand subjects. Man not against himself but against the gods. For us, now in the twentieth century, the gods are still unknown. Man against disease. Man against premature death. Man against mass hatred. Man crying for security, or solitude, or love. Man against war or poverty or misunderstanding. Man against greed or corruption. Man against his own ignorance. A new kind of Faust. In this kind of drama the protagonist, the hero, would once again assume a heroic stance. His failures against unknowns, and not the failure of his own petty misfortunes, would assume the grandeur of real tragedy.

One of the unknown gods of the twentieth century, whom no one paid much attention to in 1966 when those words were written, was the god of the environment. Twenty-first-century tragedies caused by global warming, many of the earth's oceans becoming warmer than they were twenty years before, and sea levels increasing two inches or more, breeding hurricanes, flooding, poverty and hunger, are the subjects of tragedies that will always be beyond man's control.

But, now, baby boomers, living into the twenty-first century, long past middle age can, with their children, dare to visualize a world they can control as they usher in the final sexual and education revolution that will transform America and give the rest of the world a really brave new world to emulate.

Visualize a world where kids grow up seeing human beings of all ages naturally naked, and are aware of, because they have been taught to appreciate it, the changing beauty of the body from youth to old age. Visualize a world where mom and dad, still married, or single, or married again, have made videos of themselves when they were younger, making love, playing together with friends naked. Visualize a world where mom and dad happily show the videos to their kids, and even pictures and videos of gramps and grandma, naked when they were in the flower of youth, and kids can be proud that their parents once were shapely and pretty as they are now. Visualize a world where Americans, no longer hiding behind clothes, realize that with good diet and exercise they can, well past middle age, maintain firm and pleasingly erotic bodies.

Visualize a world where teenagers are able to ask their mothers and fathers, without embarrassment, when they first made love, and did they wait until seventeen, as they do now? Visualize a world where parents can tell their teenagers their experiences with the joys of sex. Visualize a world where mothers and fathers, in extended families created by amicable divorces, are able to discuss with their children and with each other the mental incompatibilities and sexual problems, or emotional blocks that undermined their first marriages.

Visualize a world where mothers and fathers and their children can watch caring men and women making love together in movies, and on television—naked, but in no hurry with lots of verbal communication, in many different environments. And the kids can coolly discuss with their parents caring sexmaking like this, or in SDH (Sexually Devaluing Historical) films, comparing people in past centuries who presumably suffered from mental and sexual hang-ups, which psychiatrists like Sigmund Freud and his followers foolishly believed were buried in man's genes or inherited from his childhood.

Visualize a world where a boy or girl in their early teens, thirteen to fifteen years old, can tell mom or dad, or a single parent, that their boyfriend or girlfriend is going to stay over tonight so that they can do their homework together, and sleep together. And they assure their parents "Don't worry, we won't have intercourse, but we may hug a bit." Visualize a world where your son or daughter discusses with you his or her work/study undergraduate education, and if he or she is in the ROSP program, brings home her or his current roommate for the holidays, and you are happy that you have an extra bedroom or private space for them, and you're fascinated with their charming, loving, sexual sophistication.

And you can keep visualizing a new generation who has learned that caring sex is a gift of a loving God—a laughing, dancing God, a spiritual and erotic God who didn't invent marriage or monogamy, or how and when men and women will make love, but rather knows that in the act of love we are expressing our oneness with him, and the fertility of the earth—even when we refrain from procreating. And visualize a new generation that knows that there is no God who will stop us from overpopulating, or provide us with enough food, or all the material things man has invented, nor will God stop us from creating human tragedies in our lives where no tragedy should ever have existed. But there is a loving God who constantly gives us the experience of him, as he did Jesus, Buddha, and Mohammed, in our caring love for each other, a God who celebrates our sexual mergers because they are a merger with him that all men and women can learn how to experience.

Just past mid-century, in 1961, J. H. van den Berg, a Dutch professor of psychology at the University of Leyden, wrote a prophetic book, *The Changing Nature of Man,* in which he explored the fallacies of Freudian solutions to man's neuroses and expanded on Emile Durkheim's study of suicide which Durkheim traced to "anomy"—society's state of "normlessness" and its failure to regulate the individual. Berg cites a *Unesco* study of the healthy community:

> First, all aspects of life are integrated—work for instance is not something separate and distinct. . . . This means in a healthy community there are no gaps between work and recreation, work and play, work and religion, faith and desire, life and death, youth and adulthood. Everyone is bound together in one coherent totality, with no splits anywhere. Second, social belonging is automatic. Everybody belongs to a community. Third, change is slow and continuity is sustained by attitudes, customs and institutions that are stable. And lastly, important social groupings are small. If these qualities are absent, "social sickness" will appear. Neurotic and psychosomatic diseases will appear along with divorce, criminality, and suicide.

Van den Berg explores these in a mid-twentieth-century context. His book will be required historical reading for the twelfth-grade liberal arts education, and this requirement will not change until NSME legislation is enacted, which, as a byproduct, along with Future Families of America, will recreate twenty-first century versions of healthy communities.

Before you put this book down, or cruise through part 2, which will give you some entopian, "ahead of its time" perspectives on the twenty-first century, let's face a question you have been probably asking. Can we indoctrinate a new generation with a need to love and a need to know? Will we be creating a more dangerous sexual environment than the one that developed so haphazardly in the twentieth century? Would we be creating a new generation of Richard Specks, Ted Bundys, David Berkowitzes (Son of Sams), Wesley Dodds, and other males, all of whom became sexually berserk murderers? Many religious leaders in the twentieth century believed that these men became serial killers and mass murderers because they were obsessed with pornography. What will happen when young men grow up seeing men and women, naked, or in the arts, making love? Will the misfits really run amok?

Of course, there will still be misfits, but there will also be a sexual safety net, in later life, in the form of Stress Relief Clinics and federal drug clinics, and a secondary school environment where young people having sexual problems will be easily identified in the later years of the K-12 human sexuality seminars. And more likely, the mass murderers and serial killers of the twentieth century were created by a pervasive, sick sex environment. In the twenty-first century, a combined school/church/state consensus on human loving will give all young people a healthier indoctrination than they would have received in the past.

Rape and serial murders are less likely in a world where children aren't taught to hate—a world where magazines like *Soldier of Fortune,* with a substantial monthly circulation, provides a periscope on human hatred and xenophobia. There was no pornography permitted in Hitler's Germany or visual sex in Serbia, but there was rape and millions of murders committed by Catholics and Protestants who had been indoctrinated that Jews or Muslims weren't like them—children of God.

Mention indoctrination, and Americans think "brainwashing," and they cringe in horror. But keep in mind that the indoctrination proposed in the new sexual morality is to not create an "evil empire" but a loving one. One way or another, a new generation will be indoctrinated—either into healthy human sexuality, or into a new-style Christian/Judaic orthodoxy of the conservative right that will continue to be a breeding ground for sick, devalued human sexuality.

18

Late Twentieth-Century Advocacy Organizations and NSME Legislation

In his book *The Activist's Almanac,* "The Concerned Citizen's Guide to the Leading Advocacy Organizations," David Walls details the activities and personnel of more than a hundred nonprofit groups actively trying to influence public policy on the crucial issues of the late twentieth century. Walls details the activities of some of these groups, which are listed below in greater detail.

In the following listing, you will find names of groups that may be sympathetic to some, if not all, aspects of the NSME legislation, or that may be challenged to present other alternatives. Also included, with an asterisk preceding their name, are many groups affiliated with the religious right, that could resolve most of the twentieth-century sexual malaise and devaluation problems, and the byproducts they inveigh against, if they could agree that the best solution is to deal with sexual realities in an upbeat manner and bring caring, joyous sex back into the church in a new kind of "God Is Love" worship.

Also listed are many smaller, not-so-well-known organizations that are very definitely advocacy groups. Many are headed up by children of the baby boomers who, like their parents in the 1960s, are still experimenting with different lifestyles, but not in a utopian way. In the 1960s, they were called alternate lifestyles and they included some far-out attempts at communal living combined with unstructured sexual freedom. If nothing else, in the mid-1990s, the children of the baby boomers have discovered that lasting sexual merger is only achievable with one or two persons and not at the same time! In the 1990s the search continues and a reasonable guess is that ten million people in United States are living/loving nonmonogamously but, at the same time, are functioning in some kind of viable, committed family grouping.

One problem for many people living on the outer fringe is that they have lit-

194

tle or no moral support from children, parents, or friends and communities in which they may live. Unlike sexual rebels of the 1960s or the homosexuals and lesbians in the 1990s, they don't seek publicity, or even want "to come out the closet." In most respects they are model citizens, your next-door neighbors, and their bedroom is still private even though more than two people might be in the same bed, or those in one bed or another are not with their spouse. Many of those who live more dangerously and publish newsletters often indulge in too much navel gazing, or they are hooked on Freudian and post-Freudian complexes and neuroses that they think can be alleviated in group endeavors. Some make no attempt to relate their sexual lives to potential stable family environments.

In 1993 at a lifestyle assembly of several hundred people at Kirkridge in the Poconos (Pennsylvania), I suggested that a national magazine, possibly called *Loving More,* and with an editorial point of view that reflects the New Sexual Morality Education legislation, could rapidly gain a big circulation from a majority of Americans who will endorse NSME. Such a magazine could offer articles on new approaches to marriage and the family, as well ongoing experiments in the economic and interpersonal problems of people who are searching for a full life based on the Five Ls—Living, Loving, Laughter, Learning, and Ludamus!— all of us playing in ways together that may or may not include multiple relationships. It has happened. See below.

So here with a chuckle is a listing of some strange bedfellows who may ultimately have to agree that NSME legislation is the only possible twenty-first-century route to sexual sanity.

ABUNDANT LOVE INSTITUTE, P.O. Box 4322, San Rafeal, CA 94913, and Island office, P.O. Box 6306, Ocean View, Hawaii 96737. If you believe that alternative life style was a 1960s phenomenon and everyone has now returned to monogamy, then you'll be happy to know that for the past ten years, two young women (both in their forties)—Deborah Anapol, in California, and Ryam Nearing, in Hawaii— are in contact with thousands of people in the United States and worldwide who are living successfully in many variations of marital relationships from monogamy, to serial monogamy (divorce and remarriage), open marriages, closed group marriages, and what they call "polyfidelity." Both women have written detailed books. Deborah's is titled *Love Without Limits* and Ryam's *Loving More.* The chart on the next page condenses the many relationships in which humans are involved. Polyfidelity, or polyamory, is described as "a new marriage form that is based on individual choice. No one chooses polyfidelity because he or she can't affort a spouse of his or her own. We are an international organization of people who believe in family groups in which all partners are primary to all others partners and sexual fidelity is to group and the shared intent

These represent the basic relationship-style choices available. **Which best describes your current style?** Some people simply "find" themselves in a particular style, while others made a specific choice based on their experience and other considerations. **Which are you?**

ONLY ONE PARTNER/SPOUSE AT A TIME:

 Traditional monogamy: only one partner who is a lifelong mate; primary intimacy and sexual fidelity only with this partner.

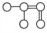 **Serial monogamy:** a succession of monogamous partners over time; overlapping sexuality only in the transition from the current "monogamous" partner to the next.

MORE THAN ONE PARTNER/SPOUSE AT A TIME:

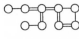 **Open:** varying numbers of sexual partners at any time, depending on availability and circumstance; all relating is secondary level or less and no shared future assumed. For most people this is an interim or exploratory phase.

 Intimate network: individuals who desire friendship and perhaps sex with their lover's other friend(s) and lover(s), forming a web of varying connections within a social circle.

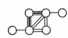 **Open marriage/partnership:** includes one primary spouse bond, and other secondary or tertiary lover(s) depending on availability and circumstance.

 Open group marriage: a group of individuals who describe themselves as married, but may or may not be all primaries, and who are open to outside sexual relationships.

 Closed group marriage: a group of individuals who describe themselves as married, but may or may not be all primaries, and who are closed to outside sexual relationships.

 Polyfidelity: a group in which all partners are primary to all other partners and sexual fidelity is to the group; shared intent of a lifelong run together.

Take a look at the charts on the left. Beginning with how many intimate partners you desire and proceeding logically, this determines where your choice will appear. Once you've found your appropriate chart, follow it out based on your preferences about primary and secondariness. For example, if you want more than one partner and are therefore looking at the bottom chart labeled *More Than One* and you have decided that in addition to your one primary partner, you want some secondary contacts, then open marriage would be the right choice for you. **Please remember that for your relationships to work smoothly, you need to find partners who want the same thing.** It is very difficult to be in an open marriage and find that the lover you want as a secondary in your life wants you as a primary in his, etc.*

ONE

Traditional   Serial
Monogamy   Monogamy

MORE THAN ONE

Open: Closed:
Open Single   Closed Group
Intimate Network   Marriage
Open Marriage   Polyfidelity
Open Group
Marriage

---

*Adapted from Ryam Nearing, *Loving More: The Polyfidelity Primer* (1992).

of a lifelong run together." Anapol details the forms that responsible non-monogamy can take. They include open marriage, or open relationships, intimate networks, group marriages, or multilateral marriage. I was delighted to discover Deborah and Ryam, and happy that after long rejection by publishers that my novels *Harrad* and *Proposition 31,* and many others, offering alternative-style relationships, were still very alive in the 1990s. I convinced Deborah and Ryam to join forces, and instead of individual newsletters to their thousands of believers, they now publish a magazine called *Loving More.* I am sure that there are a potential million or more subscribers. The first issue appeared February 1995. It's now on a quarterly basis. It lays the groundwork for a Future Families of America Commission. I'm sure if you sympathize with the ideas in this book, you'll want to become a subscriber.

AMERICAN CIVIL LIBERTIES UNION, 132 West 43rd Street, New York, New York 10036-6599. Should be pro-NSME since the legislation will only affect first Amendment rights by reeducating Americans to a greater awareness that freedom of expression carries with it social responsibilities and speech.

*AMERICAN FAMILY ASSOCIATION, 107 Parkgate Drive, Tupelo, Mississippi 38803. Tackles violence and vulgarity and nudity on television programs like "NYPD Blue" with full-page advertisements in major newspapers. Dr. Daniel Wildmon, in charge, may shudder at NSME but like other religious leaders listed below, it gives him a religiously oriented alternative.

AMERICAN FEDERATION OF TEACHERS, 555 New Jersey Avenue N.W., Washington, D.C. 20001. Albert Shanker, president, who editorializes weekly in a paid advertisement in the Sunday *New York Times,* should be in favor of NSME and GLUE since it will make teaching the prime occupation of Americans, and could resolve unemployment, not only in the United States, but in most of the G7 nations who met in Detroit in 1994 at a job conference but came up with no real solutions for a total of thirty million unemployed in their nations.

*AMERICAN CENTER FOR LAW AND JUSTICE, P.O. Box 64429, Virginia Beach, Virginia 23467. Pat Robertson's organization wants to combat "religious cleansing" and have all Americans "stand up against the ACLU, Planned Parenthood, and the National Organization of Women." NSME resolves Robertson's attack against "pro-lifers" since teenage abortion will no longer be a big issue. But concerned Christians will have to change their attitude toward K-12 sex education and make room for a really loving God in their sanctuaries.

*AMERICANS FOR RESPONSIBLE TELEVISION, P.O. Box 627, Bloomfield Hills, Michigan 48303. Terry Rakolta, who heads up this group, worries about sixteen-year-olds seeing fifteen thousand sexual acts on television, in the framework of "casual sex, wife swapping, rape, incest, and prostitution." Will she approve of FFAC's self-imposed rating system on the arts, which solves these problems but permits caring, one-to-one male/female sex portrayals?

AMERICAN SUNBATHING ASSOCIATION, 1703 N. Main Street, Kissimee, Florida 32743. With thirty thousand or more members they should endorse NSME legislation. But, of course, "being naked where it is convenient to be naked" with certain restrictions, will eliminate the need for a nudist resorts and gatherings.

ANTI-DEFAMATION LEAGUE OF B'NAI B'RITH, 832 United Nations Plaza, New York, New York 10017. Among other things they keep a close watch on the Christian Coalition and the Coalition's goal to build a Christian-controlled society. One of their 1994 reports describes "the movement's drive to return society to its Christian values" as "evangelical romanticism" that prompts leaders to create scapegoats out of feminists, gays, lesbians, and Jews. They should approve of NSME legislation.

AQUARIAN RESEARCH FOUNDATION, 6620 Morton Street, Philadelphia, Pennsylvania 19144. Working on a shoestring, Art and Judy Rosenblum have for many years published, sporadically, a newsletter of what they call a "prophet making organization dedicated to facilitating an age of world peace and brotherly love." They deserve funding from some foundation with the same objectives but with more capitalistic bucks!

*CENTER FOR AMERICAN VALUES, P.O. Box 91180, Washington, D.C. 20090-1180. Headed up by Deborah Stone, the center's values should accept that God is Love, but probably won't in the context of NSME.

CENTER FOR LIFE DESIGN, 7843 Girard Avenue, Suite C, La Jolla, California 92037. Peggy and James Vaughn are firmly committed to "people making their world a better place to live." Peggy has published several books describing her life with James, and how she coped with his extramarital affairs, and held their marriage together.

*CHRISTIAN ACTION NETWORK, P.O. Box 606, Forest, Virginia 24551, Martin Mayer, President. Basically pursuing the same objectives as the Christian Coalition, they were at war in 1994 with the Clinton administration over First Amendment rights.

*CHRISTIAN COALITION, P.O. Box 1990, Chesapeake, Virginia 23327. A mid-1990s transformation of Jerry Falwell's Moral Majority, this organization runs multimillion-dollar mail-order, radio, and television campaigns against abortion, homosexuality, lesbianism, sex education, and condom distribution that goes beyond basic biological information. Extolling biblical moralities, it presumably has 10 million members or contributors. Pat Robertson and Robert Reed who head it up believe that "America has become a largely anti-Christian, pagan nation—and our government has become a weapon of the radical left which is being used against Christians and religious people." Can Robertson and Reed abandon their quixotic battle against the sex wind mills, and see that NSME could reunite the church and state and give all Americans a new sense of national purpose?

*CHRISTIAN LEADERSHIP MINISTRIES, 100 Support Lane, Orlando, Florida 32809-7875. J. Stanley Oaken is director of this organization, which is a division of Campus Crusade for Christ, and believes that "Christians are under the most vicious attack ever on college campuses," and millions of young Americans are being raised as atheists or agnostics. Will they endorse a new sexual morality that affirms the sacramentalizing of human sexuality and the message that God is Love?

CHURCH OF ALL WORLDS, P.O. 1542, Ukiah, California 95482. Otter G'Zell publishes a monthly magazine, *Green Egg*. The mission of his church is to evolve a network of information, mythology, and experience that provides context and stimulus for reawakening Gaia and reuniting her children through tribal stewardship and ever-evolving consciousness. A pagan or wiccan religion, it has thousands of covens and believers, many of whom are Tantric sex enthusiasts. Pantheistic, they celebrate human sexuality and panfidelity (sacred sex) with earth goddesses. It is a modern religion that blends sex and sexuality but offers many different varieties, too many of which get involved with ancient rituals and occult practices. Nevertheless, in many areas it is a forerunner for NSME.

COMMON BOUNDARY, P.O. 445, Mt. Morris, Illinois 61504. A magazine which "builds a bridge between the two most vital areas of human life: psychotherapy and spirituality." Featuring writers like Charles Tart, M. Scott Peck, and Virginia Satir, the editor should be sympathetic to NSME legislation.

COMMUNITIES, JOURNAL FOR COOPERATIVE LIVING, Route 1, Rutledge, Missouri 63563. A quarterly journal covering the activities of more than five hundred intentional communities where the participants and their children live communally, but only in a few cases are they involved in multilateral relationships. A wave of the future for those who have completed GLUE Roommate of the Other Sex undergraduate education.

*CONCERNED WOMEN FOR AMERICA, 370 L'Enfant Promenade S.W. #800, Washington, D.C. 20024. Beverly La Haye believes that "Clinton's unconditional embrace of the militant homosexual agenda is a radical assault on traditional values in America." NSME legislation accepts homosexuality as a genetic inheritance, does not condemn, but does not advocate freedom of visual portrayal of homosexuals making love. For those who wish to watch, gay and lesbian sex action videos will be available for rental. Will Beverly accept the exaltation of human sexuality, and visual sexmaking between caring men and women? It is the twenty-first-century challenge to the religious right.

*CORAL RIDGE MINISTRIES, P.O. Box 407137, Fort Lauderdale, Florida 33340-7137. Dr. D. James Kennedy, who heads up this group, is on the same wavelength as Pat Robertson, Jerry Falwell, and Ralph Reed. Kennedy tried to change things with a nationwide survey excoriating the sick moralities of the mid-1990s. His response to NSME will be probably be unfavorable.

COUNCIL FOR DEMOCRATIC AND SECULAR HUMANISM. 3965 Rensch Road, Buffalo, New York 14228-2713. Headed up by Paul Kurtz, the council publishes a quarterly magazine, *Free Inquiry,* which offers articles by secular humanists. Their twenty-one-point statement of principles affirms NSME legislation, particularly the following: "We believe in the cultivation of moral excellence. We believe in common moral decencies: altruism, integrity, honesty, truthfulness, responsibility. Humanist ethics is amenable to critical rational guidance. There are normative standards that we discover together. Moral principles are tested by their consequences. We are deeply concerned with the moral excellence of our children." Humanists may have some problem accepting a merger of church and state based on the sacramentalizing of sex, but Prometheus Books of which Paul Kurtz is also CEO, published *The Immoral Reverend* (See addendum).

DELAWARE VALLEY SYNERGY, P.O. Box 1551 Bensalem, Pennsylvania 19020-5551. A social club supporting open relationships in the Delaware/Pennsylvania area. "We have people of all different categories. Those who subscribe to swinging with many variations on that ranging from a kind of recreational sex to life-long friendships and involvement. There are those who remain monogamous but will become involved during a permissive party, and those who will become involved only with other couples." Obviously this group will interest Future Families of America.

*DOVE FOUNDATION, 4521 Broadmoor S.E., Grand Rapids, Michigan 49512. Director Dick Rolphe and his organization have reviewed fifteen thousand films, seeking only those that are "family friendly." As of mid-1994 only 720 have received the Dove seal of approval, which hundreds of video stores put on specific cassettes to rent. Obviously no R or X. When the self-imposed ratings become law Dove may have to change their views on what is "family friendly."

DOWN THERE PRESS, P.O. Box 2086, Burlingame, California 94011-2086. Headed up by Joani Blank, who says the group is "the nation's only independent publisher devoted exclusively to the publication of sexual health books for children and adults." Blank is also author of *The Sexuality Library Mail Order Catalogue,* which gives information on more than 350 sexual self-help and erotic books and videos. Obviously a resource for K-12 weekly Human sexuality seminars.

*EAGLE FORUM, Box 618, Alton, Illinois 62002. Headed up by Phyllis Schlafly, who should embrace the GLUE program since it creates the environment for sexual absintence until seventeen, but, alas, she undoubtedly believes in "no sex" until marriage, and wouldn't approve of FFAC.

ESALEN INSTITUTE, Big Sur, California 93290. Conceived by Michael Murphy who is still in charge after more than twenty-five years, Esalen and its staff have explored, and continue to explore, sexual and inter-personal relationships and the possibilities, and potential of new marital styles and expanded families. They could work closely with the Future Families of America Commission.

ELYSIUM INSTITUTE, 814 Robinson Road, Topanga Canyon, California 90290. Ed Lange, the director, offers to Californians and people worldwide the experience of clothing-optional living. Nonprofit, with year-round seminars, the organization explores all aspects of marital relationships and encourages overall body healthfulness and the enjoyment of the natural human body. A quarterly magazine, *Journal of the Senses,* offers articles such as "On Being in Love All of the Time."

FAMILY ABUNDANCE NETWORK, P.O. Box 7766, Portland, Maine 04122. A Northeast regional resource, headed up by Wes Nickerson, dedicated to celebrating family diversity, including extended families, same-gendered families, intentional families, cooperative households, coparenting, nurture networks, and polyfidelity. Obviously, rooters for NSME.

FAMILY SYNERGY, P.O. Box 3073, Huntington Beach, California 92605-3073. Founded more than twenty years ago, the group is "non-profit, volunteer-run, educational organization for people interested in non-possessive, caring interpersonal relationships. We believe that people can live fuller, more rewarding lives, achieving more of their potential, if they develop the awareness of their freedom of choice concerning interpersonal relationship styles, and that given an increased awareness, many will select open, multiply committed relationships. In the mid-1990s Family Synergy was experiencing organizational problems but is sure to survive in some form.

THE FEMINIST MAJORITY FOUNDATION, P.O. Box 96780, Washington, D.C. Headed up by Eleanor Smeal who, among other goals, is trying to resolve the anti-abortionist war against RU 486 and make it generally available to eliminate pregnancies up to 63 days after impregnation. But NSME approaches are a better solution to eliminate teenage pregnancies, and RU 486 is not a completely private decision since it requires medical supervision.

FOCUS ON THE FAMILY, Colorado Springs, Colorado 80995. Promoting teen sexual abstinence before marriage, they may be in agreement with the idea of NSME legislation but probably will be totally shocked by the GLUE approach and sexual Rite of Passage at seventeen, which is more realistic and bridges a five-year delay or more before a wedding ring.

GANAS FOUNDATION, 135 Corson Avenue, Staten Island, New York 10301. A group of people who consider themselves "a family of love" organized in groups of varying size. Currently sixty of them live together in five large adjoining Victorian houses. Ganas's social and political goals are (1) the capacity for autonomy, (2) the ability of individuals to govern actively and well, and (3) the willingness to care about one another and the world at large. Obviously, Ganas is the vanguard of the twenty-first century.

HARPER-SAN FRANCISCO, 151 Union Street, Suite 4, San Francisco, California 94111. A publisher whose many books in print (price of their catalogue $2) reflect the growing search of millions of Americans trying to find both sexual and spiritual answers. Harper offers books with Christian, Gnostic, and Asian religious answers.

HEALING ARTS, Box 2939, Venice, California, offers a six-hour video based on Margo Anand's book *The Art of Sexual Ecstasy* in which "you can learn unique ways to awaken your sexual energies based on ancient Tantric practices . . . and honoring the sexual union as a bridge between body and soul." It is a video that will be used in both GLUE programs during the human values seminars.

HAELIX-PLUS PUBLICATIONS, Box 265, Suite 93, Scotland, Connecticut 06264. A center for wholeness and transformation of consciousness created and organized by Genia Pauli Haddon, a minister of the United Church of Christ. Her 1993 book *Unifying Sex, Self and Spirit* should be a source book for the clergy who are reaffirming NSME legislation.

INSTITUTE FOR RATIONAL EMOTIVE THERAPY, 45 East 65th Street, New York, New York. Headed up by Albert Ellis, who has written many books, including a classic, *Sex Without Guilt.* He publishes the quarterly journal *Rational Living,* subtitled *Rational Emotive Theory,* which would be taught early in K-12 education and continuing into the GLUE programs. The book reveals very persuasively that most people keep harboring profound self-defeating beliefs, and rarely can change unless they learn how to act against them. Summed up by Epictetus (first century A.D.): "People are disturbed—not by things but by the views they take of them."

INSTITUTE FOR NOETIC SCIENCES, 475 Gate Five Road, #300, Sausalito, California 94965. Founded by Edgar Mitchell, one of the six astronauts who walked on the moon, the name is derived from the Greek word *nous,* meaning mind, intelligence, or ways of knowing. Noetic science studies the mind and diverse ways of knowing that will be constantly explored in GLUE human values seminars. While not a religion, the Institute explores all aspects of the mind and body interrelationships in areas that include psychic research, altered states of consciousness, and homeopathic medicine, with a continuous Gaia approach to life and the environment.

INTERFACE, 55 Wheeler Street, Cambridge, Massachusetts 02138-1168. Headed up by Roger Paine, for twenty years Interface has offered continuous seminars,and conferences with a wide array of teachers in every profession. In their words, "it is an education center to explore those trends in health, personal growth, science and religion which excite and encourage people to seek new ways of living, expand personal horizons, and join with others to create a better world. Other similar centers are the ROWE CENTER in New England, the OPEN CENTER in New York, OASIS in Chicago, and HOLLYHOCK in British Columbia. From the people who run these workshops and conferences are many potential members of the Future Families of America Commission.

KIRKRIDGE, Bangor, Pennsylvania 18013. Founded by John Oliver Nelson, a Presbyterian minister, in 1942, Kirkridge, spanning 270 acres in the Pocono Mountains, continues to "reach out, in seminars and conferences, in our media-dominated culture to value lifestyles more Celtic than Roman, more sect-type than 'church-type,' more Dionysian than Apollonian, more reformed than established—a place where praying Christians have found picketing Christians both enriching each other." An ideal place to create a new merger of the church and state with the common goal of a re-evaluation of human sexuality as the core of religion.

*LIBERTY ALLIANCE, P.O. Box 6000, Madison Heights, Virginia 24572. In 1994 Jerry Falwell, in a multimillion mailing, asked, "Should I reactivate the Moral Majority and help bring this nation back to moral sanity?"—which, by his definition, is a nation under one God who doesn't approve of homosexuals, abortion, feminists, New Agers, or humanists. Moral sanity can only be achieved with NSME legislation. Falwell and his friends have no other workable alternatives!

LIFE STYLE ORGANIZATION, 2641 W. La Palma Ave., Anaheim, California 92801. Founded by Bob McGinley more than twenty years ago, the group is the parent organization of independent swing clubs throughout North America. Life Style runs an Annual Lifestyle Convention every August in Las Vegas, at which several thousand swingers listen to and participate in workshops and seminars covering all aspects of human sexuality, run by speakers who have doctorates, like Dr. Albert Freedman, who once was copublisher of *Penthouse* and *Forum* magazines. The three-day convention features many exhibitors of sexual products, an erotic art exhibition, and a masquerade ball where outrageous, sex-enhancing clothing is the motif of the evening. McGinley also runs "Life style Cruises and vacations to all parts of the world where being naked and spouse exchange is a way of life." As with other swinger organizations, many swingers may find sacramentalizing human sexuality too inhibiting, but most will eventually discover that family stability is the sine qua non of sane sexuality.

LIVE THE DREAM, Success Center, 6454 Van Nuys Blvd #150, Van Nuys, California 91401. An organization in their words "for those originally inspired by novels written by Robert A. Heinlein, *Stranger in a Strange Land, Time Enough for Love,* and *The Moon Is a Harsh Mistress,* Robert H. Rimmer's *The Harrad Experiment, Proposition 31,* and *Love Me Tomorrow,* and Marion Zimmer's *Bradley Spell Sword* and *Forbidden Tower.* People are welcome who are ready to live such alternative lifestyles as group marriage, cooperative living and expanded family sharing." Members meet with other groups such as the Harrad Community, More House, and Expanded Families at the Renaissance Pleasure Faire, where "many long-term committed relationships have developed, and continue with current marital statuses, with both spouses' acceptance."

NATURISTS, P.O. Box 132, Oshkosh, Wisconsin 54902. Headed up by Lee Baxaendall, among other things the group publishes the full-color *World Guide to Nude Beaches and Recreation.* Very much an activist group, it has tried for many years to convince the federal government to make it official there is no nationwide law that bans nudity on federal lands.

NATIONAL COALITION AGAINST CENSORSHIP, 275 Seventh Avenue, New York, New York 10001, Leanne Katz, executive director. The group wages a continual fight against censorship that the "radical right" would impose. Of twenty-first century interest the Coalition includes the Union of Hebrew Congregations, the

Unitarian/Universalist Association, and the United Methodist Congregations, all of whom may be among the first to invite the joys and wonders of human sexuality and a loving, dancing, erotic, spiritual God back into the their sanctuaries early in the twenty-first century.

NATIONAL ORGANIZATION FOR WOMEN. 1000 16th Street, N.W., #700, Washington D.C. Headed up by Pat Ireland, NOW's purpose is "to bring women into the full mainstream of American society." This aim will take a giant step forward with NSME legislation. They should enthusiastically endorse FFAC, ROSP, K-16 education, Self-imposed ratings on all the arts, and "being naked where it's convenient to be naked."

*NATIONAL RIGHT TO LIFE COMMITTEE, 419 Seventh Street, N.W., Washington, D.C. 20004-2293. Headed up by Wenda Franz, the Committee has affiliated organizations in every state. Will they endorse the NSME legislation—and an optional federally funded K-12 human sexuality seminar that will not only teach birth control but create a new environment for teenagers to delay sexual merger until they are seventeen—a combination that will make abortion a nonissue?

NEGATIVE POPULATION GROWTH, 210 The Plaza, P.O. Box 1206, Teaneck, New Jersey 07666. Headed up by Donald Mann, it campaigns for a twenty-first-century, religious and political sexual morality that encourages couples and single parents to have no more than two children, and a worldwide approach to zero population growth. They also dream of a cabinet-level Department of Population. The purpose could be better served with a cabinet-level Future Families of America, which would most certainly have population on the agenda.

NETWORK FOR A NEW CULTURE, P.O Box 14183, Scottsdale, Arizona 85267-4183. Headed up by Stephen Davis, a former state representative, the Center is affiliated with a "sister community" called ZEGG, developed by Dr. Dieter Duhm, who in his book *Eros Unredeemed* writes,

> The liberation of love is linked to a process of insight. This is a fact that needs to be emphasized because it runs contrary to the ideas we generally have about love. Most people regard love and sex as a matter of emotions, not as something of the mind. As long as love remains merely an emotional process it cannot last. Love which goes beyond mere emotion is not blind—it always makes you see. It is the element of life that brings awakening and knowledge. In ancient Hebrew sexuality and knowledge are linguistically identical, as in the symbol the Tree of Knowledge, or in Adam "knowing" Eve. In "knowing love" you stand to see your partner in a new way, and you can also start seeing love in a new way.

Both in the center in Arizona and at Zegg University in Berlin, the key word is "Compersion"—the opposite of jealousy. "Compersion," from Latin "com," meaning "with," and "per" meaning "totally," means essentially that you have overcome jealousy, separation, control, and possessiveness of other people. The center and Zegg's view of love offers the kind of freedom with caring commitment that underlies the ROSP teaching and the exchange of roommates during the four-year work/study program. Enthusiastic members of the center and Zegg will be able to help Future Families of America experiment, and explore long-lasting approaches to marriage and the family, monogamous and otherwise.

OMNIFIC DESIGNS WEST, P.O. Box 459, San Dimas, California, or 204 East 2nd Avenue, #407, San Mateo, California 94401. The group publishes *Loving Alternatives,* a bimonthly magazine that is a contact point for swing clubs, similar to Sandstone detailed by Gay Talese in his *Thy Neighbor's Wife.* Many people think that after the demise of Sandstone in the 1970s, plus a nationwide fear of AIDS, high-class catering to "swingers"—and presumably several million Americans who expand their sexual encounters with multiple partners, before and during monogamous marriage—is no longer a way of life in United States. Omnific Designs offers a series of X-rated videotapes under the label *American Connection Video Magazine,* which show that there are many very attractive resort-style swinger environments available in the mid-1990s in California, Washington, New Jersey, Michigan, and other areas. Swingers will endorse NSME legislation, but whether they are too sexually amorphous and could live within strong, committed family structures is questionable. On the other hand, in later life most gravitate toward mental/sexual merger with more structured groups.

OMEGA INSTITUTE FOR HOLISTIC STUDIES, RD 2, Box 377, Rhinebeck, New York 12572. Stephen Rechtschaffen, M.D., a co-founder, heads up Omega, which has been offering as many as two hundred summer workshops from June through September covering eleven aspects of body, gender, relationship, and family health. A perennial question to which the group seeks answers is, "How will we have to change, individually and collectively, to achieve a more balanced place for human beings in the web of life?" The NSME answer is that it won't happen except in dreams until we go beyond freedom and dignity and create a sexually sane moral and educational environment.

THE OPTIONS INSTITUTE, 2080 South Undermountain Road, Sheffield, Massachusetts 01257. Headed up by Barry Neil Kaufman and Samahria Lyte Kaufman, the group offers year-round programs in an idyllic environment for families and groups seeking to improve the quality of their lives by using the "Option Process—exchanging a negative outlook for a positive one," which has some relationship to Albert Ellis's rational emotive theories. In the twenty-first century, when K-16 education becomes a way of life, the various centers to explore emotional and sexual relationships will take on a different dimension as a new generation learns to cope with multiple relationships.

PEOPLE FOR THE AMERICAN WAY, 2000 M Street, N.W., #400, Washington, D.C., originated by Norman Lear, of television fame, headed up by Arthur J. Kropp. In its words, "People For is a leading force in efforts to defend pluralism, individuality, freedom of thought, expression, and religion, a sense of community and tolerance for others." The group publishes a monthly report, *Right Wing Watch*, that keeps track of the activities of what it calls the "radical right," most of whom are listed here with an asterisk as potential foes of NSME legislation. But, who knows, before the year 2000 they may see that they have no sane alternative. But Kropp is worried that in the short term the religious right is trying to "Christianize" the public schools . . . with an intermediate agenda of clearing the libraries, gutting sex education, and making a mockery of biology instruction."

PLANNED PARENTHOOD FEDERATION OF AMERICA, 810 Seventh Avenue, New York, New York 10019, headed up by Pamela J. Maraldo. While the NSME legislation is pro-choice, in a sexually sane society the reality-based sex education that Planned Parenthood has fought for many years, coupled with total teenage awareness that participating in the additional four-year GLUE programs means no children, will defuse the abortion problem. But during the twenty-first century, Planned Parenthood and the Future Families of America Commission will be working nationally and globally to guide family-planning efforts. A man and woman who wish to have more than two children are natural candidates for expanded families.

RESIST, One Summer Street, Somerville, Massachusetts 02143-9957. Funding groups working for peace and social justice for more than twenty-five years, among many other projects Resist has funded the Coalition for Positive Sexuality (Chicago), a group dedicated to getting "meaningful, effective, peer-oriented, positive and safe-sex information into the hands of teens and creating a debate about the lack of meaningful sex education in the schools."

THE RESPONSIVE COMMUNITY, 714 German Library, George Washington University, Washington, D.C. 20052, created by Amitai Etzioni. With coeditors and an editorial board composed of professors in the major American colleges and universities, the publication promotes the concept of communitarianism. Basically, communitarians are searching for a new national consensus "beyond rights, beyond selfishness, beyond little me." The issues are saving family structures, providing moral education without indoctrination, building neighborhood communities, and the role of values. "Is our culture being devalued and vulgarized? How can it be enabled without censorship? How can morals be revised without busybodies meddling in personal affairs? How can we recommit moral values without personal excesses?" Communitarians will find most of the answers in the NSME legislation.

*RUTHERFORD INSTITUTE, P.O. Box 7482, Charlottesville, Virginia 22902, headed up by John Rutherford, who contests the ACLU and other organizations, which he believes are undermining our religious freedoms. With a common church/state point of view that New Sexual Morality and Education legislation proposes, more harmony should reign.

SECRET GARDEN, 1352 Yukon Way, #20, Noavto, California 94947. Publisher Ray Stubbs offers beautiful, erotic, quality paperbacks. They include *Tantric Massage: An Illustrated Guide for Meditative Sexuality, Sensual Ceremony,* and *Sacred Orgasms,* three separate books, lovingly illustrated with joyous sexual action. These books comprise the Secret Garden trilogy. He offers many other books that could also be used in K-11-12 sex-education courses including *The Clitoral Kiss: A Fun Guide to Oral Sex* and *Women of Light: The New Sacred Prostitute* (which contains his fascinating autobiography), as well as an extensive Tantric Massage videotape during which the masseuse, female or male, doesn't neglect the genitals of the person being massaged.

SEX INFORMATION AND EDUCATIONAL COUNCIL OF THE UNITED STATES (SIECUS), 130 West 42nd Street, #2500, New York, New York 10036, headed up by Debra Haffner, a Unitarian Universalist, (see below). According to Haffner, in the mid-1990's "90 percent of Americans want sexuality education for their children—because only about 20 percent postpone sex until marriage." Using the K-12 Guidelines for Comprehensive Sexuality Education, the NSME legislation offering optional federal funding goes a giant step further and teaches the history of sexual devaluation. Will SIECUS approve?

SIRENS, A VISIT TO A POLYFIDELITOUS COMMUNITY, by Robin Hill, 454 Dodge Rd., Frewsburg, New York 14378. Robin describes an intentional community of women who invite specific men to live with them in their carefully planned household. She never gives the location but her forty-five-page, single-spaced description of the day-to-day workings is well worth reading.

TARCHER, JEREMY, 5858 Wilshire Boulevard, Los Angeles, California 90036. Jeremy is the West Coast publisher of the *Art of Sexual Ecstasy* by Margo Anand—a book that all K-11-12 students will read in their sex-education courses and will want to own. In his catalogue you'll find many other fascinating books on sex and loving.

TOUCHSTONE NETWORK, 27 Music Square East, #169, Nashville, Tennessee 37202. A contact service for people exploring alternatives to monogamy. A late twentieth-century straw in the wind.

THE THIRD MILLENNIUM ADVOCATE FOR THE FUTURE, INC., 817 Broadway, New York, New York 10003. In its words: "The mission of the Third Millennium is to provide a voice for the post-baby boom generation by advocating solutions to economic stagnation, social fragmentation and environmental deterioration so that all Americans may enjoy prosperous and promising lives in the next millennium." The group publishes a quarterly newsletter, *Slacker,* and runs an on-line network transom.

UNITARIAN/UNIVERSALIST ASSOCIATION, 25 Beacon Street, Boston, Massachusetts 02108-2803. The only organized religion that has dared to offer a sexual-related course, *About Your Sexuality* (first in 1971 and revised in 1994), that can be taught in the church as a part of continuing religious education. The course, which runs between thirty and forty sessions, goes far beyond the SIECUS K-12 recommendations, and what is offered in the mid-1990s in most secondary schools. In all probability Unitarian/Universalists will be among the first churches to champion NSME legislation.

UTNE READER, published bimonthly by the Lens Publishing Company, Inc., 1624 Harmon Place, Minneapolis, Minnesota 55403. Headed up by Eric Utne, the *Utne Reader* publishes what it calls "the best of the alternative press." In every issue there is an extensive description of hundreds of magazines, newsletters, and books produced by many more advocacy groups who will be fascinated by and will endorse NSME legislation.

WAY OF THE MOUNTAIN LEARNING CENTER, P.O. Box 2434, Durango, Colorado 81302. Dolores Chapelle, publishes a newsletter that networks many writers seeking for a pantheistic road to God and personal transcendence in nature. Her book *Sacred Land, Sacred Sex, Rapture of the Deep,* offers a New Age approach to religion that should appeal to Al Gore.

Part Two

Where We've Been and Where We're Going

Utopia without reason—without dream—cannot get us out of this impasse. There is only one way left with reason and dream, which will take us out of the bad place which is not out of place but in place—an entopia.

—Constantine Doxidias

19

Twenty-First-Century Marriage and Family Styles—Beyond Monogamy

If you are still on board, you may be dubious—agreeing that the educational aspects of NSME legislation seem practical but in the area of the new sexual morality are a bit utopian. Let me tell you about utopias. During the twentieth century, other than Edward Bellamy who wrote *Looking Backward* and a fascinating sequel, *Equality,* there have been few utopias in the complete sense of proposing a completely new society from the top down covering every aspect of life from economics through interpersonal relationships of all kinds. I tried it in one novel, *Love Me Tomorrow,* but the publisher got so incensed with the lengthy description of my new economics that he put a footnote in the book and told the readers, who he assumed would be bored, to skip the next twenty or thirty pages if they wanted to get on with the story.

Actually, I'm not a utopianist, I'm a futurist—proposing what I have, with a chuckle, called achievable utopias in the areas of premarital and postmarital relationships. My proposal for a cabinet position for Future Families of America with a secretary of FFAC who is actively trying to involve all of us in the problems of marriage and family, is futuristic thinking that must happen! Strong family structures of some kind are just as essential as national defense. Maybe more so. Without families who believe in a future for their children—and that includes education and some upward financial ability—there is nothing much to defend. We spend trillions on defense. Spending on families and education will give us a nation worth defending and emulating.

You can go over the statistics, which I have repeated more than once in part 1, and if you are young enough to be alive in the next twenty-five years you can start worrying. Just as worrisome as the disappearing nuclear family is the over-worked structure of the late- twentieth-century family, which for economic survival requires husband, wife, and older children to work. Equally dangerous to the family is crowding, families who can't afford much personal space or who live in buildings where touching earth can only be achieved by getting in an automobile and driving miles. What happens when there are a hundred million more of us? As in China, sooner than we think, we may be forced to redefine some of our beliefs on human rights.

A Future Families of America Commission is inevitable. In addition to reinforcing monogamy, it can set up "game plans" for possible new-style families—invite people to participate for periods of five years or more, and in the process, with the help of the participants, discover and evaluate the problems, and whether certain new family groupings should be legalized or even given tax preferences.

During the past twenty-five years, in my novels, I have envisioned many possibilities. Here is a survey of some of them. Keep in mind that the various proposals are interwoven into story lines that explore the interpersonal problems, and will keep you reading. In the late 1960s and 1970s millions of readers were intrigued. As I write this in 1994, most of the novels are out of print, but they all appeared in large paperback editions and you may be able to find them. So beginning with *The Rebellion of Yale Marratt,* here's bigamy, which I prefer to call:

Ménàge à Trois

In the novel, which takes place between 1939 and just after World War II, Yale Marratt is very much in love with Cynthia. They both graduate from the same college but she's Jewish, and neither family approves the marriage. Cynthia breaks off the engagement tragically, and ultimately marries a college instructor.

During the war in India, Yale is stationed on a base in the Assam Valley (now Bangladesh) where the Air Transport Command is ferrying pipe over the Hump into China. With our allies, the premise was that we might have to fight the Japanese (who had already occupied most of China) on land, all the way back to the Pacific. The pipe was the first step—to supply oil and gasoline to our planes, trucks, and tanks on the Burma Road. Still in love with Cynthia, not knowing why she left him, Yale meets Anne, a Red Cross worker on the base, falls in love, and marries her in a Hindu wedding ceremony. War-time marriages in combat areas were not permitted, but the marriage is legal in the United States. Yale is transferred to China, and loses track of Anne. Although, unknown to him, she is pregnant, she never contacts him. She thinks he's still in love with Cynthia and she was a convenient war-time "shack up." The war is over. Yale searches for Anne but learns that Cynthia, whose husband was killed in an automobile accident after the war, is pregnant.

Yale marries Cynthia, then discovers that Anne is alive. He brings the two women together, and after a long, tip-toe relationship, they decide that living together in a ménàge à trois is preferable to divorce. In essence, they all really enjoy each other as people, and simply have to solve the problem of sharing one man. Charged with bigamy by Yale's father, the novel begins and concludes in a Connecticut courtroom where Yale and his wives try to change the laws and legalize bigamy.

This is obviously not the story of a guy who marries two women who don't know each other, or who is a Mormon—one whose ascent into Heaven, in the old days, was predicated on the number of wives he had. Rather, it's about three people who could have divorced, or lived together illegally, but love each other and want to bring up their children in a family structure that has the same legitimacy as monogamy.

As an aside, filmmakers, right after the book was published, had it on option for ten years, but no one has yet dared to film the story. The assumption was, and still is, that American women detest the idea, and would never accept another woman in a triadic relationships with their husband. Times change. I have since updated it as a screen play to the Vietnam War. Eventually, some filmmaker will realize that twenty-first century women for multiple reasons are intrigued with ménàge à trois—either way, two women and a man, or two men and a woman.

While I have no actual figures, ménàge à trois relationships are a family pattern for hundreds of thousands of households. During the years that *Yale Marratt* was in print, I received thousands of letters from enthusiastic readers, male and female, young and old, living together as one man and two women, or two men and one woman.

Threesomes are an ideal solution for older women who live longer and in many cases can find a reasonably able man to join them in one of their homes, or vice versa. When my mother was in her nineties, her only husband dead for many years, she would have married a man in his late eighties, but they were better off in terms of Social Security to stay single, proving that many twentieth-century laws have to catch up with twenty-first-century reality.

Writing in 1978 in the *Los Angeles Times* (the article is reprinted in a collection of my essays, *The Love Adventurers*) Susan Haggerty, a young black woman, suggested that "polygamy is an alternative worth examining for the black race." She based her belief on the facts that there were many more black women than black men and that there was a high black divorce rate caused by infidelity. Haggerty believed, "a polygamous relationship would be a more honest relationship with a man being able to acknowledge his children by other women."

But, despite Mormon successes in the nineteenth century, polygamy, or bigamy, is not a practical twenty-first-century solution. On the other hand, triads, or ménàges à trois are workable and are a form of marital relationship beyond monogamy in which the FFAC cannot only fund experiments but lay the groundwork for legalization. Why legalize? Because all of us want and need some kind of structure and commitment with others in our lives, and monogamy is not the only way possible to achieve it.

Many highly educated women, career oriented or not, may discover that sharing a husband with another woman is an ideal solution. Highly motivated women often have a problem finding a man whose interests or hobbies, particularly in the humanities, parallel their own. Many career-oriented women would be happy to share a husband with a second wife who might be quite willing to be daytime mother to both of their children. Or two working wives, along with their one husband, would have three incomes, thus making it possible for any one of them to take a work vacation, or work on different schedules, or hire a nanny to take care of young children during the day. Keep in mind, too, that there are ten million unmarried or previously married women in the United States who, with or without children, would be happy to live in an group marriage and escape their single household lifestyle. Legalizing ménàge à trois relationships creates an approving environment for them. In reverse, many women would be happy to take care of two husbands sexually, and with any two out of three working they would be stronger economically than a monogamous family.

Corporate Marriages and Families

In my novel *Proposition 31,* I proposed the legalization of group marriages of up to three monogamous couples, past the age of 33, who could combine their families into a family corporation in which all adults and children are equal shareholders. In the story, two couples, each with two children, live next door to each other in San Pedro, California. For many reasons they are on the verge of divorce. Within a plausible story line, one of the husbands, a professor of sociology, trying to find a solution to their marital problems, which includes his wife being pregnant by the other husband, reads to all of them from Christopher Alexander's essay, "The City as a Mechanism for Maintaining Human Contact." It offers insights for FFAC.

"What social mechanism is required to make contacts intimate?" Alexander asks.

> In preindustrial society, intimate contacts were sustained by primary groups. A primary group is a small group of people characterized by intimate face-to-face association and co-operation. The three most universal primary groups were the

family, the neighborhood group, and the children's play group. Many anthropologists and sociologists have taken the view that man *cannot live* without primary groups. But the open society is no longer centered around placebased groups, and the very slight acquaintances that do form around artificial neighborhoods [created by city planners and architects in modern high-rise apartments and condo developments] are trivial; they are not based on human desire. The only vestige of the primary group that still remains is the nuclear family [Alexander wrote this in 1967]. The family still functions as a mechanism for sustaining intimate contact. But where the extended family of preindustrial society contained many adults, the modern nuclear family contains two adults. This means that each of these adult-child relationships has at most *one* intimate contact within his family.

Alexander goes on to exclude children as adequate intimate contacts because the adult-child relationship is essentially one-sided in this area, but he sets the stage for group marriages:

> *I believe that intimate contacts are essential for human survival* and indeed each person requires not one, but several given intimate contacts at any one time. I believe that the primary groups which sustained intimate contacts were an essential functional part of traditional social systems, and since they are now obsolete, it is essential that we invent new social mechanisms consistent with the direction that society is taking, and yet able to to sustain the intimate contacts that we need.

Offering another view of the major problem of the disappearing family in his book *The Rise of the Unmeltable Ethics,* Michael Novak writes: "The ethnic culture seems to offer all the things that rebellious young Americans now seem to be seeking—[the book was written in the 1960s] a denser family life, a richer life of the senses and instincts." By contrast, Novak points out, in many typical American families "no culture was ever so systematically based on solitariness; for each child a separate room, a separate tv set, separate everything to the full extent of possibility. The constant search for the authentic self reflects this solitariness. When you have to seek your roots, you have already lost the battle."

Novak wrote those words before the "information superhighway" became the futuristic dream of the mid-1990s. None of the enthusiasts for this futuristic nightmare seem aware that it would be a breeding ground for mental sickness. Family grouping, nuclear family or not, will be inundated with five hundred channels plus interactive television and computers. Individuals in small families will no longer need anyone except the tube, a mouse, and a keyboard to make contact with other humans. It won't happen, of course. Even in a diminished, far-from-soul-satisfying way, people seek other people. During the late twentieth century, they tried to make "safe" communal contact in movies, restaurants, and shopping malls without threatening their privacy, or growing inability to share their thoughts and emotions with others.

Combining two families as I proposed in *Proposition 31,* resolves the human need for deeper friendships with more than one person. In this novel I envisioned Future Families of America, which is created by the two couples who have become activists. Agreeing to share their lives, determined to create a family structure in which their children can function proudly and happily, they try to make corporate marriage legal in the state of California. Here's the basis of the proposition:

> To the Secretary of State of the State of California: We the undersigned, being duly qualified voters, and registered voters in the State of California, and constituting no less in number than eight percent of the votes cast for candidates for Governor in the last election, hereby petition the Secretary of State and request the following proposed law, to be known as the California Corporate Family Law, be submitted directly to the electors of the State of California for their adoption or rejection at the next succeeding general election provided by law. The text of the proposed law is as follows:
>
> The people of the State of California enact an act to permit not more than three married couples, past the age of thirty, to join together in a joint form of marriage to be known as group marriage or corporate marriage, establishing a family unit that will exist independently of the individual members and have all the rights now permitted under the existing laws of corporations, such as family corporations to appoint their legal members by marriage, or from the issue of these marriages, directors to govern the affairs of these family corporations and to continue with their full human powers to carry on the purposes of corporate living, which will be construed as follows: To create a joint family environment for the financial security and independence of its members, and to provide all members an environment that fulfills their needs, both emotional and economic, so they can live fully self-actualized lives and develop to the full limit their abilities as human beings.
>
> It further being a provision of the law that such Corporate Families, once established, may on a vote of a majority of the directors past the age of twenty-one dissolve the Family Corporation, if there are no children under the age of eighteen within the unit, and if there are children under the age of eighteen, that the Corporation may be dissolved by a majority vote, if any of the original incorporators shall undertake to assume responsibility for all children under the age of eighteen, and to maintain a suitable home environment for them that shall be in conformity with the original purpose of the corporation. It is further permitted to the incorporators to assume for legal purposes one surname for all

members of the corporation, which may either be a single agreed-upon surname, or a new joint name combining the surname of the original incorporators.

A few years after *Proposition 31* appeared in print Lloyd Barbee, a state representative from Milwaukee, Wisconsin, tried to legalize corporate marriages and homosexual marriages in the state of Wisconsin, and introduced a bill that would permit a man or woman to marry more than one spouse. Barbee's bill never came up for vote (the entire bill is included in *The Love Adventurers*), but it has elements that will interest the Future Families of America Commission. Here's a brief excerpt:

> Monogamy is not a sacred edict or natural law. It is a reactively recent statutory standard set up and enforced against the will of a large number of individual human beings. Thus the State has adopted one ancient cult, or religious view, over another. . . . Adults are capable of building private and personal healthy and rewarding relationships between one another, or groups. Unless the specific terms of such an arrangement pose a significant threat to the public well being, society should exercise restraint in applying any control over these arrangements. There is no social purpose served by our present laws, which force people to live monogamously or heterosexually.

There are many aspects of corporate marriage that can be explored by FFAC. One of the beneficent effects for children is that a group marriage of two or three husbands and wives could not only provide security for the children but offer them different male or female role models in intimate day-to-day relationships that they could obtain in no other way. Couples willing to experiment with funding from FFAC could gradually determine whether a three-couple family with children would be a better arrangement than a two-couple family and might mitigate potential jealousies.

In reality, the living arrangements should be adaptable, and an agreement should be reached so that at least one adult is at home each day. Corporate families could expand smaller homes, or take over complete floors in some high rises, or portions of them, and they could even organize space in older, nineteenth-century-style homes that were built to accommodate many relatives so that an older generation of parents could live with the families, thus eliminating the necessity of day care centers and, ultimately, nursing homes. There are many fascinating twenty-first-century-style family environments that FFAC can fund with the participants maintaining an ongoing record of joys and trials and tribulations.

Young people past thirty who have completed the GLUE ROSP program are ideal candidates to experiment with the many facets of corporate marriage, and the significant economic and tax advantages that will occur when it is legalized. Those who have completed GLUE but not ROSP, should experience at least a year of "courtship" during which couples of the same age discover their similarities and differences. After a few years of marriage most couples have met at least one other husband and wife with whom they have much in common, and they spend much leisure time together. The women often become mentally more intimate than their husbands, but both men may find the other wife attractive. In corporate marriage, both men, who probably directly or inadvertently play the male power role with their wives, must learn how to cede the power role between themselves and the women. Once they've made the big break into separate sexual encounters with each other's spouses, they should avoid discussing the sexual action, or make sexual comparisons: "He/she is more fun in bed," etc, that devalue the relationships. Couples who really learn to like each other in corporate marriages will discover, as a group, how to appreciate each other's good and bad traits, and that being lovingly, laughingly, noncritical with each other is a great learning experience.

Confamiliums: On the Road to New Family Structures

In my novel *The Premar Experiments,* you'll find the seeding ground for GLUE and the ROSP option. Unlike in *Harrad,* I envisioned a group of students from low-income families living with their roommates of the other sex in tenement houses in a racially mixed area of Boston called Topham's Corner, similar to the real-life Uphams Corner. The Premar students get involved with the families living in the area and as a part of their human values studies create what they call "Confamiliums"—meaning "with family."

A Confamilium could comprise any group of cooperative households. It is another approach to stabilizing families that will be explored by FFAC. In the novel, a Confamilium is proposed by the undergraduate students that would be composed of sixteen families living in "three deckers" (tenement houses) in this area of South Boston. These houses were built around the turn of the century in the Eastern Seaboard cities and there are many similar ones in San Francisco. In the mid-1990s hundreds of thousands of these buildings are still standing with three families living on separate floors. They are actually superior accommodations, providing more intimacy between families, and closer to the earth (with small backyards), than any high-rise apartments.

But the concept of Confamiliums could be developed in different-style housing arrangements. In the particular Confamilium I explored, the cooperative grouping of forty-eight families comprised ninety-six adults and eight-four children under the age of eighteen. Together they owned (with mortgages) forty-eight apartments in sixteen separate buildings as a Confamilium corporation. If the original incorporators moved or died, their shares could be sold back to the corporation or inherited immediately by family members. The value of the shares could be determined at any one time by dividing the total shares into the net worth, or current market value of the entire property, and with continuing inflation should increase in value.

Confamiliums would be more communally oriented than condominium developments. As I projected it, the Confamilium shareholders would agree to assign a predetermined portion of each shareholder's income to cover not only housing costs but the cost of food. A well-organized Confamilium would be able to build or buy a separate building that could be used for everything from a gymnasium to a meeting house and communal dining room for the members.

Each Confamilium member, which would include the children, would be assigned one week a month to communal kitchen and cooking duties, and youngsters would wait on tables on a rotating basis. In this respect, a Confamilium is equivalent to an urban kibbutz, except that the members do not work communally, but earn their living in regular working environments. Privacy of living is maintained in a Confamilium. Members of the Confamilium would run a cooperative food store or take advantage of wholesale purchasing at chains like Costco. Within the community building, the Confamilium could run an English-style pub for members that could have areas for children and teenagers with ping pong tables, pool tables, and a soft drink bar.

Day care would be provided by older Confamilium members at minimal cost, and there would be space in the communal buildings set aside with a few beds for simple nursing care, offered by members to other members who are ill but don't require hospitalization. A teenage dormitory environment might also be offered to give young people a loosely supervised opportunity to escape the domination of their families and to give them an area where they could do their homework together with friendly help for older Confamilium members.

I also envisioned, as a part of the Confamilium proposal, which could function with new housing as well as rehabilitated housing, that eventually a network of Confamiliums would make it possible to change jobs or swap ownership for Confamilum apartments or housing in other areas.

This is another area in which the Future Families Commission could lay the foundation for extended families by the merger of monogamous couples who in this case would still maintain sexual privacy, with an older generation of cooperating families, merging young and old in smaller environments. This is the only solution to huge, impersonal, government-operated or funded day care centers, senior citizen centers, and nursing homes. There are many organizations and groups in the United States involved in cooperative family ventures who will endorse Future Families of America and the entire NSME legislation, which is designed to create new-style, sexually sane family structures. Those willing to experiment need help and guidance.

Synergamy in a Sexually Sane Society

All of these potential postmarital relationships have two features that do not prevail in swinging, open marriage, or adultery today. They presume that the participants are not "one-night standers" and because they are on the same brain level, they are absolutely sure (even by prior testing) that they are not carriers of STDs, and the relationships are long-term, structured commitments of various kinds. Enjoying a sexual relationship beyond monogamy that is socially approved by the church or state is another aspect of *The Cry for Myth*, which Rollo May explores in his most recent book (W. W. Norton, 1991). I will say more about this later but first let's take a look at synergamy, which I proposed in my novel *Thursday, My Love*.

Angela and Jonathan Adams, in their late forties, are not unhappily married to Jim and Janice. They have grown children in college or just married. How they meet on Thursdays and fall in love is the subject of the novel. Divorce and remarriage is not what they are seeking. In his Canadian printing plant, Jonathan has discovered a book the company is printing, called *Synergamy*, written by a Jesuit priest, Father Je Songe Lereve, about a new marriage form that he is offering—synergamous marriages. Based on the word "synergy," defined by Buckminster Fuller as "the behaviour of whole systems unpredicted by separately observed behaviour of any of the system's separate parts or any subassembly of the system's parts," and made from the Greek words *syn,* meaning "together," and *gamos,* meaning "marriage," Father Lereve has proposed that some of the problems that now occur in extramarital affairs—such as divorce—could be resolved in a new, structured comarital commitment for those who wished to undertake it. Synergamy and synergamous marriages would bring the second relationship out into to open not so much as a legal form of marriage, but as an emotional commitment, in a church ceremony, in which the adulterous or extramarital relationship is given a status approximately equal to the first marriage commitment.

In a perfectly operating synergamous marriage, the spouses making the second commitment would be responsible for any children emerging from the second marriage, though in most cases synergamous marriages would be childless as a matter of preference as well as population control. Financial responsibility for the second family embraced in the second marriage would be optional. Thus the original husband and wife would be able to relate to a second wife and husband without destroying the original monogamous marriage.

Father Lereve points out,

> The contemplated relationship in a synergamous marriage, unlike a group marriage, would be two separate dyads . . . two males relating to two separate females and vice versa, but with no necessity for a complete family relationship, as would occur in a group marriage. It would be assumed in synergamous marriages involving two couples who previously knew each other that the spouses would change households, or basic home environments, a few days each week, and enjoy complete involvement with the children of the second spouse equivalent to the love and involvement with their blood children. Synergamous marriages might lead to corporate marriages, but not necessarily.
>
> Synergamous marriages are predicated on the fact that most individuals can find a member of the opposite sex with whom they can relate fully, but it is considerably more difficult for a monogamous couple, a dyad, to effect a mutual relationship with another monogamous couple not only in the areas of sexual exchange, but in simultaneous, multilateral, interpersonal encounters of a quartet or sextet.

The vows that a couple would take are given in the novel. Angela and Jonathan are synergamously married by Father Lereve:

> Angela and Jonathan . . . as lovers you come to this humble church to consecrate your love in a form of marriage which has no sanction in laws of the State, nor, as yet, of the Church. Yet the truth is that the marriage or commitment of two human beings to care for each other has neither strength or stability because of any divine origin, nor sacramental quality, nor pronouncements of man, but rather because individuals dare to transcend their own egos and in the process be each other."
>
> Father Lereve smiled as he noticed that Angela and Adam were holding hands.
>
> "There is no ring in this ceremony. The words I ask you to repeat after me are only as strong as your joy and love for each other as interacting human beings. Repeat after me this synergamous bond you willingly assume. 'I, Angela . . . I, Jonathan . . . with no less love for my present spouse and my family do accept the commitment to love and to cherish . . . , You, Jonathan . . . You, Angela, repeat after me, I am aware that my love for you does not modify my prior commitment to my husband . . . to my wife. While our relationship to each other is supportive, it should also grow in strength because it reinforces and strengthens and adds perspective to the nature of our love both for each other and our first spouses and children.' I pronounce you man and wife. May God love you!"

"LovXchanges" in a Sexually Sane Society

Once NSME becomes law and major churches reevaluate their teachings about sex, marriage, and the family, some form of synergamous-style relationships could be condoned and celebrated in church ritual. But "LovXchanges," as I detailed them in my novel *Come Live My Life,* could become the province of marriage counselors and family advisors who could easily create the kind of "dating" network that would make them a real adventure for many couples in different time frames of their marriages.

Here's the advertisement that Shari and Mark Silverman, a Jewish couple in their mid forties—he a professor at Boston University, she a social worker—and Charles and Roberta Atwood—he a millionaire radio/electronic chain store operator, she his former secretary—respond to. Both couples have been married fifteen years or more and have children, and the wives make the first household exchange.

> LovXchange. A guilt-free, postmarital adventure for carefully selected couples between thirty and fifty years of age who wish to "open" their marriages and experience an intimate, loving relationship with another couple. LovXchanges are arranged between couples living in different cities or in homes at least twenty miles apart in larger metropolitan areas. LovXchanges are arranged between wives and husbands who are free to make the household exchange for two-week periods at least twice a year. It is up to the LovXchangers whether or not their primary husbands and wives will meet each other. Unless otherwise requested, most matches are made on the basis of common interests, life objectives, and similarity of ages and income. The object of a LovXchange is a potentially long-lasting satellite relationship, and the growth experience of a modern, expanded family.

As a prelude to the novel, the *Manpars,* marriage counselors who run a LovXchange, answer the replies to this advertisement with a prospectus. Here is an excerpt from it, which should intrigue the Future Families of America Commission.

> We must warn you that LovXchanges, like monogamous marriage itself, are not for every one. LovXchangers must pass a Love Test that reveals a person's educational background, current interest, sexual adjustments, and parental conditionings, and the kind of marital adjustments that have been made in their marriages thus far. Individual questionnaires for each husband and wife must be accompanied by standing naked photographs. LovXchangers will not meet for three months prior to the two-week household exchange—thus heightening the

adventure—but each husband and each wife must write several letters to the other spouse and talk with them on the telephone. In the beginning they only know that they have been matched with people of approximately the same age and income level (although, as the Silvermans and Atwoods are aware in the novel, a professor and a social worker's income could not equal a businessman's income). They will not have seen each other's naked photographs nor exchanged any pictures of themselves or family, but they will be assured that they have been matched with people approximately the same weight (based on the Manpar's belief that couples who are mismatched weight-wise could "undermine the ultimate success of LovXchanges developing into long-lasting satellite relationships and expanded family commitments." LovXchangers agree in advance that sexual intimacy may or may not occur during the two-week exchange, but if it does occur it will be the mutual desire of both the husband and wife. LovXchanges are not arranged between couples who may be seeking divorce. They are between couples who are emotionally and intellectually able to enjoy another intimate postmarital relationship. LovXchanges will not only provide the adventure of original 'courtship,' but may lay the groundwork for corporate marriages, which would be legalized. In a twenty-first-century world, where adventure is not easily obtainable except through structured world travel and cruises that insulate the travelers from people involvement, LovXchanges offer exciting changes of environment as the exchangers adjust to strangers.

Love Groups in a Sexually Sane Society

In 1978, when I was writing *Love Me Tomorrow,* the story of an unhappy young woman (Christina—patterned after Sylvia Plath) who tries to commit suicide but is kidnapped by a cryobiologist and frozen, I made the time of her return to life the year 2050. At that time she would look exactly as she did when she was thirty years old. But my publisher insisted that the date was too far in the future (okay for science fiction but not for this work), so I changed the action so that it could end in the year 2000. The novel introduces Newton Morrow, who thinks that he is a reincarnation of Edward Bellamy.

If you can find the novel, you'll be amused by the fact that I didn't anticipate Reagan or Bush or a temporary return to Republican presidents. But with this exception, most of the novel is still on target for the twenty-first century and has become a collector's item for many people who are intrigued with a new religion, Unilove, which I describe in detail, and Love Groups, which I predicted would develop rapidly in the twenty-first century and would comprise about three million households and at least thirty million adults involved in complete new family styles. Future Families of America can fund experiments with Love Groups within the framework of five years, but in reality they would be lifetime ventures. Here they are—described by David Convita, the doctor who froze Christina and explains to her what has happened while she has been, unwillingly, hibernating for twenty-five years.

"Many Love Groups, like ours, as distinguished from Care Groups, are an incorporation of four families and their children. The goal of these new-style families is to try and maintain approximately a ten-year separation between the original pair bonds. Paul and Carol Thomas, who you see working in our garden, are in their seventies. The basic reason that Congress finally legalized Love Groups and Care Groups is that we do not depend on nursing homes. We're committed to care for ourselves, no government subsidy. Paul and Carol are the only members of our group who are legally married, separately. Ruth Wirtz and I, who are in our fifties, are the next oldest couple bonding. Then come Jag Rayne and Zara Schmidt, who are in their middle forties, and finally Chandra Convita, my daughter by my first marriage, and Ralph Skolnick, who are in their early thirties. Jag and Zara have two kids, seventeen and fifteen, Chandra and Ralph have two youngsters who are eleven and thirteen. This week, when we will be all together (they have a summer home in Cape Cod), there will be fourteen of us. We are an old-style pioneer family except that here there are no patriarchs or matriarchs—we're all androgynous.

"You are going to discover," David tells Christina, "that for many of us, the sham morality of the late 1970s and 1980s has given way to a new kind sexual honesty. The continuous struggle to survive financially in a world that is plagued by worldwide inflation, unemployment, and heavy taxation has created a new sense of human solidarity and community sharing. . . . Gradually, millions of us realized that we could pool our resources, share our automobiles and homes, and instead of trying to hack it alone and try to own our own private quarter of an acre in surburbia, or living in small apartments or townhouse clusters, we realized that four couples and their children—people like us—could share a summer home like this or combine our apartments in a highrise building. It was simply a saner way of economic life—floating with the tide rather than fighting against it."

Love Groups are a clear illustration of how sex and family styles can reorient the industrial and political direction of society. Love Groups are totally opposite responses to the necessity for ever-increasing capitalistic national income growth. They are a pooling of larger forces than the vulnerable one husband, one wife family can ever muster. On the other hand, they are fiercely individualistic responses to the human depersonalization that has been created by the capitalistic system. Love Groups are dedicated to the idea of protecting their members from ever becoming dependent on an anonymous bureaucracy.

Later, another member of the group explains to Christina,

As politicians and educational leaders finally became aware of the continuing disintegration of the family they followed the recommendation that Sol Tax, a professor of anthropology at the University of Chicago made in 1976—that Congress should authorize a new type of legal entity, family corporations that could be voluntarily chartered and would, initially, extend vertically over generations, with new members acquired through birth and marriage.

The main impetus behind the legislation was the impending breakdown of the social security system, and the inability of the younger generation, which had declined in number, to carry the increasing tax burden. Even then there were more people over sixty-five than teenagers, and people eighty-five or over constituted the fastest-growing age group in the United States. It was expected that by the year 2040 there would be one million Americans aged one hundred years or older, and the level of Medicare spending for this group alone would be $212 billion in 1987 dollars.

The new corporate family law permits a monogamous family to incorporate, if it has at least one child. Other family corporations, including former ménage à trois and various equal or unequal distributions of adult males and females, up to a total of eight, can now be chartered. Voting shareholders in any family corporation must have passed their eighteenth birthday.

"In Care Group corporations," David explains,

> The people are all of approximately the same age and there are no dependent children. Care Group corporations are formed mostly among people past sixty. Using our Love Group as an example, the four children are equal shareholders with all of us and can vote when they are seventeen. The value of their shares when they leave the corporation will be an equal pro-rata share of the net worth of the corporation at that moment. Right now our Love Group has a net worth of $400,000. Keep in mind that these are 1996 dollars which keep declining in purchasing power. Thus Raynor, Zag and Zara's boy, who is now seventeen, may be the first to leave the corporation. If he left right now he would receive about thirty-two thousand dollars, or one twelfth of our net worth.

Carol also explains to Christina why Paul and Carol, or even David and Ruth, who have no dependent children, are willing to share a portion of their net worth with the other two couples who do have children.

> It's a two-way street. We originally pooled our resources with the others because eventually this corporation, as a total family, will take care of us. Love Groups are offered a great many state and federal tax advantages. Hopefully, the eight of us, as a corporation, will be able to provide for our complete social security. Paul and I, as well as Chandra and Ralph, are relative newcomers to this corpo-

ration. When David and Ruth, and Zag and Zara, first incorporated, there were only four of them. To improve their tax situation they needed a couple like us in an older age group. When Paul and Chandra became thirty, they joined us on the youngest age side—thus completing this corporation.

If I should die first, Paul will have a home and loving friends, and in all probability, if he wishes, an occasional younger female bed companion. When anyone dies, their shares revert to the corporation. If it is me, then my shares can be sold to a widow in the same age group." She smiled. "Whoever is the survivor in a particular age group must approve of the new shareholder. But Congress has now passed a law giving us the legal right to die whenever we wish. You may be sure that none of us will permit ourselves to end our lives in nursing homes or become an unusual burden to the other shareholders. The corporation can sell the shares of any of us who die to another of the same sex and in the same age group. With the eventual death of the oldest couple, a place for a new young couple opens at the bottom, thus keeping the corporation intact indefinitely, unless a majority of the incorporators, for one reason or another, decide to disband.

How the Love Groups meet, and how they adjust to each other, is explained in depth in the novel, as well as a completely new tax system F.I.S.T. (the Floating Instant Skim Tax)—on all purchases, adjusted up or down monthly, to meet all state and federal needs, eliminating *all* other taxation.

Eventually some publisher may reissue the novel, which was published in an original paperback in 1978.

Marriage Contracts in a Sexually Sane Society

During the past twenty-five years, marriage contracts have received a passing vogue. But in the 1990s, most of them provide in advance for a potential divorce, and hence have an element of cynicism and distrust. Most lovers about to be married, sure that it will never happen to them, (and some aspects of a contract may not be legal anyway) never write or sign one.

In an unpublished novel called *The Trade Off,* I proposed a very different kind of marriage contract, which Karen Bradford offers to her husband, Hank. They have been married eighteen years, have three children, but are on the verge of divorce. Karen hopes the contract will be a solution to their marital problems. They are en route to a vacation at Club Libre in Guadeloupe. It's a vacation that Karen and her lover, Tony, have arranged in the hope that Hank and Tony's wife, Gina, a very beautiful but sexually hung-up Catholic woman, might discover each other.

Based on the Equalog Contract devised by Janette and Paschal Baute, marriage counselors, the thrust of the contract is equality in interpersonal relationships for the female spouse, which, despite the efforts of many feminists in the last half of the twentieth century, still quickly disappears in many marriages. Here is an excerpt from the contract.

> Whereas we affirm that we still love each other and therefore want to make our relationship stronger, more open, and more enduring; whereas we appreciate that each of us has a personal frame of reference and a world view different from each other, that differences are therefore inevitable, and these may be the occasion of either blaming and bad feeling or mutual acceptance and maturing; whereas we understand that we grow and develop as persons in a changing environment, and that because of personal and societal change, agreements set at one period of our lives may not be appropriate at a later time; whereas we acknowledge that sustaining a mutually satisfying relationship is a continuing conversation requiring an ever-increasing openness and responsiveness to the other; whereas we love our children, and deeply feel our commitment to them as parents, and would like to provide them with love and security until they leave the nest; therefore we now agree, as it states in the Equalog Contract, to make our intentions and expectations explicit.

The Equalog Contract has numerous clauses that most couples premaritally or postmaritally would respond affirmatively to, but now Karen expands it in areas where she feels that she and Hank have both been negligent.

> Each of us agrees to give support, comfort, and nurture when the other needs, and asks for such, though never fostering an unhealthy dependency. Each of us agrees not to expect the other to guess his/her feelings, wants, intentions, and therefore will ask directly everything he/she wants from the other. We recognize that the relationship gives no rights of possession over the other, and no one has the right to tell the other how he/she should behave.
>
> Hank agrees, for my own peace of mind, that I must have some occupation outside our home [unlike the majority of American women of the time, Karen did not have to work because Hank earned more than enough to support a nonworking wife]. Whether this is a part time job or full time, you agree not to object, and we both agree to make every effort to share the joys and sorrows of our work.
>
> Finally, while I know it is probably illegal to make written marriage agreements that might include an extramarital relationship, I believe that if we should meet the right couple, it might be an interesting experiment if we could integrate our marriage and family by expanding it. Like millions of Americans, we have few relatives, and are thus deprived of much of the emotional support and deep

intimacy that closely knit families often achieve. Within the next few years our children will probably have left the nest. When that occurs we will often be alone trying to divert ourselves with many superficial acquaintances who we now call friends.

So without knowing, as I write this, whether we could together or separately find two other people with whom we could blend into a total new relationship, I have dreamed up a name for this kind of future marriage,—*a Succeedaneum Marriage.* If you look up "succeedaneum" in the dictionary, you'll discover it means "a thing which serves in place of another." Traditionally, the word refers only to things, but some authors have used it in reference to people. It's a lovely word, Hank. A succeedaneum husband or wife, if we find one, would not replace either of us but would function within the fabric of our marriage, as we would in theirs. If we opened the doors into ourselves and our lives, we could share our joys and wonders and sorrows in a way that we can never do alone or with casual friends.

This kind of marriage contract (which, in the novel Karen devises to serve her own interests and to keep her marriage together) might serve as guide for young people in the twenty-first century who have grown up in a sane sexual environment and have been educated in their undergraduate years in the Roomate of the Other Sex Program and wish to experiment in new-style Future Families of America.

20

Goodbye to the Work Ethic, Hello to the Five Ls

In his book *The Cry for Myth,* Rollo May points out that the American dream (and myth) grew from a belief in America as a new frontier where our forefathers shook off the corruption and sins of European emperors and kings. Relying on sheer willpower and self-reliance, they created a world where, blessed by God and hard work, a man (women were still trapped in the Adam and Eve myth) could rise from poverty, educate himself, and eventually become rich.

The myth of male "rugged individualism" was reflected right from the beginning in the New World by the Puritans and their religious teachings, which insisted that good work (even though it might be for the individual good, and only indirectly for the public good) was the high road to salvation, and a way of life approved by a not-too-loving God. Three hundred years later, the myth was encapsulated in the stories of Horatio Alger, but disintegrated a bit during the 1960s, after the Club of Rome's dire prophecies about the future. There was a short-lived attempt to create a new myth, "small is beautiful," but rugged individualism was restored, in spades, by the "greed is good" and "supply side" philosophy and economics of the Reagan/Bush era.

Sinclair Lewis took a shot at the bitch goddess success in his novel *Babbitt,* and so did Arthur Miller in the play *Death of a Salesman,* and John Steinbeck in his book *The Grapes of Wrath.* But Americans prefer the syndrome of *The Great Gatsby,* and in the mid-1990s the most popular stories and dreams were about the rich and those who are "bound to rise" and become rich and famous.

Discussing the myth of Sisyphus—the poor guy Zeus forced to roll a heavy rock uphill, a rock that kept rolling back on him endlessly, because he deceived the gods, Rollo May agrees with Albert Camus that we must consider Sisphyus happy because, fighting against odds, he never gave up. My own feeling is that

231

Sisyphus won his battle against the gods because he discovered that he was no longer working. He was playing!—and laughing up his sleeveless arm. Zeus thought he was suffering but Sisyphus transformed work into play.

Millions of Americans hate to admit it, but the greatest joy in many people's lives is their work. No matter how menial it may be it gives meaning to their daily existence. But to suggest that work can be metamorphosed into play is heresy. In the mid-1990s our seeming productive failures against the Japanese were explained by the claim that "Americans don't work hard enough." Yoshio Sakurauchi, a Japanese lawmaker, responding to President Bush's visit to Japan in 1992, stated bluntly, "If America doesn't watch out, it's going to be judged finished by the rest of the world." Amusingly, by 1994 many Japanese needed more leisure and time to spend money to buy things and thus get their domestic economy going again.

It's my belief that with a new kind of job training much of what is now conceived as work, including all education, both K-12 and GLUE, can be redirected. A new generation, discovering the five joys of life—Living, Loving, Learning, Laughter and Ludamus—will be playing together during the day, and at night in bed!

Take a look at Webster's definition of the key words "work," "play," "game." You'll quickly discover one truth—most people will work harder at play than they ever will at work. Webster defines "game" as: "1. Sport, any kind of play, frolic or fun. 2. An amusement or diversion. 3. A scheme or art employed in pursuit of an objective. 4. A contest, physical or mental."

"Work" is defined as: "1. Exertion of strength or faculties for the accomplishment of something important. 2. Effort directed toward an end, toil, labor, as the work of the teamster or a doctor which requires much exertion or effort."

Some work today still requires physical exertion, but much human muscle power has been replaced by machine power that usually requires mental faculties of exertion. But can thinking really be called work? At lower levels, learning a skill or doing a repetitive job may be tiring or boring or even "brain fatiguing," but only because the owner of the brain involved has not been taught (or has not discovered) how to let his or her brain play! At the upper levels of thinking, when one uses one's mind to solve a problem or to create something new, no matter how many hours are spent in the process, one is really playing—and the person doing so usually knows it.

Using one's brain to acquire information and to retain it or pass it along to others is automatically its own reward. In the process one can feel creative—and creativity in any form is not only mentally satisfying but also a form of play. Test yourself. If you are fixing an automobile engine, papering a wall, painting a room, making a dress, building a birdhouse, fixing a broken appliance, baking a cake, writing a letter, drawing or painting a picture (even by the numbers), are you working or are you playing? In the same way programming a computer, typing a perfect letter, adding one or more components to a product, running a lathe, driving a bus, filling a tooth, filing a legal brief, selling a product, or even making hamburgers at a fast food franchise—no matter what the task may be, it can be transformed into play by discovering how to make it creative. Or, if it is mechanical work that can be done with only part of the brain, one can learn to play with the other part.

To transform work into play, we must get rid of the derogatory definitions of play that have evolved because most religions have put play in the same category as human sexuality. Playing and making love isn't something that God ever does in the Bible. The Christian/Judaic/Islamic god is not a Hindu dancing god. He's a latter-day Zeus who believes that rolling a rock uphill is good for your soul.

Here's how Webster defines the major aspects of play: "1. To move swiftly, or erratically [not the implication of untrustworthiness in this definition]. 2. To engage in sport or lively recreation, to amuse and divert oneself [obviously diverting oneself from more important occupations like work is frowned upon]. 3. To contend, or take part in a game [contending is not really nice either]. 4. To dally amorously, to have sexual intercourse [Having sexual intercourse doesn't fit the work ethic. In a sexually dishonest society most sexual mergers are fifteen minutes of work. Making love is goal-directed and rarely just play, or letting come what may including the orgasmic touchdown].

The common expressions that evoke "play" are practically all suspect and prove that playing is not nice. Here are a few: play around, play at, play a trick, play away, play both ends against the middle, play down, play fair, play hooky, play one's cards, play politics, play possum, play the ponies, play up, and play with fire. If you read through all the various interpretations of "work," you'll soon discover that work wasn't held in high esteem in the ancient world. Both Aristotle and Plato made it clear that work was for slaves. The ancient Greeks believed, along with Judaic rabbis and early Christian philosophers, that a life of contemplation and service to God should be the ultimate goal. During the Protestant Reformation Martin Luther and later John Calvin equated work with a moral life. Opening the way for Karl Marx and what became a basic concept of the Russian revolution—"He who works eats"—Hegel and Fichte stated bluntly, "Everyone should make his living by work," and "Work is a necessity and by it man creates wealth." But Johann Huizinga, in a book recommended by Martin Buber, *Homo Ludens: A Study of the Play Element in Culture*, will convince you that in most cases when you think you are working, praying, or even making war—essentially you are playing.

In my novel *The Byrdwhistle Option* (alas, as of 1994 it has yet to appear in paperback) Byrdwhistle is a multimillion-dollar mail order company run by a former professor of philosophy, H. H. Youman, who believes in the five Ls. Byrdwhistle only hires husband and wife teams and pays them equally the median salary plus substantial bonuses based on the company's profitability. In addition, Byrdwhistle provides complete child care on premises in different locations and mothers and fathers can take time off from their work on an alternating basis to take care of all the Byrdwhistle children. All jobs are rotated. There are Love Rooms where spouses, with each other's prior consent, may relax with an alternative spouse.

H. H. Youman has an entirely new theory of management which combines Abraham Maslow's *Theory Z,* Herbert Marcuse's "Pleasure Principle," and Albert Low's *Art of Zen Management* into a play ethic. It is a concept that is missing from any books on management technique that I have ever read. Nowhere does there seem to be any understanding of play versus work. Even today most owners or directors of capital equipment employ labor and machinery on an interchangeable basis. In 1957 Douglas MacGregor, in his book *The Human Side of Enterprise,* labeled this common management style "Theory X." MacGregor proposed a "Theory Y"-style management that counteracted the old beliefs that workers disliked their work, wanted to avoid responsibility, and consequently had to be treated as children by patriarchal, autocratic owners and managers who devised all the rules governing work. Feminists are aware that "Theory X"-style relationships still dominate many marriages.

MacGregor admitted that he was drawing heavily on Abraham Maslow's thinking. Later Peter Drucker elaborated with his theory of "management by objectives," in contrast to management by control. MacGregor points out, "People are accustomed to being directed, manipulated, controlled in industrial organizations, and finding satisfaction for their social, egotistic and self-fulfillment needs away from their job. By contrast *Theory X* places exclusive reliance on external controls, whereas *Theory Y* relies heavily on self-control."

Discussing Maslow's theory that we all have "a hierarchy of needs" and that man lives by bread alone when there is no bread, MacGregor points out that when the need for bread is satisfied it is no longer a motivator of human behavior. The need for safety (job security,) association, acceptance of fellow, friendship and love, self-esteem, and recognition are all frustrated by "Theory X"-style management. But MacGregor never equated work with play. By the 1970s some companies recognized that the Japanese approaches to organized "quality circles" at least gave employees the impression, that they were participating in management. But *playing* instead of working was and is still a dangerous concept.

William Ouchi, a Japanese, wrote a book, *Theory Z,* on Japanese management techniques, but Abraham Maslow's *Theory Y* preceded Ouchi's by twenty years. Maslow envisioned a totally new kind of work environment. In his *Theory Y,* Maslow explores twenty-four basic differences between people he calls "self actualizers" and merely healthy people, and after analyzing the different needs of job applicants he concludes that many people live at a "Theory Y" level. "They are seeking work environments that offer more than just pay for work. These people are seeking working environments with friendly coworkers, good surroundings, a source of future challenge and growth, idealistic satisfactions, responsibility, freedom, an important product or service, compassion for other, helping mankind, helping the country, a chance to put one's ideas into effect, and a company of which can be proud."

Maslow added: "I assume that greater psychological health would make these kinds of pay more valuable, especially with sufficient money, and with money held as a constant variable." He concluded, *"Of course, a large portion of self actualizing people have probably fused work and play, anyway"* (emphasis added).

As NSME education takes hold, teachers and managers of people in various businesses will gradually diffuse the twentieth-century work ethic myth into a holistic perception of life that combines the five Ls into a play ethic, and a new realization that all of us are players. Much of what we call study, learning, and later a job, or work, will be melded into a total lifestyle. The process of earning one's living in company with expanded families, and a new sexual morality will give each person a sense of purpose and more "meaning" in their lives, and the opportunity to be aware of and to experience from day to day what Matthew Arnold called "The calm soul of all things."

In 1994 multimillionaire Michael Huffington, age forty-six, a congressman running for senator and a possible presidential candidate in the twenty-first century, along with his wife Arianna, also very wealthy and a Cambridge graduate who at the age of twenty-three had already written several books on the lives of Picasso and Maria Callas, are potential believers in NSME legislation. Proving that the rich are not always the idle rich, Arianna has written a book called *The Fourth Instinct,* which she calls altruism. The first three instincts, she believes, are survival, power, and sex. Like Hillary Rodham Clinton, Arianna is searching for a "politics of meaning" that is rooted in "spirituality," the need for which she expects will spread like an epidemic in the twenty-first century. Whether you define spirituality as a search for God or Gaia, the reunification of church/ state made possible by the NSME legislation is the key factor.

But the environment for "spirituality," with "sacramentalizing human sexuality" as one aspect of it, is dependent on complete work/play jobs and full employment. In the mid-1990s major manufacturers from General Motors down restructured their organizations. With thousands of smaller companies following suit, millions of jobs were eliminated. James Baker, a vice president of General Electric in the 1980s, saw the handwriting on the wall. "U.S. industry has three choices . . . automate, emigrate, or evaporate." By the mid-1990s all three things had occurred.

With increasing billions of people worldwide gaining skills to manufacture anything that has been formerly manufactured in the United States, we must create a new generation that is even more skilled vocationally. Keeping young people seventeen to twenty-one out of the prime workforce in work/study programs, and keeping teenagers under seventeen out of the service industry workforce, will open up service jobs for millions of healthy people past seventy, who need a work/play environment to give their lives meaning.

Reducing unemployment in the twenty-first century, combined with the need for work/play that provides some income, will be even more difficult as Social Security purchasing power diminishes, actually or by inflation. But there is a way to keep unemployment down, or practically eliminate it. Giving millions more Americans a complete education will require millions more teachers. Teaching, at minimum wages, can be a retirement profession. And as time passes, a new generation with many new skills can not only teach in those retirement years, but rejuvenate the living arts with live theater and hundreds of thousands of live actors and musicians performing in thousands of communities—and not only offering lots of people contact, but proving that the five Ls can't be found on the computer screen or the information superhighway.

In my novel, Ronald Coldaxe, vice president of W.I.N. Inc. with a Stanford MBA, is trying to acquire Byrdwhistle, which, percentage-wise is much more profitable than his own multibillion-dollar conglomerate. Marge Slick, vice president of Byrdwhistle, along with H.H. Youman, attempt to indoctrinate Coldaxe with Theory Z and give him some further insights into a new sexual morality based on the five Ls. Here's what Marge tells Coldaxe:

> H. H. is experimenting with Freud's pleasure principle versus his reality principle, which presumably govern man's behavior. Freud was convinced that such a things as a nonrepressive developing civilization was impossible. He believed that civilizations advance because man has learned to control his sexual and erotic compulsions. According to him, the Eros instinct has been deflected by the Oedipus compulsion. The patriarchal male prevented his male offspring from possessing his mother. When the son finally kills his father so that he can fuck his mother, he is overcome with guilt. The necessity to repress this guilt has become a way of life for all men.
>
> Gradually the patriarchal father lost power and was replaced by a new myth—the Protestant and Jewish work ethic, and by the capitalistic system that fertilized it. Then man's alienation was complete. He started living a joyless life

and rejected his basic instincts, and in the process began to believe that suffering instead of the pleasure principle was the path to heaven. Natural genital joy and living in playful, unrepressed receptiveness with one's own mind and body—as well as the bodies of friends—was sinful and dirty. Unable to communicate their need to please one another, men and women became distrustful. People discovered that it was easy to hate each other, because hating another person fortifies your petty ego and you're not forced to surrender it.

H. H. Youman is convinced that Freud's reality principle, with its reliance on delayed satisfaction and unnecessary restraint of human pleasure and play, combined with a life of unremitting toil, along with pressures for increased productivity, does not have to be a guiding force in our lives. Byrdwhistlers reject the Judeo-Christian work ethic and its morality. We believe that a total emphasis on making money and earning one's bread might have been necessary in the beginning of human development, but the philosophy and psychology that has dominated Western civilization and is woven into Freudian thinking is no longer viable. H. H. Youman is determined to prove, here at Byrdwhistle, that giving full rein to man's basic loving nature and a play ethic cannot only eliminate the anxiety, neurosis, and insecurity that plagues Western man, but can prod the donkey much better than guilt, suffering, and a work ethic based on Freud's reality principle.

In his essay *New Dimensions in Human Sexuality,* taking the play ethic into religious areas, Francoeur points out that Alex Comfort agrees with Marcuse's "pleasure principle" as a way of life rather than Freud's reality principle.

> The acceptance of sensuality and the widening of its focus to include not one but many others will likely be correlated with a new sense of social justice, non-possessiveness, non-exploitation, ecological concerns and the eroticization of friendship.
>
> What lies behind play, fantasy, imagination and the free exploration of possibilities but the ecstasy and epiphany of the Transcendent Other?

Francoeur asks, "Incarnating human sexuality in an aesthetic paradigm is an open attack, not just on patriarchal values, but also on the power structure these values have supported. It is thus an attack on both consumeristic capitalism and authoritarian governments both civil and religious."

Many religious leaders will challenge the play ethic because as Ann Lammers, assistant professor of theology at Church Divinity School, in a rebuttal to Francoeur, insists,

> It would seem necessary for a Christian to confess that the shadow of sinfulness pervades all of life . . . sin affects our sexual relationships as it does the rest of

our lives. People are especially vulnerable to the wounds inflicted in sexual relationships, and our anger and grief about such wounds sometimes prompts us to
sin against those whom we most want to love. Thus considered as sexual moral
agents we are both creative and destructive, both innocent and cruel.

Unfortunately, this is the kind of past thinking that has dominated religious
morality. It posits a God out there to whom we must pray that we won't sin but who
will forgive our sins because they are inevitable. By contrast, in the twenty-first
century, the kind of education that NSME sets in motion puts the challenge where
it belongs—on individual men and women. And, if God is interested—you know
that He knows—you can't really sin against Him, or any person, because you have
learned never to let your emotions blow your mind/brain. And God will be delighted when all of us really show each other from childhood how to play God.

It isn't as difficult as it may sound. In *The Cry for Myth,* Rollo May points
out the charm of morality, and the story of Amphytrian, wife of a Greek general
with whom Zeus has fallen in madly in love. A God in love with a human? Zeus
is so distraught with his love for Amphytrian that Mercury cooks up a war that
keeps her husband busy and Zeus finally has the lovely lady to himself. But afterwards, when he promises her immortality in appreciation, she sighs. Living forever is not the answer. Amphytrian tells Mercury, "I would miss the poignancy of
the transient—the sweet sadness of grasping for somethings we cannot hold."

It's getting back to basics—but our schools are not teaching it to children.
Underlying a joyous approach to life should be an awareness of the shortness of
life, and how much we have to learn, and how much we need to love and be
loved. It is not undercutting a young person's feeling of immortality to make her
or him aware of the contingency of each us as human beings.

You are going to die. You are going to disappear forever from this planet. The
person you are arguing with, in a fury over, completely disgusted with, who is not
measuring up to your ego ideas—that person, too, is dying (unless he or she is
under fifteen) right before your eyes. Now, really—how in the world can you hate
any person who is so fragile, and who, like you, holds such a tiny claim on life?
If you were immortal *maybe you'd have the time* to hate someone, or to be jealous of someone, or "wannabe" someone you're not, or just generally be "pissed
off" at someone. Wouldn't it be better for you to think and even say, "You know,
a minute ago I was so mad at you, I couldn't think straight. Then, I thought of you
naked, alone, tears in your eyes because you weren't feeling well, or sitting on
the toilet and trying to have a bowel movement, and you were alone and no one
was watching you, but I loved you, because we both knew if you couldn't shit,
you'd die."

I'm sure that you've looked at the body of the opposite sex, or your own sex, and thought how lovely it is, how lovely the shape you are looking at, that face staring at you, and how it is all so dependent on so many variable coexisting function under that skin, and how the person who is that body doesn't really own it—and most certainly *you* as husband, wife, friend, or lover can't own it. Think about it, once you know you really can't own something, or control someone, you not only begin to see them in a new light, but you yourself start to live.

So an integral part of the new sexual morality and new-style education for Americans—one to twenty-one—will be to teach a new generation not only to plumb the depths of every phenomenon, explain it, analyze it, until, if possible, the mystery is dispelled, but at the same time to maintain a balancing awareness that there is no end to the mystery of why we are here, and not to be ashamed but dare to be awed, or to wonder and experience tears of joy at parts of life that are ineffable. That essentially is the religious experience. To make this possible for a new generation we must create a society where people not only know how to play, but are deeply aware of human history and aren't so much concerned with seeking one's own particular genealogical roots, but rather all of our amazing, intertwining roots as human beings.

The new-style liberal arts education made possible by NSME legislation will give teachers the opportunity to teach history from the viewpoint of the average "everyman." Using the five-volume *History of Private Lives* will show a new generation how people ate, slept, dressed, married, raised their children, and treated their spouses from early Greek to pagan Roman times and through the Middle Ages, the Renaissance, the Industrial Revolution, and the Great Wars. Seeking "the riddle of identity in modern times," it gives clues that bind all humanity together and show us how it is possible for the new great White, Hispanic, Black, Asian and other peoples to be GLUEd together in a small American mixture that blends our amazing human roots, religious roots, and the neverending wonder of human sexuality.

Sacramentalizing human sexuality, along with the interwoven ecological significance and the realization that "life is social" is a thesis that James Lovelock explores in his books *Gaia* and *The Ages of Gaia*. It is an aspect of "spirituality" that Arianna Huffington believes will become endemic and it can easily be incorporated into most theologies. With Gaia—from the Greek, meaning "earth goddess," Lovelock proposes that the earth, and the universe itself, is a living interrelated entity that includes all of us. It is a myth for the twenty-first century that is beautifully epitomized and brought to life by the photograph of earth taken by the astronauts. As Rollo May points out, "The myth and the immortality of the true myth are captured in that photography . . . an indelible impression on people's minds that the earth, emblazoned in dark blue and gold, turning serenely in its orbit, should be populated by people who are brothers and sisters."

And, as James Lovelock adds, "This view of earth from space gives us a personal sense of a real live planet on which living things, the air, the oceans, and the rocks all combine in one as Gaia."

Many years ago, standing naked on the hearth of one of the many fieldstone fireplaces at Sandstone, rapping with about fifty naked or partially naked men and women who were lounging on the thick broadloom carpets or making love while they listened to me, I told them, "I came into this world with a full share of male drives flooding my genes. Standing here enjoying the sight of your naked bodies, both male and female, I am in awe—and as a man I feel like a kid in a candy store." Everywhere I looked women were following my words, smiling at me, listening expectantly, stretched idly on the floor, sitting with their hands clasped around their knees—breasts and vulvas completing their identity as persons.

Here and there in the sinuous firelight, dancing on the logs, I could see guys with erections, joining with a particular woman, or having their cocks held or lightly tasted by their companions. "I am a man," I told the ladies.

> You are women. I want to kiss and taste all your mouths, all your breasts, and your bellies. I want to bury my face between the legs of each of the women and sense your femaleness and the soft warmth of the middle of you that leads to the source of new life. I want to put my tongue on all your labias and taste the firm swelling of all your clitorises. *I am man, and I love all women,* but only for one or two of you can *I be me, or with me, can you be you.* And that is the process of life for me. Sex as exaltation. Sex as a merger with you because I am making a merger with me possible, and neither of us is any longer encased in our bodies, and we know that we can float into a laughing, loving, recurring orgasm because we have displaced ourselves.
>
> And that relationship between Thou and I is dyadic. While it surely can be experienced with more than one person in a lifetime, it can't be experienced with more than one person in one day or night, or perhaps even in the same week. So be careful in your life. Don't devalue the sexual experience, or you may come away wondering how or why you took the trip without becoming deeply aware of the scenery.

And that's the essence of NSME—leading to a twenty-first century with a new sexual morality, kissing the joy as it flies, kissing goodbye to a life of endless, repeating, joyless, television sound bites, and daring to jump in and enjoy the delightful rhythm and occasional chaos of the everflowing stream of Living, Loving, Learning, Laughter, and Ludamus.

21

X-Rated Movies
Before and After NSME

If you study the self-imposed rating system of the arts that I have projected in chapters 8 and 9, which would be monitored by the Future Families of America Commission, you will understand that the intent is not to censor X-rated films as they are now being offered for sale or rental in video stores, but to eliminate interest in them as the complete NSME-style education takes effect and human nudity, K-12 sex education, men and women enjoying one-to-one caring sex (in all the arts with SN ratings) is a common experience. Early in the 21st century, as that occurs, the sick-sex subject matter and interpersonal sexual devaluing of X-rated videos will appeal only to a small fringe group of males who, like cigarette smokers in the late 1990s, finally became ashamed of their addiction.

Since much of the sexual sickness and hang-ups of the twentieth century were both catalyzed and crystallized by adult film producers with some good and some dangerously bad results, which I will cover later, let's take a look at the nearly twenty-five-year history of the porno industry.

In the mid-1990s *Adult Video News,* a glossy, glamorous monthly magazine, continued to lead the safari of multimillion watchers through the swamps and jungle of devalued human sexuality. They reported that in 1993 the number of adult tapes to hit the market was 2,475, and that the industry grossed $2.1 billion. The first adult tapes were released to the video market about 1979 (and provided the first fodder for VCRs—and the only reason to own one for several years). My guess is that from 1979 to the present at least twenty thousand different hour or longer X-rated tapes have been produced. Averaging about ten thousand copies each, by now they provide at least one tape for every adult American.

But this is only the tip of the sexberg. Rentals of adult tapes were close to five hundred million in 1994. Assuming that the average rental is ten tapes annually, fifty million Americans have watched, or watch regularly, men and women who have become X-rated "stars," as well as their next door neighbors (amateur and pro-am, as the label may state), enjoying (?) every possible kind of sexual action anyone has ever done, or dreamed of doing.

Reading like an index to the study of sexology, you can watch feature films devoted entirely to *anal sex,* presumably something every heterosexual male dreams of with a woman whose anus provides a tighter fit than her vagina (there are also many all-male homosexual films where the sexual merger is anal, but in the heterosexual variety you rarely see a macho male getting his asshole penetrated—rather, this is the female gift to her lover, and presumably many women enjoy it and climax in the process).

Practically all sexvids, as I call them, offer separate sequences of *oral/vaginal sex,* and *bi sex,* which in the heterosexual videos is usually two or more women tonguing and fingering their breasts, vaginas, and anuses, and using dildos and other "sexual toys." They may also include bisexual guys who enjoy each other's mouths and anuses as well as female vaginas and assholes. Run-of-the-mill sexvids usually have a *masturbation* sequence, with a single woman masturbating alone, but occasionally a man and woman watching each other masturbating. They always offer *threesomes,* either two men and one woman, or two women and one man. And many of the directors, following whatever story line has been concocted on which to hang together the sequences, wrap up a story with *group sex,* or orgies, during which most of the cast participate in variations of the above including *DPers* (double penetrations—some of the women accepting up to three cocks in all of their orifices at the same time).

But this is not all. There are many specialty tapes devoted entirely to one of the sexual actions listed above as well as tapes featuring *big-busted women,* or *lactating, pregnant women,* or *grossly fat women.* Some of these had twentieth-century merit. Seeing big-breasted, naked women in action and comparing them with their smaller-breasted friends, who often compensated with sensuous, pear-shaped behinds; seeing how a young woman actually looks pregnant and able to suckle her child; or seeing very heavy-fleshed women naked before marriage— all this can be educational. By contrast, after NSME, a new generation will grow up not only to see pregnant women naked on beaches, but see the birth of children, and women of all shapes and sizes both live and on film and television in SN story lines.

On the other hand, *gang bangs,* one woman taking on many men, sucking five or more cocks in a row, and taking on three guys at once in DPers, one in her mouth, and two in her anus and vagina at the same time, are totally Sexually Devaluing.

In the mid-1990s *amateur tapes* flooded the market. Made by hundreds of "swinging couples," they featured young women and wives and husbands reselling their "home made" tapes for distribution by the established "professional" industry. In a series like *Dirty Debutantes* (with twenty or more tapes) they offered an entry into "pro-amateur" and possible sexvid "stardom."

And finally there are thousands of *bondage and discipline* videos, featuring consensual bondage and whipping of mostly women (but a few with masochistic men). Many of these tapes border on the sadistic, with women naked or partially naked being gagged, tied hand and foot, hung spreadlegged against a wall or from a ceiling by their wrists, being spanked, being whipped with specially designed whips, or having clothespins and clamps attached to their vaginal lips or nipples (or penises, where the woman is the "slave master"). There is no sexual merger in the B/D tapes, since this might be construed as rape, but orgasm is achieved by the slave as she begs her "master" for *more*—presumably ecstatic—of the mixture of pleasure and pain.

Despite the radical right insistence that child pornography is rampant, this has not been a product of the X-rated industry for the past fifteen years. During the early days, independent producers made little or no effort to determine a young woman's age, and there were a few films with girls under eighteen. The famous Tracy Lord films and videos, produced when Lord was only fifteen (and by any standards very much a full-blown woman), created an uproar in the industry and were totally withdrawn from the market. During the 1970s there were quite a few X-rated tapes in which the women in the story line were raped (*A Dirty Western, Abduction of Lorlei, Expensive Tastes*). But most of these have been withdrawn, and now rape—never shown graphically—is confined to R-rated films. Child pornography is still being produced in some European countries. There is an underground market for videos showing men and women having sex with animals. Many of these originate in Argentina.

As you may know, I have been reviewing X-rated tapes since they first arrived in video cassettes. The first *X-rated Videotape Guide* was published in 1984 and covered all of the films that had been transferred to video up that date. In passing, I should mention the *Better Sex* videos offered by two different companies during 1995 and advertised, in of all strange places, in full-page ads in the *New York Times* Sunday book-review section, along with three tapes offered by Adam & Eve, in Carrasboro, North Carolina (a multimillion-dollar sexual mail-order business from which you can buy everything you ever wanted to see or use to jazz up your sexual life)—Kay Parker's *Guide to Tantric Sexual Potency* and Nina Hartley's *Guide to Better Cunnilingus and Fellation* (two separate tapes). Each of these videos as well as the Better Sex series are performed by porno actors and actresses on tapes that run about an hour and a half.

They could all be shown in K11-12 sex-education courses. They prove several things. Although Kay Parker (a gentle former porno star, now in her forties) is mistress of ceremonies, you'll soon discover that the joy of extended tantric sexmaking can never be revealed on film or video tape. The ecstasy and potentially transcendent experience of making love for several hours or longer can only be experienced by lovers who know how to prolong the mental/genital merger. Such lovers can talk, self-disclose, and reveal themselves to each other as they walk the razor's edge before climaxing or not at all. A writer can describe this experience with words but it's impossible to convey visually since the viewer is a voyeur and not a participant. Young people on the verge of seventeen and their rite of passage will learn this in the final years of their high school sex-education courses. They will soon discover that learning by doing, emulating writers who can express the many aspects of their sexual/mental surrender in words, and learning how to become the other person, is far more fun than watching Nina Hartley try to teach her pupils the short-term boom/boom of sucking and licking each other's genitals.

In volume one of the *Guide* (they are all still in print) I explained how and why I got interested in sexvids. Essentially, it's because, like most males, I enjoy seeing naked women walking, running, playing, and reacting to men as normal sexual persons, and I enjoy watching and listening to a man and woman (not in real life—that would be too inhibiting for them and me) making love graphically, playing with each other's genitals, kissing, tasting, and above all *talking* and trying to communicate with each other with no game playing, and thus revealing themselves in some depth. Alas, very little of this kind of joyous sexual action occurs in most sexvids.

As I write this in April 1995, Prometheus Books has recently published the fifth edition of the *X-Rated Videotape Guide*. I was completely involved in the first four editions, having reviewed all the sexvids in volumes 1 and 2, and about half of those in volumes 3 and 4. All of them offer a unique letter-rating system which will help you pinpoint the relatively better sexvids with a Collector's Choice rating or, depending on your interest, identify the sick, ugly, and horrible. When it came to volume 5, I decided that my remaining time was too precious to devote about an hour and a half each to watching and writing a review of each of the continuing flood (more than 2500 in any one year). I agreed that Pat Riley, who I discovered in 1992 (see introduction to volume 3), could continue by himself with volume 5 and subsequent volumes. But he couldn't use my rating system. He didn't want to, anyway, and was champing at the bit with an approach to reviewing sexvids rather different from my own.

I never would have gotten involved in reviewing X-rated films if publishers had continued to accept my new novels with open arms. But in the past ten years I have written four of them—*The Trade Off, The Oublion Project, The Way to Go* and *Dreamer of Dreams*. Thus far in 1995, after reviewing my synopses, all main-line publishers of fiction have refused to read the manuscripts—no doubt on the untrue premise and belief that men and women in the 1990s aren't seeking, via novels as they most certainly are in pop-psychology nonfiction, solutions to a more joyous marital life.

Thanks to about twenty of the major porno producers who enjoyed volumes 1–4, I still receive many review tapes. I'm sure that Riley has reviewed most of the 1994 crop. But unless this book strikes home and awakens publishers to my unpublished novels, I may finish my remaining years keeping "The Journal of an X-Rated Video Watcher"—in which I can sadly reflect on American sexual hangups and insanities, all of which are interrelated with a democracy that will not survive unless it finds a unifying sense of national purpose.

In passing, I disagree with most of the male reviewers of adult films, who believe that "porn films exist primarily for sexual arousal" and no one (male) cares about the story line, or "fuck films are good or bad based on whether they give you a boner." Actually, the character development vis-à-vis the age and background of the viewer is the sexual turn on. For example, older men remembering their youth, and an actress who reminds them of the girl they dreamed about then, or women responding to a male actor who seems genuinely to like a particular woman, makes a particular sequence more erotic than slam-dunk sex. One by-product for me was watching sexvids with *The Anatomy Coloring Book* and learning, as I colored, more about the amazing muscular, bone, and genital structure of the male and female bodies. I also coined more loving dirty words, kissing good-bye to the old ones that devalue sexual mating. In addition, I discovered in books like *Slang and Its Euphemisms* and the *Historical Dictionary of Slang* the thousands of words, many now obsolete, used in the past thousand years to describe human sexuality and mating.

My reviews offer a rating system that attempts to define the contents of particular tapes with the following letters—CC ("Collector's Choice"), NN ("Normal Non Committed"), Bi ("Bi-sexual"—meaning that the women involved engage in same sex action because they are paid to do it, but are probably heterosexual), NR ("Normal Romantic" or caring sex), NL ("Normal Laughing"), which in most sexvids is contrived humor or dirty jokes and not spontaneous laughter, DK ("Deviational Kinky"), not including caring threesomes, which seem to be a widely held sexual fantasy; unfortunately, in most sexvids there is rarely any personal involvement evinced between the participants. There is also a DS ("Deviational Sadistic") rating on which the B/D tapes walk a razor's edge.

If you have read any of my fifteen novels, you may be aware that the long, descriptive sexual encounters are mental/sexual mergers, during which the participants are discovering each other and themselves in the joy of extended sexmaking. I am extolling caring, one-to-one sex. Although my characters may enjoy more than one sexual partner in the course of their lifetimes, they never are involved in group sex, or bizarre variations on penile/vaginal sex. Thus, if you read my reviews, you'll discover that, without too much success, I have tried to redirect and convince some of the better- known directors to offer upbeat, even romantic, sexual involvement.

This happens occasionally, but in the more than three thousand X-rated films I have reviewed there are less than two hundred that have a sequence (and this is not usually the thrust of the entire tape) that I have rated NR. This is interesting because *AVN*'s survey of "Who rents adult tapes" proves that women are still reluctant renters of X-rated films. In 1994, 59 percent of the renters were men alone and 19 percent women renting a tape with a man. The rest were 15 percent men renting with men, and 6 percent women renting alone. Of course, these rental figures for men don't reveal how many are watched by the men's wives or female friends.

In volume I of the *X-rated Videotape Guide* I offered twenty-five conventions or characteristics of practically all porno films which, in the absence of any sexual value training K-12, or even in the undergraduate years, I deplore; they have contributed to the sexual devaluation that permeated American society in the late twentieth century. I think it would be informative to revisit them here:

25 X-Rated Sexvid Conventions

1. The male actor rarely ejaculates inside the female.
2. When he does ejaculate, it is on her breasts, lips, or stomach. Without the friction of his penis and often using her own fingers, the female actress seems to be climaxing herself while she ecstatically rubs his jism into her flesh.
3. If the male actor is being sucked off, he ejaculates so that not only the female can be seen swallowing his jism or letting it dribble over her face, but in addition her facial expression indicates that it's good to the last drop.
4. Females never feel embarrassed and rarely indicate that they don't know how—or don't enjoy—sucking a male cock. In fact, they often initiate the procedure by grabbing the male and unzipping him.
5. Most actresses, not to be outdone by Linda Lovelace, manage to go down on the entire length of the male penis (the only possible exception being Johnny Wadd's thirteen-and-a-half-inch unerected member). Actresses manage to do this for quite a few minutes without gagging.
6. Rarely do actors and actresses say, "I love you" to one another, but via moans and groans and occasionally via speech they tell each other, "It was a great fuck!"

7. There is very little conversation between male and female before or during the act of love in most films produced prior to 1978, but it's becoming much more common in recent films.

8. There is very limited foreplay. The male is usually aroused orally by the female. He may take a quick lap or two of her vulva, but when he enters her she is apparently lubricated, waiting and right on the edge of an earth-shaking orgasm—all of which occurs because she enjoyed sucking his penis so much.

9. There is rarely any afterplay or any friendly cuddling. When the male ejaculates, the plot, if there is any, will finally continue until the next fuck scene (the fast forward button on videocassette players is a great convenience in helping the viewer to get past the "ins and outs" and back to the story).

10. Jealousy and most other human emotions (except fear and lust) are rarely expressed in most adult films. In practically all films, two (or more) women work over the hero and share his penis from mouth to mouth, vagina to vagina, or even anus to anus, with no apparent jealousy—or worry about sanitation.

11. All sexvids have at least one scene of lesbian sex, during which the women enjoy each other often more than they have enjoyed the hero.

12. A very large percentage of sexvids have one orgy scene (Mazola party) involving at least four or more naked couples screwing together.

13. Practically all sexvids have one scene in which two women work over one man, but rarely are two men ever seen sexmaking with one woman. (*Cosmopolitan's* 1980 sex survey reveals that 23 percent of *Cosmo* girls had sex with more than one partner at a time, and these were male partners.)

14. Anal sex occurs in many sexvids, with the female being penetrated but never the male. Keep in mind that male homosexuality is not a factor in sexvids and is rarely shown, unless the films were specifically produced for gay males.

15. Women rarely get pregnant. If they do (see filmography on *Beach Blanket Bango*), it is treated humorously. Women practically never menstruate, or wear sanitary pads, externally or internally. There's also rarely any discussion of birth control. No condoms are ever used and are rarely seen. Women never admit if they are on the pill.

16. Men past forty rarely appear naked. If they do, they are paunchy, lecherous, can't get it up, and are usually cast as simpletons or villains.

17. Sexvids rarely show a woman past forty naked, let alone sexmaking.

18. The age limit for female lead actresses is between twenty and thirty. Georgina Spelvin, who is in her forties, now appears in supportive roles. Since a great many sexvids are teenage-oriented, both actors and actresses often look older than the ages they are portraying.

19. Practically all lead roles in sexvids are between unmarried or formerly marrieds. If extramarital sex is treated, it is usually from the standpoint of swingers (uncommitted spouse exchange). An amusing exception is *Babylon Pink* which won a best film award in 1980. If a male actor seduces a woman who

is married in the sexvid plot, usually both are totally guiltless. If the husband appears, he is often flaky or some kind of dud.

20. Most males are circumcised. A fascinating exception is John C. Holmes (Johnny Wadd), but you rarely see a scene in which the female plays with his foreskin, moving it over his glans.

21. Many of the 1970s sexvids commence with a genital sexmaking scene that continues through lengthy film credits. This entree is slowly disappearing.

22. Many recent sexvids commence with a real "class" ambience that equals or exceeds many regular Hollywood productions. But after the first ten or fifteen minutes, complying with most of the conventions listed above, the director frequently loses the plot. In some cases it never returns.

23. Sexvid stories, with a few unique exceptions, rarely revolve around a single male-female or even a two-couple sex relationship. And the male actor must have sex with at least three different females, and often many more, during the course of a particular sexvid.

24. Female stars, such as Vanessa Del Rio, rarely have breasts that hang normally on their chests. You can tell a woman's silicone breasts by their impossible perkiness when the actresses are standing, lying, or being touched. It's interesting to watch sexvids for exceptions.

25. A very large percentage of adult films cater to the male fantasy of having a virgin—or a sexually inexperienced woman—who learns all she knows from him. See how many films have a "teenage" or "high school" or "young" reference in the title.

Keep in mind these conventions were written in 1984. During the past ten or more years there have been a few changes. Largely because of the fear of many actors and actresses (despite the protests of the aficionado viewers) the use of condoms is much more widespread (not in oral sex). In the mid-1990s too many of the female actresses have had breast implants and shave their vulvas completely or leave a delta moustache—thus in total creating a Barbie doll, or embalmed appearance that is far from reality.

Not all of these sexvid conventions fly in the face of twentieth- century "normal" human sexual reality. Like many sex manuals, sexvids give the impression that the joy of sex is based on many environmental variations—*where* (not in bed) and *how* you do it—with little verbal communication or mental intimacy. Moaning dirty words is the acme of great sex. Almost all of the male climaxing is genitally visible. Men spraying their lovers, or the ladies happily imbibing or swallowing male jism, undermines and devalues human sexuality, as does anal and group sex. Sadly, people get conditioned, "brainwashed," by movies that portray this as a normal way of life.

While most sexvids don't offer bondage and discipline as a part of the story line, thousands of specialty tapes were offered in the mid-1990s. Whether men have it built into their genes— their nature—or not, there's no question that millions of men are stimulated by a helpless female. Most of the slice-and-dice R-rated movies produced by the score since 1970 are based on this premise. Both these and the X-rated B/D videos may act as catharsis for many men who repress their fantasies, but they are a potentially dangerous conditioning that will gradually disappear as the NSME legislation and the self-imposed rating system take effect.

In a larger sense, X-rated films and videos are socially immoral. The lifestyles they portray undermine the monogamous family fabric. Along with many R-rated films they portray an easygoing sexual lifestyle where sexual sharing is rarely a cause for lasting jealousy or divorce, and of course there are never any children to contend with, and sex is for the young. The "starring cycle" for women in X-rated films is approximately three years, after which they are swiftly supplanted by a younger "crop" of eighteen to twenty-five-year-olds. Many older male actors survive into their forties, but sexmaking past thirty for women and forty for men is rare. In many reviews, with no response, I wondered why no producer/director would make sexvids with former stars such as Kay Parker, Georgina Spelvin, and Judith Anderson, to mention just a few. Henri Pachard finally did in *American Garter* with Seka, some ten years later. But, unfortunately, while she was featured on the box, she wasn't too involved in the story line, since she had put on weight and become quite matronly appearing. Like their Hollywood brethren, filmmakers in the late twentieth century assumed that sexual merger after age forty is no longer a way of life—except offscreen.

The worship of youthful sex wasn't always so apparent in the deluge of amateur sexvids, which are closer to reality than the so- called fantasy motivations of professional porno films. But these homemade videos offer a swingers' view of reality that is totally sexually devaluing, with husbands and wives (many in their late forties) graphically exploiting their sexual abilities with each other and with friends—all with little or no intimacy or mental involvement, except camera placement, as they manoeuvre to give genital closeups.

By contrast, in the twenty-first century, when all the X-rated offerings must prominently display an SD (Sexually Devaluing) self-imposed rating, the SN ratings which will appear on thousands of new films and videos will not only offer joyous oral and vaginal sex, but will do it within story lines that may even include sex with other persons in mental sexual mergers that reveal real people, making love premaritally or after marriage, experimenting with family styles beyond monogamy. Not only will the sexual mergers portrayed be happily, lovingly upbeat, but the participants will have much to talk about before and after the loving.

So, while the X rating will change to SD, in retrospect X-rated films and videos not only paved the way for NSME legislation but they made millions of Americans aware that seeing human beings naked together is not pornography, or even erotic, that oral sex is natural and women enjoy it as much as men and that despite the claims of hard-line feminists, X-rated women actresses, for the most part, aren't sex objects. In a majority of the sexual encounters in X-rated films, women are in total command of their mouths, vaginas, and anuses—deciding whether they will or won't give blow jobs, or have anal sex. Physically and mentally they are taking command of the male penis.

Perhaps one valuable by-product was that sexvids provide warnings for many men who have watched ball-busting porno stars like Sharon Mitchell, Sharon Kane, Seka, Judith Anderson, Erica Boyer, Nina Hartley, Tori Welles, Ashlyn Gere, Jeanna Fine (to mention a few) in action. They may become aware that this is the kind of woman who they may be happier watching on their television tube than living with. Revealing mentally different styles, females (and males) will be carried over into the future via SN (Sexually Natural) story lines. Men and women who haven't taken the ROSP undergraduate GLUE program can thus get further insights into the kind of man or woman with whom they could spend a lifetime. Another aspect of twentieth-century X-rated movies that reflects twenty-first-century sexual sanity is that there never was any racial discrimination. Blacks, Whites, Asians, with no seeming racial feelings (except occasionally in a few sexvids where a white woman wants to experience the presumably larger cock of a black man) enjoy each other as human beings without thought of color or ethnic background.

Watching sexvids, also, has probably helped millions of young women in the late twentieth century, before and after marriage, to overcome their religiously indoctrinated fears of sexmaking and enjoy themselves as much as any man. In the mid-1990s, perhaps a majority of women past forty were turned off, or horrified, by X-rated tapes, and too sexually graphic X- and R-rated sequences. They were sure that their husbands were fantasizing sex with younger, more nubile women. In the twenty-first century, after NSME legislation has taken hold and a new generation has grown up seeing videos of their parents naked, and even making love when they were young, older women and their lovers and spouses will extol the beauty of youth and have the joy of comparing themselves when they were in the flower of their youth, and be happy to reminisce, and admit their joy in remembering, or fantasizing sex with younger people. And unlike the late twentieth century, many story lines will offer lovers in their sixties and seventies in happy sexual mergers. In a sexually honest society the human body will be a source of wonder and joy in both youth and old age.

In 1991, well aware that a very large percentage of Americans were watching adult films, Oryx Press, a well-established publisher of textbooks, offered a new book for libraries. Written and edited by Martha Cornog, it is titled *Libraries, Erotica and Pornography.* In the mid-1990s libraries were inundated with books and audiotapes that the radical right was quick to label pornography. But editors Martha Cornog and Timothy Perper point out in the introduction to this three-hundred-page book,

> A central aspect of America in the 1980s and continuing into the 1990s is to debate sex loudly, publicly, and often. By politicizing sex—not merely secularizing it, but actively bringing it to the forefront of politics . . . *the debate is the message.* It is virtually a minor detail that Pastor A is saying homosexuality is right while Father B is disagreeing. . . . The major and all important fact is that they are *both on television.* And while Pastor A and Father B busily neutralize each other's arguments with rhetoric and passion, the message comes across: it is acceptable and inevitable to talk about homosexuality, abortion, pornography, teenage pregnancy, and AIDS.

Amusingly, my contribution to this book, requested by the editors, was a listing of fifty of the best X-rated tapes that I thought librarians should offer for rental to adults. The belief that "once you've seen one adult film, you've seen them all" is completely wrong. Here's the list of tapes that is in the book, with the year of release and a few additions. They are worth viewing once. Actual reviews are in various volumes of the *X-rated Guides.* After passage of the NSME legislation all but two or three of them will carry an SD label (Sexually Devaluing), and some may be used in K-12 human sexuality seminars to show students the sexual sadness and dishonesty of the late twentieth century:

Alice in Wonderland (1975); *Angela, the Fireworks Woman* (1975); *Beauty and the Beast* (1989); *Blonde Ambition* (1981); *Cafe Flesh* (1982) *The Dancers* (1982); *Every Woman Has a Fantasy* (1984); *In Love* (1983); *Justine 2* (1993); *Love You* (1980); *The Masseuse* (1991); *Night Trips* (1989); *Opening of Misty Beethoven* (1975); *Pretty Peaches* (1978); *Ribald Tales of Canterbury* (1985); *Raw Talent* (1984); *Rising Star* (1986); *Roommates* (1982); *Sensational Janine* (1979); *Slave to Love* (1993); *Taboo,* vols. 1 to 6 (one story line on six tapes running close to seven hours); *Taboo American Style,* vols. 1 to 4; *Talk Dirty to Me* (1983); *Three A.M.* (1975).

An aspect of X-rated films that has been overlooked by most sociologists, sexologists, and psychologists is that the annual output of X-rated videos reflects every conceivable sexual hang-up of the religiously conditioned American male, and by reflection of male desire, those of the average American female. Underlying practically all X-rated sexual portrayals (except the stylized sex education videos, or the glamorized *Playboy* and *Penthouse* releases) is the

Christian/Judaic/Islamic indoctrination that sex is dirty. The producers speak with forked tongues trying to convince you in some of the quick/zip and fuck sequences that this is normal female reaction (no doubt about the erect male). But verbally, male and female sexual excitement is heightened when the action includes "talk dirty to me," a title that was given to a series of award-winning sexvids.

As you can see, my interest in sexvids goes far beyond particular porno tape offerings to the much more interesting cultural phenomenon in the twentieth century that created an environment in movies of X and R and NC-17 ratings. The continuous sexual devaluing has in the past 20 years induced thousands of young women, and a few hundred guys (at any one time the adult film family is about 150 women to 50 men) to expose not only their bodies, but what most of us consider a private sexual surrender, to be observed by God and no one else.

Other than Jerry Butler's book, *Raw Talent,* and Mistress Jacqueline's *Whips and Kisses,* which Cathy Tavel and I cowrote with them, there are still very few first-hand whys and wherefores, or "this is the way it really is" revelations of men and women who have purposely or inadvertently stumbled into the three-ring porno circus. In recent times, Richard Rhodes, a Pulitzer Prize-winning author, in an amazing autobiographical book, *Making Love,* opened the door on his private sexual drives and motivations, but as yet no one in porno land has published her or his true sexual confessions, not even Jerry Butler. We know little about how porno actors and actresses feel and survive in a world where they are breaking all the traditional moral rules of human sexuality.

During the past few years, I have tried to convince a 1993 actress like Alex North to let me help her write her autobiography thus far in life. But she finally backed off. Thus far in 1995 no female porno star has written or cowritten such a book. If they would answer the following listing of fourteen questions in some detail, the book would not only be a twentieth-century bestseller, but it would be read well into the future by a new generation comparing a twentieth century with a saner twenty-first century where the church, state, and schools had combined to reevaluate the wonders and joys of human sexuality.

But making truthful, unhyped confessional contact with any of the hundreds of women (past or present) in the X-rated industry isn't easy, and as yet no one has accepted the challenge.

Here are the questions:

1. How you got into the business. Your feelings when you made your first adult film. Presumably, you weren't a virgin, so your pre-porno sexual experiences will also be interesting to the reader. Include childhood experiences and aspirations, what kind of student you were, what other occupations you held, and where you grew up, if you'd like. In short tell us about *you!*

2. Describe your religious background and beliefs, conflicts with your early conditionings and fear (or not) of family exposure. Include some details of how you overcame these fears, or haven't. If you family knows about your involvement in erotic films, how did they react and how did they find out?

3. Tell us the kind of woman you are sexually, easily aroused or not? And what arouses you?

4. If you're married, or have a relationship inside or outside the porno industry, how do you differentiate the sex with them? Or do you?

5. Describe a typical shooting day. Do you ever climax with a guy on camera? Which actors do you particularly enjoy working with, and why?

6. Do you ever experience any sexual embarrassment during the make of a film? Have you ever refused to perform a particular sexual act? Are there costars you don't enjoy having sex with or have refused to work with? (Feel free to name them.) Please tell why.

7. Have you ever participated in a D. P.? Tell why you do or don't like anal sex and what type of lovemaking really turns you on.

8. How do you take care of your body to stay in shape, and minimize sexual diseases? What preparation is necessary for anal intercourse? In the age of AIDS, have you ever refused to do an anal scene? Are you frightened about the possibility of getting AIDS?

9. How do you feel after an orgy sequence or threesome? A lesbian scene? In what sexual situations do you feel used?

10. All contributors should deal with the following question: After a few years of making adult films, and having genital and oral sex with different men (how many, in your estimation?), do you feel you could ever settle down into simple monogamy and forsake all others? Can you envision a world where human beings, premaritally and postmaritally, could enjoy more than one sexual partner in some kind of open marriage that allowed more sexual freedom? (You may be aware that most of Bob's thirteen novels address that very question and the possibility of a sexually utopian society.) Visualize the kind of loving, sexual world you prefer we lived in. One with fewer hang-ups about nudity and sex?

11. Relate the importance of sex with the deeper needs of companionship that you may desire, including your own needs (or not) to have children. If you already have kids, how would you, or do you, explain yourself to them, both now and in the future, when the films and videos you've appeared in will still be available.

12. We've heard a great deal about the abuse of drugs (cocaine, especially) and alcohol in the industry. Has either ever made its way into your life? Why do you think the abuse is so common in the field? Could society's condemnation of erotica be a reason?

13. In your own words, describe the nature of the porno business. Is it really like an extended family with some security? After working with a particular guy more than once, do you feel like old friends?

14. Talk about your fears of sexually transmitted diseases (syphilis, gonor-
rhea, herpes, AIDS). How do you feel when your mate on a shoot is a guy
you've never seen before?

Before he died prematurely in an automobile accident in December 1991,
Robert Stoller was professor of psychiatry at the University of California. In his
book *Porn, Myths for the 20th Century,* he offers what he calls "an ongoing piece
of ethnography—or an adventure in porno land." In one chapter in this book,
titled, "Where Are the Men?" he explores with Ron (not Ron Jeremy), a writer
who is much involved with the porn industry, how the male performers react to
their profession. (This was written before Jerry Butler's book was published and
confirms why even Jerry Butler, despite much prodding from me, was never able
to really evoke his feelings.) Ron, speaking on tape, says: "I find male porn performers to be among the most close-lipped, guarded, remote individuals, I have
ever known. They really keep to themselves and each other much more than the
women. . . . The girls mix much more . . . they schmooze, they fool around and
chat and flirt."

Ron points out,

> As a man I can understand. If I'm going to have two orgasms in eight hours, the
> erection in my second session is probably not going to be as strong as in the first.
> But at another level, it is something psychological that he's saying: "I want the
> maximum physiological advantage for dealing with this thing." That seems to be
> the pattern of male performers. The male performers do not seem to identify
> with the culture of pornography. . . . You don't see them do promotional stuff. .
> . . I think the most common false pretension of male performers is that they are
> just horny guys. With lots of false jocularity they try to act like fraternity broth-
> ers."

In both *Porn* and *Coming Attractions,* Stoller advances his theory: "The people who create pornography embody the communication systems that make up
the culture's avowed erotic desires." Previously, in other books, Stoller has made
extended studies of women who "think and feel erotically, and have done so con-
sciously since childhood. They are profoundly exhibitionistic, always feeling that
they are being watched, and they spend hours highly focused on cosmetics, fash-
ion, sexy underwear, and watching themselves or performing in highly erotic
movement."

Bill Margold, a well-known porno actor and director, tells Stoller in a
lengthy interview: "All porno queens are born this way." Stoller, a tourist in a
strange land, listens to Margold tell him why he loves the industry: "It's an anti-
social, highly immoral, utterly rebellious form of entertainment. We are the last

rebels in society. At least we're better than the stupid terrorists who go around blowing up people. No one ever died from an overdose of pornography."

In *Porn,* Stoller also recounts a taped interview with Nina Hartley (she lives in a ménàge à trois with a guy and another woman and refers to her more plebian self as Monica). Also interviewed are Happy, a nude model who had just made her first porno film; Merlin, a guy who makes bondage and S&M videos; and total egoist Jim Holliday, who knows that he is the best (even better than Margold). Holliday reveals his personal life in detail but not why Jack Nash changed his name. Holliday gives you some fascinating insights into the industry in which he has found his home "and wouldn't leave for a quarter of a million dollars." Has any one ever offered it to him?

The long conversations with Holliday and Margold continue in *Coming Attractions,* with an inside-porno-land perspective that you never see in *AVN* or any of the men's magazines. Plus there are taped conversations with Sharon Kane, Nina Hartley, Porsche Lynn, and Randy Spears, all reflecting Stoller's search to understand and know what the basis of human erotic excitement really is. He reaches the conclusion that "an element of harm energizes erotics. . . . The desire to harm, cruelty, anger, revenge, and humiliation is the grain of sand around which the pearl of erotic excitement exists."

A scary idea? You bet. Maybe all over the world males killing each other over their religious differences and raping each other's wives are finally experiencing satisfying orgasms.

In a straight-from-the-shoulder interview Porsche Lynn tells Stoller about early career and "the anger building up with me" which has made her able to rip out a male heart with her tongue. She gives one example of working and getting $14,000 for two days' work, but the check bounces. She was well aware that there were twenty other blondes with blue eyes who work more cheaply than she would, but she finally got her money "for fucking and sucking for two days."

Porsche tells Stoller, "I don't personally believe that anyone should be making adult movies until they are twenty-one . . . at eighteen most girls haven't had a lot of sexual experience. They're really not just sexually aware, although they may think they are. Younger girls get sucked in because of all the glamour around the industry, the limousines, the clothes, fancy places, the money."

Ira Levine, who put *Coming Attractions* together after Stoller's death, sums it up: "The social cost of X-rated entertainment is probably sustainable but the personal toll it exacts from its creators can be steep. In my utopian dream, society accepts the need for erotic entertainment, gives up on trying to eliminate it and mandates workplace reforms for the protection of those who provide it."

Another must-read book—if you are interested in a broader perspective on pornography from the female, and the overall cultural point of view—is *Hard*

Core by Linda Williams at the University of California. Williams tells you right off that when it comes to the question of the power and pleasure variously posed in pornography and the feminist point of view, "I am strictly on the anti-censorship side." Then, in three hundred pages, she examines the history of pornography from Victorian times, when it first became a social/cultural censorship issue, then the still photographs of naked men and women in motion of Edward Muybridge, culminating in actual naked bodies in motion in stag films. Then Williams gives a detailed analysis of "come shots" and other sine qua non of many specific porno films produced in the seventies and eighties. Subtitled "Power, Pleasure and the Frenzy of the Visible," Williams's book will convince you that the male fascination with porno is the neverending search for the feminine unknowable. In essence men, are trying, via the hard-core "frenzy of the visible," to make "visible the involuntary confession of bodily pleasure." Watching the penis plunging into the vagina or watching the come shot, according to Williams, is a surface manifestation of our need to really know "the sexually other," which is ultimately unknowable. Nevertheless, Williams believes that pornographic speculation is a valid journey into the ineffable mystery of the other person and his or her sexual pleasure.

So, too, is the attempt to really know the depths of each other's sexual needs and pleasures, which are often inexplicable to ourselves. My feeling is that beyond sexvids and the "frenzy of the visible" is written language. I'm sure that one of these days a porno actress or actor will, with the little help of a "ghost writer," attempt the impossible.

So what is the future of X-rated? There are only two possible scenarios to the end of an era of sexual decadence. Keep in mind that X-rated videos are only one facet of the continuous overt devaluation of human sexuality that has occurred in the last half of the twentieth century. The first scenario is that, ultimately, religious morality, both Christian, Judaic, and Islamic, will most certainly reassert itself. The U.S. Census Bureau is now projecting a population of 392 million Americans by the year 2050—52 percent more people than there are today, with the population evenly divided between whites and black and Hispanic minorities. At the present time, 60 percent of Americans do not attend church and for the most part live by a kind of "situational ethics" that includes consensual nonmarital sexual behavior as a "victimless crime." But irresponsible sexual behavior, including a million-a-year teenage pregnancies, families sustained by one parent, and an increasing crime rate involving mostly young men and many teenagers who have grown up in battered family structures, along with rape, sexual harassment, and pedophilia, are being traced back to an environment of noncaring human sexual relationships and commitments.

In his encyclical *Veritatis Splendor* (The Splendor of Truth), Pope John

Paul II reminds his readers of the rich young man who came to Jesus and asked, "Teacher what must I do to have eternal life?" (Matthew 19:16). Jesus responded, "If you wish to enter into life, keep the commandments." Pope John Paul also points out that life is fulfilled by knowing the truth and doing the truth. "I am the way, and the truth and the life," Jesus told his disciples.

Tipper Gore, our vice president's wife, tried to find a way in her book *How to Raise Teenagers in an X-Rated World,* but she's trying to hold back the tide. The problem, of course, is finding the way to calm the erupting sexual volcano of not only X- and R-rated films, but the degraded, devalued sex garbage that permeates television talk shows, newspapers, magazines like *National Enquirer* and *People,* and, for the upper class, *Vanity Fair* and a large portion of books being published that explore sexual insanities and moralize over them with a kind of pursed-lip prurience.

Is there a way or Tao—as the Confucians believe? More likely, as the Spanish poet Antonio Machado wrote, "Wayfarer, there is no way to go. One makes the way by going."

Dealing with reality, Linda Williams suggests that, "Sex, in the sense of a natural, biological, and visible 'doing what comes naturally,' is the supreme fiction of hard core pornography; and gender, the social construction of the relations between the sexes, is what constitutes that fiction." Williams believes that, "The visibility (seeing the action) is the source of pleasure for men, but incorporating the action into the fiction or the reality of the moment, is what makes women erotic."

So—"making the way by going"—the only way into the future is dependent on knowing where we have been. Somewhere in the 1960s Americans began to put down romance as corny and passé. In the 1940s and 1950s Lauren Bacall gave Humphrey Bogart a nice-girl kind of tease with a "pucker up your lips and blow" come-on. Spencer Tracy, discovering that Katharine Hepburn's sharp tongue was really a cover for her girlishness, fell in love forever with her long legs and impishness. Fred Astaire and Ginger Rogers found neverending romance as they danced together. All this was conditioning a generation romantically, perhaps unreasonably and often quite sillily, but in the long run offering a sounder basis for human loving than the following years of anything-goes "hot and cool" sex. Romantic love carries the seeds of twenty-first- century sexual revaluing, and the sacramentalizing of human sexuality.

Caryn James in the *New York Times* in April 1990 wrote that,

The benchmark for this turn against romance came as late as *Fatal Attraction,* the 1987 film that ended up capturing some weighty contemporary fears about sex and love . . . it is hard to ignore the social implications of this clever horror film . . . the fear of AIDS that makes a one night stand a potentially lethal proposition, the vulnerability of even the happiest seeming marriages, the panic that hit the single woman approaching middle age in a society glutted with already married men. . . . [The film] obviously reflected fears that had been festering in the minds of the audience, anxieties that are also evident in the popularity of books in the mold of *Women Who Love Too Much* . . . and the enormous social impact of the film comes in the way it distilled so many issues into one emotionally fraught scenario.

Today most Hollywood films have a cynical view about love, and there are few endings where you can be sure that a few days later the lovers, with tears of regret in their eyes, will ever see each other again. In an article, "Love, Lust, & Romance" in the *Boston Phoenix* in February 1991, Caroline Knapp explores in greater depth how Hollywood shapes our reality. "Romantic ideals are a fact of life. We all wish our lives—especially our love lives—were a little more like they are (were?) in the movies. A little smoother. A little more passionate."

But as Ms. Knapp points out, in the old days men felt lust toward women, but not vice versa—ostensibly at least. Scarlett O'Hara smiled suggestively and secretly when Rhett Butler swept her into his arms. Today all that's changed. In *Wild at Heart*, Laura Dern's character "has sexual appetite that makes most women look positively anemic by comparison. . . . She screams, she bites and moans. She grips the sheets with her long red fingernails . . . in the lust category she makes a lot of women out there feel edgy."

And that's the reason that many women detest X-rated movies, because in them the women not only take the initiative but as soon as they have a guy's cock in their mouths, they presumably make him ecstatic by telling him that they are not only "going to blow his brains out" but swallow his protein-laden jism because they love him so much.

As a friend of Knapp told her, "It's not that women don't feel lust . . . feeling lust is a private personal thing. It has to do with fantasies. When you start talking about the portrayal of lust on screen, with the exception of an occasional Woody Allen film, you are talking about performance, and not when the man and woman don't connect (mentally) or the sex is disappointing." One woman told Knapp that after seeing Meg Ryan imitate the sounds of orgasm in *When Harry Met Sally*, or seeing Susan Sarandon practically make James Spader's eyes roll out of his head, she was terrified that she wouldn't measure up for her boyfriend with regular or oral sex. But it inspired her to talk about it with him, and "it helped."

When it comes to romance and love the Hollywood message of the 1990s, according to one woman, is : "Movies always put unlikely people together. First there's friction because of their differences. But then they work out their problems, and then they live happily ever after . . . as a result many women feel we are losers when we don't work out our own problems and relationships." More lust in bed, ending on a happily-ever-after theme, is still apparent in movies like *The Fabulous Baker Boys,* but today's viewers don't buy it. Here are snippets from thirty-somethings that Knapp corralled about current thinking. "This Hollywood image really gets in the way. It's not all a bed of roses. Things aren't always romantic. A guy takes his girlfriend to see Arnold Schwarzenegger movies so they don't get the wrong idea." This from a woman: "In movies when someone has something to give to the person they love, it's rarely unconditional love. Instead, it's a lesson, it's a credit card. That's what's portrayed as 'freeing' you rather than the hardest things to give another person, which are abstract or taken on trust, values like the potential to grow and expand, be open and listen, and learn and change in real ways."

Obviously, during the last half of the twentieth century Americans were waiting, or looking for someone to provide a vision of the future, a vision that, among other things gives them art forms that the media, religious leaders, and teachers confirm. Daring to come to grips with the joys, laughter, and sheer wonder of human sexuality will provide a new kind of reality-romance, as men and women learn to look beyond themselves and share the universe with a God of Love, a dancing God! "Where there is no vision, the people perish" (Proverbs 29:18). NSME Legislation provides that vision. Will it happen. You can bet on it—there is no other way to go!

22

After Darwin Blew the Lid Off—
Past Sexual Roads and Detours

If you believe the old adage that: "If you don't learn from the past, you're destined to relive it," here's a fast trip over the high roads and low roads of human sexuality during the past 150 years. Inevitably, the roads lead to the final sexual revolution where human sexuality, which as been waiting on the doorstep of the church, synagogue, and mosque for several millennia, is invited back inside and Eros and agape are rewedded.*

Denis deRougement once pointed out, "The paradox of Christianity is that this religion of love declares that 'God is Love' but had no code of love, no sexual rites and no eroticism, either sacred or profane. As distinctive from the great Asiatic religions, it gives little or no importance to sexual love, or sentimental love, in short to Eros, instead, it antithetically bestows the highest rank on agape."

Expounding on a belief in one God, who triumphed over the pagan gods, the Christian fathers gradually transformed the bacchanal of the winter solstice (Are unrestrained sex and orgies a human attempt to triumph over death?) into the time of the rebirth of a Savior born of a virgin mother and the rebirth of the earth in the spring (another time of pagan sexual release and celebration) with the resurrection of Jesus Christ, thus offering the hope of resurrection to a mankind who had obeyed the moral pronouncements of the Almighty God.

Two thousand years later, practicing Christians and Jews and even sixty million Americans who no longer attend church, are still conditioned from early

---

*Some of this essay appears in the twenty-fifth anniversary edition of *The Harrad Experiment*, which is still in print and available from Prometheus Books, along with *The Byrdwhistle Option, The Immoral Reverend,* and *The Resurrection of Anne Hutchinson.* Written in 1990, the essay reinforces and underlines the necessity for New Sexual Morality and Education (NSME) legislation.

childhood by biblical morality and dogma. Beliefs in no sex before marriage, beliefs that the basic reason for copulation is to create children, beliefs that celibacy and following Jesus are the best way to achieve heaven and be welcomed by God; beliefs that refraining from passion for another person; loving God first; beliefs, stemming from the sins of Adam and Eve; beliefs about the Lilith character of women tempting men to lust after the flesh; beliefs about monogamous marriage (despite the polygamous style of many ancient Jewish patriarchs, along with Arabs a few centuries later); and beliefs in the shame of adultery (for women, not men)—all are at the root of most of our moral problems today. It's a morality that no longer works and which one writer, Raymond Lawrence, an Episcopal priest, calls a longtime "Poisoning of Eros."

Protestants, following Martin Luther and John Calvin's teachings about maintaining self-control and loving God first, were given religious promises that not only guaranteed resurrection, but, "All this and Heaven, too!"

Today, the work ethic for religious Protestants and most Catholics (who leave it to their priests to deal with the Old Testament) is still to somehow merge spirituality with materialism and achieve a way of life which, balanced by philanthropy, will not only assure the faithful that they will be accepted into heaven but that they will be "among that number when the saints come marching in." Most of the political and Wall Street miscreants and plunderers who have filled the pages of the media in the 1980s and 1990s with their "me first" morality, quickly repent and become born again Christians when they are caught.

Gertrude Himmelfarb, in her book *Marriage and Morals Among the Victorians,* reminds us that the sexual revolution did not begin in the 1960s but rather 150 years ago, when Charles Darwin blew the lid off the first chapter of Genesis with his theory of evolution, and Nietzsche insisted that God is dead and as a result Christian morality becomes a command. Christian morality's origin is transcendental and it is beyond all criticism and all rights to criticize. Religion possesses truth only if God is truth and it stands or falls with a belief in God.

The Victorian elite and their predecessors by a few years, those who tried to direct the thinking of the masses, such as T. H. Huxley, Jeremy Bentham, William Godwin, Robert Owens, J. S. Mill, Frances Galton (with eugenics), Herbert Spencer, and many others, tried to evoke a new kind of secular humanism with a premise that man is innately good and, whether God is dead or not, man can create his own moral parameters. But, in the area of marriage and the family, most of the eminent Victorians were unable to abide by biblical morality. They lived together unmarried, had children out of wedlock and lovers beyond monogamy.

Whether civilization would have collapsed if men and women had continued to worship many gods or whether human sexuality could have been controlled in other ways, as it was in oriental religions, is now something that should be considered. Ancient Chinese and Hindu civilization never offered the one-god idea; but their belief in the equality of the female principle sharing the universe (yang and yin) is alive and waiting to be incorporated into Western religious beliefs.

But the bigger problem is that today we are travelling without sails on an inherited moral ship that started to leak at the beginning of the Industrial Revolution and is now capsizing. Right now, we are living a future shock, even beyond what Alvin Toffler predicted twenty years ago. And morally we don't know how to cope with it. Millions of us past sixty are only dimly aware that the population of the United States has tripled since we were born. Nor do most of us appreciate that one element of future shock, one that futurists in the 1950s never predicted, is that by 1991 57 percent of all married women were working wives. In the previous hundred years, between 1850 and 1950, the growing belief was that since work had moved from the home to the factory, men were now the breadwinners. Except for isolated areas like the textile mills, where slave wages still prevailed and women and children ran the ear-splitting machinery, most women no longer had to work. Even middle-income men could support non-working wives, and the affluent, as evidenced by the big Victorian homes surrounding the older American cities, could create homes that housed several generations and solved the problem of poor relations and elderly parents. By contrast, today we have an underfunded Social Security system and nursing homes with annual costs per client running $50,000 a year or more and which most families can't afford without welfare backup.

Less than fifty years ago, the average lifespan was fifty to sixty years. Marriage for young women who could not aspire to higher education was at ages seventeen or eighteen, and many men in one lifetime had several wives, not through divorce, but because their wives died in childbirth. Be fruitful and multiply made sense. Men with mistresses were a way of life that most women tolerated because they had no choice or way to support themselves independently.

Today, women live longer than men and education takes longer. Less than 150 years ago, young men completed their education, even medical, lay, and clerical degrees, by the time they were twenty and were soon married. Biologically at least, women are ready for marriage at fifteen or sixteen and young men are able to impregnate them them earlier. But today, following the old-time religions and biblical morality, we expect that, somehow or other, 50 percent of young people who graduate from high school and try to achieve further education will abstain from pre-marital sex (true even before the AIDS epidemic) for as long as eight years, until they have completed their education, after which they will marry the only person they will ever have "safe sex" with for the next fifty years. It isn't happening, of course, and even Catholic religious leaders have reluctantly come to accept premarital cohabitation, but not with condoms or birth control.

Abstain from sex until marriage and love God is still the moral imperative for millions of Americans, but it isn't working!

Today, in most marriages, the wife is no longer chief cook and bottle washer. She must work to help support the children she bears. If she's not a high school dropout and has some sexual education, she's soon convinced that zero population growth, two children to replace herself and her husband, is the only sane way for her and her mate to live. Despite the insistence of Catholic priests and many evangelical Protestants that male sperm in her vagina should not be prevented from uniting with her ova, both she and her husband use birth control and often pray that there is no third child. If there is, abortion becomes a solution, or a moral dilemma.

Working to support their families, women soon discover there are many attractive men in the workforce (her husband may be discovering the same thing about women). Young marrieds often learn, too late, that the mate they married was not the best choice, or that they are more or less "into" sex than their mate; or, being quite normal human beings, they wonder what it would be like to really be intimate mentally and sexually with a person other than the one with whom they've made a lifetime commitment. Ultimately, in complete moral confusion, they may divorce and the wife may be left to support the children.

To add to the moral confusion, there is no longer any censorship of the written word, and little effective censorship of visual sex via movies, television, and videocassettes. Media advertising continuously offers the female as a sex object. For many young people, the sex tease becomes a shrugging way of life. Both R- and X-rated material undermines the old-time monogamous marriage morality with a tantalizing swinger-style belief that "come and go" multiple sexual relationships, without too much caring or mental involvement, is a sustainable way of life.

The popularity of soap operas, movies, and videos exploring every aspect of human sexuality (particularly the kinky and deviant) proves that most men and women are not only unable to live within the moral and sexual restraints imposed by religious doctrine, but are seeking some sexually moral basis for life that thus far eludes them.

Unless we move in the direction of the New Sexual Morality and Education legislation that I have proposed in part I, America's unmerged cultural diversity will turn us to a second-rate nation. We must prove that the American kind of blended racial and ethnic equality is superior to the relative homogeneity of the Japanese, Chinese and many European nations who are all cast in the same mold. We need not a melting pot but new kind of GLUE that is the basis of a federally guaranteed subsidized, undergraduate education.

Whether they attend church or not, millions of Americans, Catholic, Jewish,

Protestant, or Islamic, are indoctrinated with pre-marital and post-marital sexual beliefs based on the Bible, the Koran, or the Torah. In many cases, Catholics will defy papal doctrine when it comes to birth control or divorce, but will join with Southern Baptists on the right to life and try to eliminate their agreed upon versions of pornography whether it reflects a wide range of sexual behavior that others consider normal or not. Nevertheless, in a democracy, they have to accept laws passed by a more liberal majority, along with the judicial interpretations of the First and Fourteenth Amendments guaranteeing rights to privacy and freedom of speech.

Sixty million Americans do not attend church, but many of them also are caught up in the same moral whirlpool when it comes to making value judgments about sex before marriage, masturbation, sex with a nonmarital partner after marriage, homosexuality, abortion, nudity in the home and in public, portraying sexmaking on television and in the arts, and what constitutes obscene and criminal behavior.

Now, at the end of the twentieth century, we have arrived at the crossroads. Our religious leaders are unable to come up with the new moralities without getting into interdenominational warfare over the validity of their beliefs in premarital sex, birth control, abortion, adultery, and the visual presentations of human sexuality.

When *The Harrad Experiment* was published by Bantam Books in paperback in 1967, the subtitle was *The Sex Manifesto of the Free Love Generation.* I had seen the artwork before the paperback appeared and I protested. I thought I had made it abundantly clear that the Harrad concept, which was the first approach to the Roommate of the Other Sex Program, was predicated on caring sexual relations and commitment and most certainly wasn't "free love."

In the long run, there is no such thing as free love and the so-called sexual revolution of the 1960s was not a revolution but a rebellion by a different generation against the old-time religions, during which many women, led Betty Friedan and the growing feminist movement, discovered in nauseating detail the extent of male patriarchal domination that has held women in subjection for thousands of years. The self-appointed male leaders of the tribe were "poisoning Eros" as Raymond Lawrence claims in his book of the same title. Using Christian, Judaic, and Islamic religious laws that carefully define the good and the bad in nonmarital, premarital, and postmarital sexual relations, men closely defined the boundaries of socially acceptable human sexuality. In the process, women became chattel. To protect males from themselves and the libidinous temptations of women, and to make sure their progeny came from the male owner's seed, adultery, in the laws of the major manmade religions, became a sin. But thanks to their male vision (and recognition that they as well as most men were compulsive maters) Mohammed and, much later, Joseph Smith interwove the need for many wives (polygamy, a male approved adultery) with a love of Allah/God.

Today we are still trying to live by religious moralities that no longer work in a Western world of growing populations, vast economic change, and much longer active sexual lives. We must reinvent marriage and create new approaches to normal human sexuality, where new-style families can lead more varied sex lives and expand their interpersonal relationships with and underlying belief, and a God-approved morality, that loving other persons in a lifetime marriage can be "in addition to" and not "instead of" the primary bonding. Male/female equality will inevitable and finally prevail.

The greater sexual freedom that many women enjoyed with the pill was lost with the fear of AIDS; and before that with herpes, which, although it didn't cause death, seemed to be incurable. But the problem of AIDS and STDs can be minimized for a vast majority of the population if a new-style sexual sanity prevails. A historical perspective on the need for a democratically approved new sexual morality shows that it is the direction in which the Western world has been moving for the past four hundred years. Controlling human sexuality by various means has been explored in utopias from Plato in his *Republic*, to Sir Thomas More in the seventeenth century (who invented the term "utopia," to mean "no place"), to Robert Dale Owen, Charles Fourier, and John Humphrey Noyes in the nineteenth century, who less than 150 years ago were trying to make their utopias a communal way of life. Some of their approaches surfaced once again in the 1960s as the solution to the problems of human sexuality as well as capitalism. On the negative side, a vocal minority in the English-speaking world had discovered sexual censorship and legislating morality as the means to keep their versions of religious morality intact.

As G. Legman points out in his article "The Lure of the Forbidden," sexual censorship began in England in the early eighteenth century, when Alexander Pope, in 1725, published an expurgated edition of Shakespeare's plays. Legman is famous for his explorations of human sexuality and particularly his hundred-page monograph, *Love and Death,* in which he asks, "Why, over many centuries, has sex been considered a crime on paper, though legal and permissible in fact, and why per contra, are sadism and murder, which are illegal in fact and on paper, in fact our "best sellers"? Legman wrote this before visual sex on film and video had replaced the problem of written sex, but the question remains the same.

In their book *Intimate Matters: A History of Sexuality in America* (which could be required reading in the senior year of the K-12 course in human sexuality) John D'Emilio and Estelle Freedman survey the very different Protestant sexual climate that prevailed in North America for more than a hundred years, in contrast to Central America and South America, which, after Columbus's first voyages, was divided between Catholic Portugal and Spain and almost completely reflected Catholic sexual morality and still does.

While the Puritans condemned adultery and nonmarital sex, they wanted many children and they actually accepted sex for pleasure within marriage. But, as D'Emilio and Freedman point out, "The English rejected the Catholic condemnation of carnal desires that had required the celibacy of priests and associated all sexual expression, even in marriage, as a fall from grace. The idea that marriage was accepted primarily as a way to channel lust and prevent sexual sin gave way to a belief that marital love, as well as the need to produce children, could justify sexual intercourse."

But the Puritans were utopians, too, and believed in an undeviating theology based on the Decalogue, the Ten Commandments. People like Anne Hutchinson and Roger Williams who defied their biblical interpretations became known as antinomians or enthusiasts. They believed that since Christ had already sacrificed himself for human sins, if you acknowledged "enthusiastically" that Christ was within you, you were absolved from all sins, past or future. Some of the religions, like the Family of Love and the Anabaptists, laid the foundations for wife-sharing and family groupings that were anathema to the Anglican and the Puritan (Congregational) denominations.

Hutchinson, Williams, and many others were banished from John Winthrop's utopian "city on the hill." As Winthrop's journals reveal, there was plenty of voyaging into sexual waters in the Massachusetts Bay Colony beyond monogamy. Women were publicly punished for adultery; but, mostly men got away with it. Then, and until the past fifty years, there were few books in print dealing with sex. Rabelais, Chaucer, Boccacio, and even Shakespeare were for the few who could read. There was little erotic art even seen by the general public, no photography, no movies, television, or X-rated videocassettes. Other than the Old Testament stories, there was nothing to undermine the prescribed morality.

Nearly four hundred years later, the conflict between the Catholic and Protestant views of human sexuality continues in America. In the areas of divorce, birth control, abortion, nonmarital sex, pornography, and human nudity, liberal Protestants and Jews are aligned against the Catholics and the Southern Baptists.

Long before the new sexual direction taken in the 1960s, from 1880 to 1930 there was continuous probing of the problems of sex, marriage, and the family, which, in their days, were given wide media attention.

Unlike the sexually negative "no solutions" environment we have lived in since the 1960s, during the late 1800s there was much creative thinking about human sexual problems. It is ferment that I believe is once again brewing and will soon be ready to be bottled in New Sexual Morality Education legislation, along with healthy controversy, about better ways for people to live together and relate sexually to one another. Communal living experiments were flourishing at Brook Farm, Amana, New Harmony, Oneida, and many other places. All of them had their own approaches to living happier lives in harmony with God, nature, and one's fellow men and women. Robert Dale Owen, who tried to blend some of the ideas of other utopians like Campanella, Diderot, and Fourier, proclaimed from his commune in New Harmony, Indiana, "Man up to this time has been a slave to a trinity of the monstrous evils that could be combined to inflict mental and physical evil upon the whole race . . . namely, private and individual property, absurd and irrational systems of religion, and marriage founded upon individual property."

While the current management of the world's largest manufacturer of razor-shaving equipment doesn't like to be reminded of it, King Gillette, who invented the disposal razor blade, was of the same opinion when it came to competition and the capitalistic system, and with the help of Upton Sinclair he wrote several books declaiming the evils of the profit system. In his book *World Corporation* Gillette offered a new economic system in which all humans shared the wealth. He was not alone in this era of exciting new approaches to democratic socialism. In the late 1800s, Edward Bellamy astonished the world with his novels *Looking Backward* and *Equality,* offering visions of the year 2000 that sold millions of copies worldwide, and by today's standards were all-time bestsellers.

The Future Families of America Commission will recreate new interest in the Oneida community, created by John Humphrey Noyes, a Protestant minister. The community comprised several hundred members who, in an even distribution of males and females, practiced "complex marriage." In this community, wives and husbands, without jealousy, and after giving each other specific approval, could switch bedmates. Noyes solved the problem of birth control with his discovery of "male continence" and the ability of a man to enjoy sexual congress without ejaculating even though the female might climax more than once. Noyes probably learned this approach to nirvana from Hindu Tantric literature, aided by "coitus interruptus," "coitus reservatus," and "karezza," about which several books had been written.

With woman fighting for suffrage, as the first stage in the opening battles for equal rights, and Margaret Sanger and Anthony Comstock in a media battle over censorship of literature about sex and birth control, the temper of the times was to resolve problems that are still very much with us. How can individual dyads, a man and woman, thrive or even survive in lifelong monogamous marriage? By the mid-nineteenth century, free love became the rallying cry of the intellectuals to such an extent that in 1855 the stodgy *New York Times* ran a series of three disapproving articles on the subject.

Twenty years later, in 1875, free love was still a hot subject, lasting longer than the 1970s concept of "open marriage." Long before Betty Friedan discovered the "feminine mystique," Virginia Woodhull, an even more feisty and eloquent feminist, supported by many other prominent women of her time, ran for president of the United States on a "free love" ticket, which even by mid-1990s standards was pretty far out. Woodhull even endorsed the scandalous Rev. Henry Ward Beecher (brother of Harriet Stowe of *Uncle Tom's Cabin* fame). Stowe disclaimed Beecher when he became a national scandal. Beecher was accused of adultery with more than one young lady parishioner in his Brooklyn church, where he attracted more than a thousand people every Sunday to hear his sermons.

In her book *Tried by Fire,* Woodhull explained her platform: "I am conducting a campaign against marriage with a view to revolutionizing the present theory and practice. I have strong convictions that as a bond, or a promise to love one another, marriage is a fraud upon human happiness. The most intelligent and virtuous people of all classes have outgrown this institution, are systematically unfaithful to it, and revolt against its slavery."

Needless to say, Woodhull didn't get elected president, but she proved that a political approach to sexual morality is inevitable. Today, a political solution like the New Sexual Morality and Education bill will clarify the continuous church versus state problems of the Constitution. When the new sexual morality legislation is incorporated into the beliefs of major religions, the need for many current aspects of separation of church and state, on a political basis, will no longer exist. Priests, ministers, and rabbis, along with political leaders, will have common cause to create a new moral environment that exalts and sacramentalizes human sexuality.

Unlike the earlier believers in free love and their followers a hundred years later, the beatniks of the 1950s, followed by the hippies and flower children of the 1960s, offered no rational approach to "free love," but tried to jump on an "open marriage" bandwagon.

The K-12 sexual seminars will follow the lead of John Humphrey Noyes. He excoriated the "free love" concept. "Marriage," he wrote, "makes a man responsible to a woman [today its a two-way street] for the consequences of his love. In free love [Noyes often called it whoredom] man exposes a woman to the heavy burden of maternity, and then goes away without responsibility. [Noyes would have abhorred our million teenage pregnancies annually.] Marriage provides for the maintenance and education of children. Free love leaves them to chance. Our communities at Oneida are families as distinctly bounded and separated from promiscuous society as ordinary households. We are not free lovers in any sense that makes love less binding than it is in marriage."

Nearly a hundred years later, in books that have been labeled alternative lifestyle novels, I have been preaching a comparable version of monogamous marriage that merges one or more families. In the previous chapter I explored these proposals. There are many others being practiced today that offer a potential for both greater lifetime family stability and more intellectual and sexual variety than is currently available, with rare exceptions, in conventional marriage.

Readers who have been in college in the past fifteen years may have taken one of the marriage and family courses that most colleges and universities offer. Unfortunately, women who take these courses outnumber men two to one. There are at least twenty-five thousand-page-plus texts offered by various publishers. Written by psychology, biology, and sociology professors, they offer chapters on alternative life styles and try to deal with the realities of the 1990s. But the writers are careful to make few value judgements or offer any suggestions on how particular moral values have become embedded in religious and secular thinking.

The writers are well aware that by the year 2000 there will be 110 million households in this country with an average of less than three people, and million single households. This is a far cry from the presumed typical American nuclear family of a husband, wife, and two children of twenty-five years ago who dreamed of living in a rose-covered cottage. That was a 1940 daydream of another generation that most young Americans will never realize in the twenty-first century.

The 50 percent divorce rate, the necessity for job mobility, six million children of divorced parents, ten million widows (a very new phenomenon of the past one hundred years, because women now have greater longevity than men), the 25 percent of the American population living well past seventy years with all the problems of old age, 57 percent all wives working (not for careers, but for economic necessity), and an inflation rate that can't be resolved without creating vast unemployment—all contribute to the problems that can be greatly ameliorated by new approaches to sexual morality, which will pave the way for new-style, non-related, extended families.

In the twenty-fifth anniversary edition of *The Harrad Experiment* published in 1990, I offered a survey of the last fifty years that shows the DDD ("Democracy Drifting to Disaster") course that we have been taking since the end of World War II. The following is a recap of it which will give readers in their late teens and early twenties, and their parents, the children of the baby boomers, some historical background and a wider perspective on present problems.

During the affluent 1950s, the United States ruled the world technologically, but there was an underlying malaise. The G.I. Bill made it possible for veterans to purchase development homes with little or no down payment, and in the process created suburbia, which laid the groundwork for shopping malls, and mass traffic jams, and commuting as we know it today. The nuclear family moved into hundreds of small Levittown homes, which were unlike the large homes of a previous and much less populous generation. In the 1930s, less than seventy years ago, the population of the United States was only about 120 million people. In those days the poorhouses took care of the aged who had no family or monetary resources. After World War II, the demand for individual family privacy made it impossible to find room for the former extended families, parents, grandparents, and aunts and uncles, in the new houses that were being built. Many children of the owners became the flower children and hippies of the 1960s and they would label their homes "ticky tacky," using the words of a popular song that defined these nuclear family environments as intellectual and emotional traps. After ten years of financial prosperity during the 1950s, in the early 1960s even the upper-income, suburban "men in gray flannel suits" were identified as members of "the lonely crowd." The divorce rate was rising and millions of Americans didn't enjoy their "pursuit of happiness."

Jack Kerouac hailed the new "beat generation." According to him this was composed of "people who never yawn or say commonplace things. Instead they burn, burn, burn like fabulous Roman candles exploding like spiders across the stars. In the middle you see the blue center light pip and then everybody goes 'Awww.' " A few years later the beatniks would become hippies and flower children. By this time they had discovered pot instead of the booze used by their parents to escape reality. In the late 1960s the only sense of national purpose, aided by smoking marijuana, was to "turn on" and "drop out."

Life magazine, then selling millions of copies each week, recognized the problem and called upon national leaders to discover a national purpose for the United States. From a series of articles came many platitudes as well as the recognition that man, "satisfied with good," needed more from life than the pursuit of happiness. But no thinker in the United States seemed able to propose a unifying concept for this country and/or Western man.

By contrast, the English Puritans who arrived in the New World in the seventeenth century, and the "huddled masses" who arrived over the next two hundred years, had much better defined purposes. Trusting in God, they were going to improve their lives and make a better and more affluent world for their children. By the middle of the nineteenth century, hundreds of thousands of new arrivals from Europe and China were being exploited by the textile and railroad barons who employed them at very low wages in the cloth mills of Massachusetts and laying rails across the country. America suddenly had a new "royalty" based on wealth: the Astors, Vanderbilts, Goulds, Morgans, Cabots, Lowells, and their progeny, plus some later money achievers, were soon making up the 5 percent of Americans who controlled 95 percent of the wealth of this country.

Their leaders convinced these first generation Americans that they could make the world "safe for democracy" and in 1917 and 1918 they tried to stop Germany from the never-ending rearrangement of the borders of Europe, which continues for other reasons in other parts of the continent because of racial, ethnic, and religious differences to this day.

The sense of national purpose that motivated the country during World War I dissipated in the Jazz Age and was completely wiped out by ten years of depression in the 1930s. But then, in 1941, when the Japanese attacked Pearl Harbor and we faced the grim necessity of ridding the world of Hitler and his master race, Americans were once again united around a common cause. Our entry into World War II cured the economic malaise for many years. But it is worthwhile to remember that in the mid-thirties hundreds of thousands of Americans were singing the song "Brother, Can You Spare a Dime?" and thousands were listening to Marx and Lenin. They became "card carrying" Communists, hoping to eventually create a revolution. The *Communist Manifesto* provided the missing sense of purpose. You may be sure that a severe depression with much unemployment among vast numbers of unskilled people could still, today, create the environment for a new savior.

Completely educating all Americans during the first twenty-one years of their lives is crucial in a capitalistic system that is treading on the razor's edge. In the late 1960s our political leaders tried to create a sense of national purpose around Vietnam. But the "domino theory," the theory that the loss of South Vietnam would lead to world communism, didn't convince the younger generation. If we could not save Hungary and Czechoslovakia from Communism in the 1950s, the "domino theory" and the imperative that we must defend our right to trade anywhere in the world didn't make much sense in 1964 nor for many people twenty-seven years later in the Gulf War defending the Saudi Arabians.

In 1967, the younger generation rejected the international political belief of our leaders. But they did believe in "the greening of America" and the Club of Rome, who, well in advance of the current ecological movement, predicted the demise of the planet. Some of the generation who now have the reins of power in their hands were living in Haight Ashbury, San Francisco, or in the East Village of New York. Or they were living in communes in New Mexico, where they called themselves "love children" or "gentle people."

President Bush later hoped that they had become the "kinder and gentler people." In the 1990s, now called the "aging baby boomers," they've long forgotten that many of them extolled love and smoked marijuana, and that a few believed, as one male communard suggested: "All the girls are my wives, the guys are my brothers and all the babies are mine. . . . It's true love."

Unfortunately, their brains weren't so able to adjust to the conflicting demands of interpersonal relationships as their genitals.

In the words of Mick Jagger, they were "all together" and tried to prove it at Woodstock where four hundred thousand gathered in 1969 still seeking a sense of purpose that eluded them. In addition to smoking "grass," they tried to find their true selves and a new kind of spiritual uplift with LSD, or else they sought "soul experiences" in communes like Drop City and Hog Farm, which offered "hog consciousness."

It was a mind-blowing world where the true color was psychedelic. It was the "Age of Aquarius," and a time for gurus like Maharishi Mahesh Yogi and Bhwagan Shree Rajneesh, who, ten years later, would try to create the Rajneesh Puram in Eugene, Oregon, and die in 1990, claiming that he was poisoned by the CIA. It was the age of Free Universities, with the students deciding to set up their courses on campus, and Esalen at Big Sur, where the groundwork for the Human Potential Movement, no longer an expatriate who wrote dirty books, was being lauded at his home in Nepenthe. It was the age of the "generation gap" (still persisting via heavy metal rock, MTV, Madonna, and Michael Jackson into the 1990s). You couldn't trust anyone over thirty. If you were under thirty and "with it," you adopted the "mod" look from Carnaby Street. Women flattened their breasts and men grew long hair and beards and wore ankh symbols and love beads. Psychologists were proclaiming that sexual differences were disappearing and the world of unisex was just around the corner. It was also the time of student strikes against the Vietnam War, of the Black Power movement and a conviction that a free style of education developed by the students themselves was superior to anything offered in university catalogues. Compare the 1990 fervor of "political correctness" in university teaching and "multiculturalism," both determined to equate African civilization with Western civilization . . . and minimize the long social, cultural and political contributions of Western thought.

It was a time of awakening to the direction that the U.S. government was taking. The country was spending billions of dollars annually on defense to achieve military superiority and dissuade the Soviet Union, whose billions combined to make a world total of trillions of dollars, that use of nuclear power was a "no win" situation. We were blithely interfering in other people's civil wars in the name of democracy and napalming innocent victims. It was a time of realization that no one knew how to stop the military establishment, or if we were ever to achieve an agreement with the Soviet Union, how we would lower military spending and employ millions of Americans in peaceful and, perhaps, less profitable endeavors. It is a problem that may never be solved in a laissez-faire, capitalistic economy . . . but we still reject higher taxes and our slow, but inevitable socialization, which is proving whether we like it or not, that we are our "brother's keeper."

Today, few who are alive remember General Douglas MacArthur and his retirement speech, in which he declared to congress, "Old soldiers don't die, they just fade away." He deplored war as a solution to problems between nations. Later, President Eisenhower warned the nation: "Every gun that is made, every warship launched, every rocket fired signifies, in the final sense, a theft from those who hunger and are not fed . . . and those who are cold and not clothed . . . this world in arms is spending the sweat of its laborers, the genius of its scientists and the hopes of its children."

Nearly forty years later, we seem to be slowly moving to curtail the "high tech" arsenal of missiles, rockets, and nuclear bombs. But now, many of the so-called Third World nations, India, Pakistan, North Korea, Brazil, along with China, Israel, and possibly Syria, have nuclear capacities. With their help and plenty of American assistance, the arms merchants of the world become billionaires aiding and abetting internecine hatreds in the former Yugoslavia and many of the newly liberated Eastern nations. America may be the world's superior power, but, as the Gulf war, Somalia, and the tragedy in Bosnia proves, we cannot police the world alone.

But we can show the world we believe that men and women can redirect human sexuality and create a nation of people who believe that human history is not ending, but just beginning to take a great leap forward, as we give the upcoming generation a complete education and a new sense of wonder . . . and thus make living a lifelong process of loving, laughter learning, and ludamus (playing together).

In the early 1960s, the "feminine mystique" had been discovered and it gave birth to the equal rights movement, still a long way from reality. But there still was no national sense of purpose. Dropping out, living communally, giving up certain kinds of material goods (with the exception of fast automobiles and hi-fi equipment) were the messages. The designations "hot" and "cool" applied to books and television as well as sexual relations. It was a world of "future shocks" and the realization that no one knew how to cope with the implication of our scientific breakthroughs or absorb the vast avalanche of new information acquired by data processing and pouring out of computers, a problem that continues unabated into the 1990s.

Those who tried to lead with new "trendy" ideas quickly discovered that the commercial business world could quickly co-opt their ideas and that they became obsolete or "dated" almost as soon as they got off the ground. With multimillion-dollar advertising campaigns "living healthfully" became identified with jogging, high-fiber diets, certain kinds of breakfast cereals, and even getting thin by ingesting "dream tablets" and special powdered formulas.

All the surface confusion produces billions of words of interpretation, with the Clarence Thomas/Anita Hill affair topping the list. But more misinterpretation and misunderstanding persist in the minds of millions of Americans who watch their television an average of more than ten hours a day. Perhaps they can no longer distinguish the difference between the real world and the television world, which simply magnifies the thousands of murders, acts of violence, and sexual sorrows of the rich and poor. Or, as many writers and actors hope, maybe millions of us are being convinced that it's better to be happy and poor and monogamous than famous, wealthy and on the sexual prowl.

In the midst of assassinations (two Kennedys, one Martin Luther King), ghetto riots, and wars, in 1969 astronauts landed on the moon. Thanks to the blurring effects of television viewing, some people still think it never happened, but was a television spectacular designed to keep people's minds off their troubles. We discovered lasers, DNA, and the possibilities of genetic manipulation. Computers moved from tubes to transistors, silicon chips, and man's new ability to compress a world of information on less than a pin point. But the vast majority of Americans, with insufficient education, are unable to understand that the Faustian quest is only beginning. Inevitably we will have artificial intelligence in the form of computers who (yes, we'll personify them) will regulate our daily lives, for better or worse. Today we are presumably on the road to an information superhighway and even more automated manufacturing which, along with free trade, will eliminate most industrial unskilled labor and create continuing unemployment in many areas as Third World nations raise themselves by their "bootstraps" and take over many of our manufacturing jobs at lower wage rates.

After Vietnam, the drift toward disaster continued. We discovered that we were consuming most of the world's energy and were dependent on the Arabs and other nations, who didn't like us very much. Inflation, exacerbated by the rise in the price of oil, plunged the country into some long-needed soul searching. It was "Bye, Bye, Miss American Pie" in more ways than one. For a few years, with the help of a grim President Carter, we almost had a sense of national purpose. We began to worry about energy shortages; we could stop wasting fuel; we could build smaller automobiles and return to the stick shift that consumed less gas per mile. Some people became enthusiastic about nuclear power and the vast potential for solar energy. We began to believe that the Club of Rome prophecies might be true. Many were sure that we were exhausting the planet's natural resources. We were travelling on Buckminister Fuller's "spaceship earth." "Small is beautiful" became a slogan for those who wanted to return to the simpler ways of our forefathers. Ecology and Earth Days gave us some common bond.

But it didn't last long. We elected a famous movie actor president. He didn't think negatively (except toward the Soviet Union) and supply side economics became the new password to the future. Just let the rich get richer and the poor will become less poor, as excess money trickles down to them. For nearly eight years, the Reagan presidency seemed to work; but then we woke up to the horror. It was all a glorified kind of pump priming. The well was dry and we had a national debt of close to three trillion dollars. We were (and still are) importing much more than we are exporting and our trade deficit is so horrendous that many middle-income "ugly Americans" had to stay home because they couldn't afford to travel in Japan and most of Western Europe.

During the 1980s, the Japanese and West Germans were underwriting our

Epicurean, "I gotta be me . . . live today, tomorrow you die" philosophy. But in the 1990s, Third World nations were climbing on their backs, too, with a continuing global shift of manufacturing to lower wage rate countries.

With credit cards expanding our purchasing power, millions of Americans "owed their soul to the company store." Theoretically, nations like Japan and Germany grew rapidly because their people were great savers. But if Americans save too much, most economists get alarmed. We have to keep spending and spending to keep everyone employed. On top of that, every year the dollar buys 3, 4, or 5 percent less than it did the year before, so why save? As for the national debt, that's no problem since economists assure us that we owe it to ourselves and international debt is no problem either, according to other financial wizards. The Japanese, the West Germans, and the British may own a very large percentage of our factories and employ hundreds of thousands of us indirectly, but they can't afford to flush the economic toilet because they might go down the drain with us.

In the past century, with the exceptions of wars, the only sense of national purpose that most Americans had that still motivated most of us was summed up by the gestalt psychologist Fritz Perls, in the following lines, which he was happy to recite at Esalen (home of the "get into yourself" movement) while wearing a jump suit with nothing else under it so that admiring females could see his dickie): "I do my thing, and you do your thing. I'm not in this world to live up to your expectations, and you are not in this world to live up to mine. You are you, and I am I, and if by chance we find each other it is beautiful. If not, it can't be helped."

Twenty years later that was the political philosophy of the Watergate conspirators, of the behind-the-scenes dealing so that Reagan and Bush could contravene the law and supply arms to the Nicaraguans fighting the Sandinistas, of Iran fighting Iraq, of Donald Trump, Leona Helmsley, Imelda and Ferdinand Marcos, Ivan Boesky, Michael Milken, and many of the savings and loan bank presidents and many of our congressional leaders today. They and thousands more, including the corporate takeover experts and the "insiders" trading on Wall Street, became the mentors of millions of Americans. It was summed up by Michael Douglas, portraying a Wall Street speculator, with the words, "Greed is good."

During these years the perversion of democracy and capitalism into a world of greed and conspicuous consumption, not all of it financed honestly, has thoroughly warped the so-called sexual revolution. We continue to devalue and commercialize human sexuality. Psychologists have told us that the big orgasm is equivalent to a sneeze. But millions of women continue to read the women's magazines searching for the "big O," the pot of gold at the end of the marriage rainbow.

Within the last few decades, we eliminated censorship of the written word. At last we can read D. H. Lawrence, James Joyce, Henry Miller, and even the Marquis de Sade. The Supreme Court finally acknowledged that the human body was not obscene in the *Sunshine* case. Nudist magazines that appeared in the 1940s no longer had to airbrush the genitals from naked men and women. But what have we gotten in return? Adult bookstores, X-rated movies, the merger of violence and sex in R-rated movies, and thousands of "how to" sex books and motion pictures that more often than not have reduced the sex act to meaningless copulation between mental idiots.

Talking while fucking, enjoying each other and the merger of genitals while each person dares to disclose him or herself, is not possible between programmed robots. Our sexual mentors try to teach us that the way to self discovery is through multiple orgasms and Kamasutra variations to enhance the joys of fucking. But rarely do they discuss, or so you see even in novels or films, two people making love and revealing to each other the kind of people they really are. Nor would anyone today write a romantic, silly song like Hector Berlioz or the "Spectre of the Rose" about a man who died happily the next day after resting the night before on a woman's breast.

As I write this, I have just finished reading *Making Love: An Erotic Odyssey,* by Richard Rhodes, who won Pulitzer prize for his book *The Making of an Atomic Bomb.* Published in 1993, Rhodes's book should be on twelfth-grade outside reading lists when the new sexual morality becomes law. "I wrote *Making Love,*" Rhodes tells you,

> to explore a part of daily life that has been cut off from open discussion for centuries. I wanted to describe honestly one man's personal experience, my personal experience of sex and physical love. I wanted to understand how that experience shaped my life from childhood up to the present and how it helped me work through the trauma of child abuse, what I learned from it about my partners, what it contributed to intimacy and coming in love. Men and women will find intimate experience here to compare with their own. Explicit description of sexual experience has long been taboo. For that reason, many readers will find *Making Love* shocking at first. Pain and shame poison the air behind too many locked bedroom doors. When the shock wears off, I hope readers will appreciate my candor.

The book reviewers didn't. They excoriated Rhodes for exposing himself as a highly sexual person. But the book is "a coming event that casts its shadow before." Most of us, educated as we are, are unable to verbalize in any depth our feelings and emotions to each other. We're too embarrassed to admit to being the deeply loving sexual creatures we really are.

So there's the sexual morass into which we are still sinking. Can we raise ourselves by our own bootstraps? Can we create a society where human sexuality and the total wonder of the human mind becomes the new foundations of the major religions? I'm sure that while sexual morality, marriage, and the family has been the province of all major religions, none of them will dare to lead the way, or, if they try, as some minor religions like the Unitarian/Universalists have, they will find few adherents. But the time has come. Americans are ready for wise leaders to dare to create an environment for a new sexual morality and a complete education for all people that will transform the United States.

Addendum

Sermon from *The Immoral Reverend*

The Immoral Reverend, a novel, was published by Prometheus Books in 1987. Despite the title, in an era when there were many immoral reverends, the novel has never appeared in paperback. The story revolves around a new approach to Unitarian/Universalism, similar to the church/state involvement in a new sexual morality and along the lines proposed in the NSME legislation where human sexuality is invited back into the church and sacramentalized. Since the novel is difficult to find and Matt Godwin's sermon may prove interesting to believers in the final sex revolution, I have included it in this book.

If you read it, please note that Matt Godwin delivers the sermon in a fictional version of the United First Parish church in Quincy, which traces its beginning back to the Massachusetts Bay Colony. In 1630, John Wheelwright, brother-in-law of Anne Hutchinson, was the church's first minister. Both were banished from Boston by John Winthrop and Thomas Dudley for questioning the morality of "God's grace," which they claimed the Puritan ministers in Boston didn't understand, or want to understand, since God's grace was for all, not just the Boston saints. The church is also the burial place of John Adams and John Quincy Adams (second and sixth presidents of the United States) and their wives.

Also note that Matt suggests that the philosophy of one of the leaders of the Unitarian/Universalist church in the 1990s, Jack Mendelsohn, is wrong. Mendelsohn stated, "We have no creed . . . our churches make no official pronouncement on God, the Bible or Jesus." Matt was, of course, hoping that U/Us would get the message, and lay the groundwork for the final sexual revolution.

Alas, when William Schultz, president of UUA at the time, read the manuscript he wasn't happy. Jack Mendelsohn was his mentor. He refused to have the

novel reviewed in any Unitarian/Universalist publication, and very few U/Us
have read this twenty-first-century approach to religion.

*   *   *

Matt rose from behind the pulpit and stared thoughtfully at the congregation for
a moment. It was an act of absorption and blending with the sea of minds and
faces, representing many different cultural and ethnic origins that were solemn-
ly concentrating on his face.

"Good morning. I love you. As loving creatures, individually and collectively you and I are God. The only God we will ever know. Indivisible and
rejoicing, we can experience Him in every moment of our lives in the many
aspects of ourselves and others. That is religion, no matter by what name it may
be called.

"I am happy to be here on the 348th year of the First Parish Church and on
this, our opening Sunday, on such a summery day in September. In New
England, despite rumors, the days never "dwindle down to a precious few."
There was a time when Unitarian Universalist churches did not close for the
summer, and in the winter the congregations did not have to move out of their
sanctuary in the Parish Hall for services. More people came to church and the
cost of heating the church was apportioned over many more parishioners.

"During this coming winter, if by some miracle we could fill the sanctuary
with as many warm bodies as we have today, and if the minister would give sermons to heat our minds, we might solve some of the financial problems of this
church. We might not have to burn oil at all—especially if the congregation
would agree to wear several layers of clothing, as our ancestors did—or thermal
underwear. The members might even agree to modify the pews and make them
more comfortable. If they did we might restore the old New England custom of
bundling. Why not?"

"Why not?" he repeated. "God is love. Why can't we have churches where
we can worship love? Most Christians agree on one thing. God is love. Even Ike
Godwin, my father, who prefers Episcopalian theology, would agree that God is
love." Matt smiled serenely. "Unfortunately, like many Americans, my father
finds it embarrassing to talk about human loving in public. He believes that love
as God should be a kind of spiritual love. Philosophers call it 'agape.' Most ministers, priests, and rabbis would agree with him. They feel uncomfortable with
the human aspects of loving. They can't believe that God can be lusty, erotic,
laughing, and loving, too.

"If you want Eros in your life, you have to read *Playboy* or watch Music
Television or go to clubs like Adamsport's notorious Silly Willy's." Matt grinned
at Sylvanus Williams, whose mouth dropped open in surprise at his sudden
recognition. "During the next half hour, I want to suggest that the Western world
may be ready to embrace a new kind of God, a God who never intended to main-

tain a separate existence from his creations, a God who can't believe that He had created men and women who would not be fully aware that He and they were one and the same, an erotic God, a dancing God, a God who needs no Christ or Messiah because He is continuously giving birth Himself, a God who loves you very much—especially when you dare to be naked with Him, physically and mentally, and when you are celebrating His and your interdependence in the act of loving in all of its manifestations.

"Before I explore this new kind of God and a religion which exalts Him and you and me simultaneously, I want you to know that when I originally offered to deliver this sermon, I planned to do it in memory of my mother, Sarah Godwin. Many of you knew her personally. During the past years, she asked me many times if I might ever return to the pulpit. Sarah taught me, from my first years, the I/Thou relationship with life and death. But I wasn't, in my own mind, sure that a man who had given up the ministry for the world of business could straddle two worlds. After much thought and study, I am convinced that today, more than ever, we need a common unity between the church, the state and capitalism. We need a new understanding of the meaning of the separation of church and state. We need to understand, in America at least, that capitalism is one economic method for men and women and society to function together; but it is not so all-powerful that it can function without moral guidance provided by the church. We need a new understanding of our Constitution and a recognition that in a vibrant nation, the church and state can never be independent of each other. They must work together to give all men and women a sane perspective of themselves as a nation and a sense of national purpose which can be accepted by the majority of people. The church has a moral duty to keep the state in a continuous process of recreation for the benefit of its citizens. We need a new understanding of our national motto—In God We Trust. As God, you and I must never lose trust with ourselves.

"For many centuries the church and the state were indistinguishable. Some philosopher like Karl Marx called religion the opiate of the masses. Opiate is the wrong word. The church and its ministers and priests dramatized the bewildering interplay between good and evil in everyone's life. There were few books, no radio, no television. The Bible was the medium and the message. It offered a thousand stories of man's inhumanity to man and seasoned them with the hope of better things to come. Religion, the Church and the Good Book provided an escape route, fearful at times when it was populated with purgatory, hell and devils, but always fascinating.

"Today, the masses in Western countries have other opiates and endless escape from realities. Most of our gross national product is not for the creation of food, clothing and shelter, but rather it is a reflection of our increasing ability to be able to play instead of work. Automobiles, television, radios, books, magazines, newspapers, videocassettes and laser discs, video games, moving pictures, dining out, spectator sports, vacations all over the world, alcohol, and our never-ending fascination with our own sexual compulsions are some of the ways we divert ourselves. Escaping boredom we often act as if we were God, but in the process of celebrating ourselves and our achievements as God, we forget the more important celebration of ourselves as Gods of Love and Wonder.

"Today, no society, no nation, no group of people believe in the church or the synagogue enough to devote their entire lives and incomes to the kind of religious thinking that once dominated the civilized world. God is a handkerchief we keep in our back pocket to wipe away our tears and blow our noses should the need arise.

"If you read the invitation in the *Adamsport Chronicle* to hear me this morning, you may have detected an underlying note of heresy. My feeling is that now, as never before, the church and God needs heretics—religious men and women who dare to chart new courses and abandon outworn theologies. What is heresy? It has nothing to do with being right or wrong in the conventional sense. If everyone believes that there is a God, and I say that there is no God, that there never was one, then I am a heretic. I am reviling God, as Exodus warns both Jews and Christians not to do. Actually you may believe, since I am telling you that you and I are God, that I am reviling God. Many Jews and Christians would consider this blasphemous. I am happy to be a blasphemer. They forgot that Jesus reviled God. He declared that he was the Son of God. Long before Jesus was born, Jewish law made it a crime for anyone to say that there might be other Gods besides Yahweh. A Son of God, as every human father well knows, could destroy the father and become God himself.

"Punishment for blasphemy was stoning—not crucifixion. That was Pilate's choice. Had Jesus been left to the Sanhedrin, the Jewish trial lawyers, he would have been stoned to death. Obviously, his death in that event would not have been so dramatic. In contrast, the fate of heretics was usually burning at the stake, or, if they were lucky, banishment.

"In his fascinating book *Heresies,* Thomas Szasz reminds us, 'Just so long as there is tension between the individual and the group of which he is a member there will be heresy, whatever it might be called. . . . The individual must think for himself. More than anything else that makes him an individual. The group, on the other hand, must want its members to echo its beliefs. . . . It follows then that if the group is held together by the ideals of Christianity, then heresy is a deviation from the official beliefs and dogmas of the clergy. But when people and societies are held together, as many are now, by the images of science and technology, then heresy is a deviation from the official beliefs and dogmas of scientists and doctors.'

"This morning, as I try to convince you that you and I are God and that we should return to the religion of awe and wonder that inspired our remote ancestors before Christianity, I'd also like to revive a long-forgotten word, *antinominy,* and remind you that antinominiasts, who, in the early seventeenth century were considered blasphemers and heretics, actually erected the foundations for the religious and political liberty that in America—less than three hundred years later—we consider our rightful heritage. Antinomianism means being against the moral law, and specifically, in history, that under the Gospel, dispensation of faith alone is necessary for salvation.

"Actually, the first antinominiasts, or heretics, came just a few years after Matthew, Luke, and John. They were writing gospels of their own. They defined the Christian religion for Catholics and most Protestants today. Some of the first Christian heretics were called Gnostics, from the Greek word for "knowing." They claimed that they really knew the truth about Christ and the Apostles Peter and Paul, and they derided the Scriptures as we know them. They were unhappy that Luke, by insisting on the actual physical resurrection of Christ, was establishing the groundwork for the Catholic Church and Apostolic succession resting in Peter, the first of the Apostles. Since Peter was the first witness to the resurrection, the Pope, the bishops and the priests, whose spiritual and political power came directly from the Scriptures, would ultimately trace their lineage to Peter.

"If you study the history of the Christian religions, you quickly discover that the church and state were synonymous. Questioning the Scriptures, right through the seventeenth century, was equivalent to questioning the leaders of the state, whether they were kings or popes, bishops or priests. Questioning the leaders could lead to imprisonment, death, or banishment.

"The first Unitarians were antinominiasts. Followers of a man named Faustus Socinus, they disavowed the deity of Christ, the doctrine of original sin, and the Christian belief in atonement. The Anabaptists also rejected much of the Scriptures and believed in the guidance of an inner light derived from God and one's own conscience. The early Quakers likewise believed in the "indwelling light of Christ" to such an extent that every man and woman was the Son of God. Quakers got their name because they trembled and quaked at this revelation. One of the first Quaker leaders, a man more daring than George Fox, James Nayler, proclaimed, 'I am the Son of God, but I have many brethren,' and he told the House of Commons when he was on trial for blasphemy, 'I wonder why any man should be so amazed at this. Is not God in every house and in every stone, in every creature . . . If you hang every man who says Christ is in you, you will hang a good many."

Matt paused for a moment. "They didn't hang James Nayler for blasphemy. Under the English blasphemy laws, which, incidentally, have never been repealed, the House of Commons decreed that Nayler should be whipped with three hundred lashes, put in a pillory for many hours, have his tongue bored through with a hot rod, and be ridden through the city naked facing backward on a horse.

"That was in 1656. A few years earlier across the Atlantic in this city, John Wheelwright, the first pastor of the original church on this site, was declared a heretic and banished from the Massachusetts Bay Colony. The original church was called the Meeting House on the Mount, a Chapel of Ease, approved by the General Court of Massachusetts so that the few farmers who lived in this area who could not easily travel back and forth to Boston for religious services, could have a place where they could commune with God."

Matt was happy to note that he had the full attention of the Belchers and the Hancocks, who appreciated church history. But he was sure they wouldn't like what he had to say next. "Unfortunately for Wheelwright, he got mixed up with a woman—Anne Hutchinson, his sister-in-law, who was America's first feminist. A very well-educated woman, she dared to accuse Boston ministers of not properly understanding the Bible. She convened weekly sessions attended by nearly a hundred Boston women—keep in mind the church and religion fulfilled the lives of our forefathers—and she tried to convince these women that the Boston preachers weren't sealed ministers of the gospels. A forgiving God had given men and women a Covenant of Grace. Wheelwright agreed with her. He preached a sermon that aroused all of Boston. In Chapter 3:15 of Genesis, he told his congregation, God had actually given Adam a second covenant. The first covenant was that they must suffer and work to achieve salvation for their sin. The second was that there was a divine spirit dwelling within you and if you recognized it, saint or sinner, you could achieve Grace.

"I'm sure that Anne Hutchinson would have agreed that the Covenant of Grace is not only the recognition that God is love, but that Man/Woman is God. All we have to do to discover the truth is to transcend our petty egos and blend ourselves with the ebb and flow of the universe.

"Incensed with their heresy, John Winthrop, the governor of Massachusetts, and John Endicott brought them to trial. But they refused to admit their errors and they were banished from the Colony—Wheelwright to New Hampshire and Hutchinson to Rhode Island—where, according to the Pilgrims, she received her just punishment and was scalped by the Indians. Think about this—Wheelwright and Hutchinson were banished by a civil court, a court composed of people who had fled from England because they were considered blasphemers themselves and had refused to use the English Book of Common Prayer in their churches.

"In God We Trust. Just so long as your concept of God is my concept of God. Centuries before Wheelwright lived, Michael Servetus, who many think of as the first Unitarian, challenged John Calvin about the nature of God. Servetus insisted that God had only one identity and could not be both the Son and the Holy Spirit. Servetus was burned at the stake in Geneva, Switzerland."

Matt beamed at the congregation and noted happily that both Irene and Jill were following him intently. "In those days the true meaning of heresy, which is from the Greek word *hairesis,* 'to take a choice' was corrupted by the church leaders and applied to anyone who denied church doctrine or intimated that there might be other choices than those decreed by the church fathers. Sociologist Peter Berger has pointed out that, 'In the ancient world man had limited choice—fate and the gods determined what happened in his life. Modern man and woman by contrast have almost unlimited choices in many aspects of their lives. Thus for premodern man heresy was a possibility, but usually rather remote; for modern man heresy typically becomes a necessity. Today modernity creates a new situation in which picking and choosing becomes an imperative.'

"I have given you this background on heresy and blasphemy because today I'm asking you to join with me in a reverse kind of heresy. Separation of the church and state in this era of total overkill, nuclear war, and confused moralities has gone too far. The theory behind Constitutional doctrine is that church leaders, Catholic, Protestant, or Jewish, are supposed to take care of the spiritual and moral concerns of their believers and not shoot their mouths off when political and economic decisions impinge on moral beliefs.

"In recent years, the National Conference of Bishops and the U.S. Catholic Conference have rightfully offered official church pronouncements on many aspects of politics and economics that, in some cases, even go counter to normal Catholic moral beliefs. *Time* magazine made the statement, 'It almost seems as if the world's Roman Catholic bishops have set themselves up as a new branch of government. In country after country, they are measuring specific government programs and issuing moral report cards on what they see.' In agreement with the Moral Majority, the Catholic bishops have demanded tuition tax credits to help private schools, demanded prayer in public schools, and come out against mercy killing and sex on television. In Canada, the Bishops Commission rejected Prime Minister Trudeau's economic proposals as immoral. They accused the government of deliberately encouraging unemployment and of aiding the rich at the expense of the poor.

"The Catholic Church has taken moral positions on crime, housing, national health insurance, world food policy, the Panama Canal Treaty, the Palestinian State, Israel's right to exist, and even the redistribution of economic wealth in the United States. For the first time, not only Catholics but ministers and rabbis are questioning the nature of war and whether any form of nuclear warfare can be moral in any circumstance.

"Politicians who believe the province of the church is simply spiritual leadership and evangelism deplore what they call the secularization of the church, and they insist that the church is losing sight of its essential purpose—to preach the gospel. But they are wrong. While I don't agree with many Catholic moralities, including their uneasy stance on nuclear war, the bishops have as much right to present their moralities as the elected politicians and the media. In the last few years of the twentieth century, priests, ministers, and rabbis have much less influence on moral conduct and leadership of this country than the *Wall Street Journal*, *Time* or *Newsweek*, none of which hesitate from one issue to another to proclaim the moralities of their editors. An excellent recent example was *Time* magazine's reportorial weeping over the herpes explosion. In a kind of reverse morality, they recognized it as an overdue return to monogamous morality. In *Time* magazine's view, herpes is God's judgement on you for premarital sexual encounters.

After Brezhnev's death, both *Time* and *Newsweek* in supposedly reportorial stories advised our national leaders how to deal with the Soviets. Not a week goes by that the editors of the *Wall Street Journal* don't moralize over particular economic and political decisions of our nation's leaders.

"At the same time, the media and the politicians excoriate the intervention of the church and they try to convince you that the church is losing sight of its essential purpose—to preach the gospel. But they are wrong. This morning, as you will discover, my first heresy leads to many others.

"I believe that we must create a modern merger between the church, the synagogue, the state, and business in America, and we must offer a new kind of moral leadership. Although, in the beginning, particular religious leaders and religious sects may not agree on any particular set of moral beliefs, our combined goal should be a morally mature America. In the process, we must till the fields and sow the seeds for a new kind of religious leadership in America. We need religious leaders who will gradually establish sound national purposes and will make it possible for the vast majority of Americans to live joyous, self-fulfilling lives.

"In 1982, both the House of Representatives and the Senate passed a resolution asking the president to declare 1983 the 'Year of the Bible . . . in recognition of both the formative influence the Bible has been for our nation and our national need to study and apply the teaching of the Holy Scripture.' In my opinion, using the Bible to provide moral leadership for America so that we can muddle through into a Golden Age is equivalent to the ostrich burying its head in the sand. The old-time religion might have been good enough for daddy; but daddy is dead. He doesn't live here any more.

"Pope Plus XI suggested, 'Today, we are all Protestants.' But Protestant leaders from Sören Kierkegaard to Ludwin Feurbach to Karl Barth to Friedrich Schleiermacher to Martin Heidegger to Rudolph Bultmann were all bogged down in biblical word games that ultimately demand 'a leap of faith.' They were simply unaware that You and I, being born, living, procreating and dying, You and I surrounded by myriad forms of life carrying out the same process, You and I *are* God and the only God we ever need to know and love.

"No papal guidance based on biblical teachings has had much effect on moral behavior over the past two thousand years. If every American devoted him or herself to a study of the Bible, we'd still have abortion as a method of birth control. We'd still have prostitution. We'd still have adultery and pornography and the use of drugs and murder and theft, and we'd still have leaders of nations mobilizing their people to fight the peoples of other nations."

As he spoke, Matt was aware that many of the faces watching him had a glazed, rejecting look. Many minds were hearing, but not processing such sacrilegious thoughts in the synapeses of their brains. "Before I continue," he said with a warm smile, "I want all of you to know that you should not feel obligated to hear me through to the end. On the other hand, if you are secure in your religion, your vision of God and your moralities, I am sure that you will be able to cope with what is to come. More than a hundred years ago, Emerson asked a question for the twenty-first century: 'Why should not we also enjoy an original relation to the universe? . . . Why should we not have a religion by revelation to us? Let us demand our own laws and worship.' My belief is that all men and women are essentially religious creatures; but millions of us have lost sight of our basically loving and caring natures. We have been buried in the debris of outworn creeds and negative moralities.

"So today I am proposing to the Unitarian/Universalist leadership that it broaden its vision and create a Church of Modern Moralities. A transformed U/U church could attract millions of Americans who no longer identify with the creeds and the music and the rituals of our ancestors, who lived in an entirely different kind of world. We must provide new moralities for what is now an information society. We may never become a moral majority. Fundamentalists may denounce us as humanists; but, hopefully, many millions of Americans will hear my words. You are aware that this sermon is being televised. It is my hope that videotapes of today's service will be shown nationally at some later date. I am proposing to Americans everywhere who hear this sermon that we need a few million of you who are not afraid to help create an exciting new world. A new world where *God as Us* is a vital part of our daily life.

"I am hoping that we can create a new morally mature church on these ancient foundations. We can dare to proclaim that God really does exist in this world and that He is in constant communication with us—but only when we recognize that He is You and I. I am Thou. You are Thou. Together as God, we are in a continuous process of creation. Together, we as God have a choice. We can recognize this joyous gestalt and flow with Him in the joy and wonder and the eternal mystery of Us or we can deny Him in hateful and degrading interpersonal interactions, which is equivalent to denying ourselves.

"We don't need magic or symbols or Bibles or Talmuds that obscure the absolute wonder and miracle of life and procreation and death. We don't need to legislate our behavior with negative moralities. Rather, we need a church that offers new, modern moralities with leaders and a fellowship of human beings who recognize that our reach exceeds our grasp. We need leaders who remind us to wonder . . . to wonder at the amazement and miracle of the human brain and heart and blood and our power to recreate and transmit this miracle with penises and vaginas to future generations.

"I am well aware that many Unitarian/Universalists will not agree with the kind of leadership that I am advocating. Jack Mendelsohn, a much admired U/U leader, stated U/U philosophy as follows: 'We are believers, but beliefs centered in method, a process of religious life, rather than the closed articles of faith. We have no creed. . . . Our churches make *no* official pronouncement on God, the Bible, Jesus, immortality, or any of the other theological questions which are generally answered with unabashed finality by more traditional religious groups.'

"In my opinion, Mendelsohn's kind of hands-off religious theology and philosophy, which is reflected in the purposes and principles that Unitarian/Universalists are still trying to define for themselves, denies every sound principle of lasting organizations and sound business principles. It is equivalent to writing an obituary for a religion or a nation or any association.

"Right or wrong, lasting societies of any kind are organized around a well-fined set of beliefs on the meanings and purposes of life. Keep in mind, I am a businessman. I am proposing that the new mixture of business and religion would provide a new yeast—a new kind of manna from a heaven of our own creation. In a sense, this sermon is a trial balloon. I am not seeking self-aggrandizement. Churches with only one guru tend toward dictatorships and were the reason that our forefathers legalized, in our Constitution, the separation of church and state.

"But today the churches and synagogues of America need hundreds of men and women like myself. Not just one lone individual shouting in the wilderness but a Council of Moral Stemwinders to set the human clock ticking again. Unitarian/Universalists, humanists, feminists—in aggregate at the moment we are probably less than two hundred thousand people—should merge and create a Council of Moral Stemwinders, men and women who dare to propose a new moral structure for this country and offer moral direction that deals with current realities. Instead of the kind of divisive democracy that now exists in a thousand U/U churches, we should become a unified Church of Modern Moralities that doesn't hesitate to use the advertising weapons of the capitalistic system to attract millions of new members. Our goal should be to meld church, state and capitalism into a revitalized America.

"This morning, therefore, I would like to provide guidelines for a Committee of Moral Stemwinders. I would like to suggest that U/Us announce nationally that they have decided to phase out biblical sexual morality and return religion to its origins. Let's create a religion that is unashamed that all religion originated from sex and fertility worship. Let's dare to proclaim one basic truth. If men and women have any purpose on this earth it is to perpetuate themselves, with limits, and make this spaceship a happy, self-fulfilling place to live.

"Such a religion will not be hung up on the old rituals of any religion. During the past quarter century, beginning in the 1960s, in what was then called the Human Potential Movement, there has been a growing awareness of the joy and wonder possible in human sexual merger. Total sexual loving and religion are perfectly compatible. Sex is sitting on the doorstep of churches and synagogues waiting to be invited back in. Sex worship can be both a laughing experience and a humbling experience. Millions of men and women will be charmed to rediscover that the very beginning of religious beliefs proceeded not only from fear—fear of misunderstood phenomena such as earthquakes, hurricanes, volcanoes—but simultaneously from wonder and awe—the wonder of the sun and the moon, the tides and menstrual cycles, and procreation and the recurring birth and death of all life.

"Instead of degrading human sexuality, we need to exalt it. Instead of compartmentalizing our sexual lives and coming to our churches and synagogues like creatures who copulate with one another because we are forced to by sinful compulsions, we should make sex and sexmaking a sacrament. Sexual repression and sexual sickness are man-made diseases. For nearly two thousand years Christians and Jews have been guided by a craftily contrived sexual morality. The first pornographers were the male leaders of the tribe. Determined to gain power and hold it over their people, they invented Eve, who tempted Adam. After eating of the tree of knowledge of good and evil, not only were Adam and Eve ashamed of their nakedness, but somehow they had sinned against God, who had warned them not to eat the fruit of this tree. If you want to repress people, you must make them feel guilty. Whoever wrote Genesis laid the foundation for Christian guilt. Most of the people listening to me today probably do not really believe that God created Adam and then made Eve from one of his ribs, or that Eve, with the help of a serpent, tempted Adam. But sexual temptation and the essential nature of woman as seductress and women as temptresses have been processed into the male psyche by centuries of indoctrination. Male prophets and theologians of the Middle Ages warned men against women. Man's compulsion to merge his body with a woman's and impregnate her was evil, unless it occurred within the sacrament of monogamous marriage performed by power-hungry priests who claimed their authority from God.

"For more than a thousand years nude men and women—glorified in Greek art and sculpture—with the exception of Christ on the Cross, disappeared from European painting and sculpture. The prophets condemned the human body and its pleasures. Art critic Robert Melville has pointed out: 'When the nude finally did appear in Christian art, the body had ceased to be, as it had for the Greeks, a mirror of divine perfection. The naked body had largely become an object of humiliation and shame.' Using the medium of woodcuts, engravings, painting and sculpture, artists were permitted to show not vice itself—not the actual sexmaking—but the punishment for sexual sinning. Eves and Liliths and their female descendants became witches and seducers of men who consorted with devils and snakes and the artists of these centuries proved it by painting pictures of snakes and toads eating vulvas and breasts, or picturing lascivious women copulating with goats, and women who could only be satiated by the permanent erection of the Devil himself.

"Today, nearly two thousand years later, millions of men still regard a woman as a temptress. Men still fear her control over him and retaliate by degrading her and making her a sex object of his lust. Today, young men grow up seeing photographs of women naked and lascivious, their legs spread-eagle, exposing their vulvas, opening their labia with their fingers so that a man can't resist them and must thrust his swollen penis into them. And when he has ejaculated into this anonymous woman he feels empty and futile but he continues to exist on frustrated sex in all sizes, shape, and colors. And men profit from each other by commercializing the forbidden sight of women's breasts, vaginas, anuses, and buttocks,—or, if you prefer the common vernacular, catering to the vacillating attraction and repulsion of women's tits, cunts, assholes and asses—all existing in some forbidden land extraneous to the person herself."

Amanda Brackett suddenly stood up in the middle of the congregation and shouted, "This is disgusting, Matthew Godwin! I won't listen to it another moment." She edged out of her pew and walked out of the church followed by a scattered clapping of hands.

Matt watched her leave. "If there are any others who would like to join Amanda now or at any time during the rest of this sermon, which I assure you may be more shocking to Christian sensibilities than anything you have heard so far, please feel free to leave." He looked at the congregation with a sad smile. "If you need to save yourself from the power of mere words, for some of you, it may be even easier to make the sign of the cross."

"After centuries of sexual repression," he continued, "and sexual frustration created by ministers, priest, rabbis, and tight-lipped men like St. Augustine, who was shocked by his sexual compulsions, few people could believe that men and women could transcend their egos or find God in their own joyous physical merger, whether they were married by a priest or not.

"Denying our God-given sexuality, we have created a joyless sex world, a world of the sex tease, a sex-drenched society where the illusion of sex fulfillment replaces the reality. We have the strange phenomena of magazines designed specifically for men or women that capitalize on the frustrated misunderstandings of our mutual sexuality. They sell millions of copies as they try to explain the drives and needs of men and women to each other. Many of these articles and stories, and much of the advertising in these magazines and on television, which the average American watches six to eight hours a day, exploit a supposed continuing adversary relationship between men and women. They try to convince us that men and women have different needs and compulsions and can only coexist as if they lived in an armed camp. They ignore the truth. The adversary relationship is not real. It is built into the male and female psyche from childhood by parents, teachers, and religious leaders who are guided by sex-negative biblical moralities.

"A Church of Modern Moralities will not moralize post facto on moral problems. Rather it will lead the way. It will, for example, agree that premarital and extramarital sexual caring and loving are inevitable in many situations and that caring sex is not evil but rather is a reflection of ourselves as loving gods.

"A Church of Modern Moralities would propose new educational and post-marital structures which would offer all men and women, in their late teens and before marriage, the opportunity to experience caring sex with more than one person of the other sex. A Church of Modern Moralities would accept the fact that, in many cases, an additional caring sexual commitment can coexist with the original marriage pair bonding and not destroy it.

"A Church of Modern Moralities would propose a new right-to-life morality. It would insist that one of the most immoral things any man and woman can do is create a life they cannot, because of their youth or will, not because they feel no human obligations, be responsible for.

"A Church of Modern Moralities will insist that the right to create life is a social privilege given, not by a single God, but by men and women who are God and recognize their responsibility as creators.

"A Church of Modern Moralities, recognizing man as God, would insist that the individual man or woman has the right to terminate his own life whether it be because of debilitating illness, old age, severe depression, or simply a desire not to cope any longer with the problems of the world. The church should demand that simple medical means be provided, in a hospital-controlled environment, for this form of suicide.

"Moral Stemwinders will insist that every man and woman from the age of seventeen, until they draw their last breath on this earth, have the right to experience a full and responsible sex life. To accomplish this, a Church of Modern Moral Maturity would incorporate sexual teachings and responsibility into its Sunday School teachings and sermons. It would also advocate a state-licensed prostitution in homes run by husband-and-wife teams who arrange appointments with sexual surrogates, male or female, who could offer caring sex with regulated fees for millions of those who cannot, for one reason or another, enjoy a caring sexual relationship in their daily lives.

"A Church of Modern Moralities would bring human nudity and human loving into the church sanctuary, and, using modern visual techniques, explore the long history of man and woman's quest for love and understanding of their sexual drives and compulsions. At some services, members of both sexes would reenact religious stories and dramas and rituals from all religious traditions. A Church of Modern Moralities would propose that we change city and state laws to permit men and women to be naked in public where it is convenient for them to be naked."

Matt grinned at the surprised faces of Robert Lovejoy and Sylvanus Williams. "Thus it would be unnecessary to arrest a citizen for mowing his front lawn naked, or close up clubs like Silly Willy's, which exist only because we are so prurient about showing ourselves as naked children of God. The truth is that in a new, morally mature environment, when the beaches surrounding Adamsport are filled with young men and women frolicking naked in the sand and water and when there are naked accolytes in the church sanctuary, then magazines like *Playboy* or clubs like Silly Willy's will cease to exist.

"A Church of Modern Moralities would advocate the nationwide voluntary dispersion of black people and Spanish people and those of Asian origin, deghettoizing America and relocating these people in the white suburbs of America. To prevent concentrations of black people or Spanish or Asian groups in certain sections of predominantly white suburban cities like Adamsport, which is adjacent to heavily populated areas such as Boston, states would be compelled by their legislatures to apportion small percentages of apartment and private dwellings in various geographic areas of these cities to help these people to disperse into the mainstream of America. The survival of America depends on a melting pot that keeps melting and will produce incoming generations of a unified people with common goals.

"A Church of Modern Moralities would advocate the legalization of drugs and make hard drugs such as heroin available in state-controlled drug centers at nominal prices. It would advocate that marijuana and cocaine be sold commercially under the same kind of laws that govern alcohol. At the same time, it would continuously teach and sermonize that in a sexual, caring, and loving society, trying to escape from life by using chemically induced means is sick and immoral behavior.

"A Church of Modern Moralities would advocate the total legalization of gambling. The income from gambling would be controlled by city-licensed gambling corporations with profits and taxes regulated by individual states. This dual control would gradually eliminate criminal involvement in gambling profits. Legalizing and bringing human needs and compulsions into the light of day—compulsions such as gambling, prostitution, the use of drugs, and pornography—would ultimately minimize or eliminate the seedbeds of crime in this country. Instead of inveighing against human immoralities, a Church of Modern Moralities would guide people into more satisfying ways to express their insecurities, fears, loneliness, and need for love.

"A Church of Modern Moralities would advocate the right to bear arms, but not small arms or assault weapons. Small arms have no other purpose in this modern world except to kill another person.

"A Church of Modern Moralities would advocate nationwide experiments to rehabilitate criminals with sentences under ten years in former military locations to eliminate prison overcrowding. Prisoners would live in barracks, be given army-style physical training programs, disciplined work projects, and disciplined vocational training in service-related jobs. Prisoners would be forewarned that escapees, or those sentenced again for any crime, would have their normal future sentences doubled and would serve any future time in regular prisons.

"A Church of Modern Moralities would underwrite these new freedoms with harsh punishment for proved crimes of murder, eliminating endless appeals for men and women who have killed another person, followed by life sentences.

"A Church of Modern Moralities would advocate the death penalty, not for vengeance, or a tooth-for-a-tooth morality, but for the simple reason that you and I should not be taxed to keep these people alive.

"A Church of Modern Moralities would encourage the formation of a College of Modern Moralities, to be underwritten by a Protestants, Catholics, Jews, Mohammedans, and other religions of the world to study, create, change, and revise moral attitudes in any areas that would help all men and women to live in closer harmony with their own realities."

Matt was well aware of the growing shock on the glazed faces of many of the congregation. He saw Jill shake her head in amused wonder. He saw Father Timothy touch Irene's shoulder. He whispered something in her ear, and then, as more than a dozen others had done, he edged out of the pew, followed by Irene.

But, like a man standing on the parapet of a building, Matt knew it was too late. He had to jump. The final plunge might be to his own self-destruction, but it was impossible to pull back.

"To create the environment for this modern morality and build a new kind of church that could weave spiritual and secular concerns into a meaningful tapestry, a Church of Modern Moralities should go back to our origins and return sex worship to the church. God isn't dead! God isn't moribund! Like his creatures, during the past two thousand years God is growing! Let's worship Him as Ourselves! Let's create a sex-positive religion, not just for the young, but a life-long religion where penile-vaginal penetration, or a loving kiss, or the touch of caring minds and bodies, and the adoration and wonder and the miracle of our flesh and blood kind is a sacrament. It is the kind of sacrament a twenty-first-century God would appreciate.

"A return to sex worship would need a new kind of liturgy and eucharist. Human beings need symbols in their lives and easily graspable ritual ways of defining experiences and emotions that are beyond words. Thousands of sexual symbols and myths that have been purposely buried by Christian fathers need to be exhumed and revealed in their true origins. A Modern Moral congregation would delight in the simplicity and relevance of these early creations for our lives today.

"Above you, the dome of this church is circled by closed lotus blossoms culminating at the peak of the dome in an open lotus blossom. Was the designer of this church aware that the open lotus blossom is an ancient Indian symbol for the female vagina? Did he realize that "the jewel in the lotus" is a metaphor for the human sexual merger? Behind me is a cross without a plaster Jesus nailed to it. Regardless of its meaning for Christianity, a Church of Modern Moralities would rediscover and rejoice in the original meaning of the cross, which was also a symbol of the penis penetrating the vagina.

"In the ancient Hindu religion the lignam standing upright in the yoni was an object of veneration. Sculptured and revealed in new idealistic stylings, we should exalt human sexuality and ourselves as God with similar modern religious symbols that encourage every man, woman, and child in our new moral church to grow up fully aware of the imagery and the exaltation of life processes reflected in these never-changing fertility symbols. In such a church, men and women sermonizing on love and God and human loving would reveal the origins of phallic worship common to all religions. Our ministers, priests, and rabbis would be unashamed of the original concept of the Trinity, which is symbolized by three separate parts of the male genitals. Two testicles and one penis together form a "T," which is another form of an ancient sexual cross. So sacred is this symbol in some ancient religions that the Assyrian gods Ashyr, Anu, and Hoa were simply names of the penis and the right and left testicles.

"In our Church of Modern Moralities, we won't hesitate to explore the thousands of aspects of human sexuality revealed in the original books of the Old Testament. Our modern congregation would be delighted to know that in a male-dominated society the family jewels were so sacred that in the twenty-third chapter of Deuteronomy Jehovah advised his people, 'He that is wounded in the stones, or hath his privy member cut off, shall not enter the congregation of the Lord.'

"No man could possibly be a religious leader if he were shorn of any part of his testicles. In chapter 25 of Deuteronomy you will learn that, 'If two men fight together, and the wife of one draws near to rescue her husband from the hand of one attacking him, and she puts out her hand and seizes him by the genitals: then you shall cut off her hand: you shall not pity her.'

"Is it any wonder after thousands of years of such dictum—even if a woman is saving a man from his enemy she can't kick his enemy in the balls, or, worse, yank them—is it any wonder that even today many women are reluctant to touch their husband's penis? By exploring early sex worship we can reorient it for the twenty-first century, which has only recently discovered that the female body is better designed for survival and nonstop loving than the male body. And our new Moral Stemwinders would never run out of interesting sermons on the origin of sex worship because there are literally hundreds of thousands of sexual meanings preserved in visual art and words, not just from the past two thousand years, but from thirty thousand years of known human history and long before Christ was ever dreamed of. And the congregations would discover that the morals of these early people, who never heard of Jesus Christ as their savior, were just as good as, or better than, the morals of latter-day saints and prophets.

"Our Church of Modern Moralities would restore the original meaning of the Ark, which was the divine symbol of the earth, and hence the female principle. The Ark contained and succored the germ of animated nature. Properly understood, Noah's Ark and the Ark of the Covenant are sacred receptacles symbolizing the vagina, the divine wisdom and power, and the Great Mother from which all things come. The Ark of the Covenant contained not only the Table of Laws but Aaron's rod which sprang to life and budded, symbolizing fertility, thus making the Ark the repository of the creative deity. Our sex worshippers should discover how this symbol developed in a different but similar way in the Roman Catholic pyx, the holy receptacle for the body of Christ, and in Mary, who became the tabernacle of God.

"Amazed at the wonder of our sexuality, our new moralists would explore other religions. In Egypt, they would discover again that the Ark contains the most universal religious symbols. The Triune commences with the male testicles and harbors a phallus, an egg, a serpent. In those days, the phallus represented the sun the male generative principle the Creator. The egg represented the passive female principle. And the snake was both the destroyer and the creator. Understanding Egyptian mythology would give our modern moralists a very different interpretation of the story of Adam and Eve, which was written much later.

"Or compare this sexual trinity to the cylinder on the altar of the Hindu temple. Here the pedestal is the symbol of Brahma, the basis of all that is in the universe. The vase (the vagina) stands for Vishnu, the preserver, the female principle. The cylinder within the vase represents Shiva, the destroyer, the male god, also the lignam or penis.

"Now compare this to Adam and Eve and the serpent or the Father and the Son and the Holy Spirit, and discover that, in many respects, the snake has meanings equivalent to the Holy Spirit. In either case, they were recognized as the spirit of love between his creator and man. And our modern moralists would discover that in primitive religions where symbolism is more apparent the snake is actually a throbbing penis in the anomalous position of creating both life and the suffering and evil attendant upon it.

"And the ministers in our new Church of Modern Moralities will remind those who are about to be married that the wedding ring put on the bride's finger is really a symbol for the vagina which only begins to function when the bride has inserted her finger through it in the act of marriage. Thus a double ring ceremony has a reverse and equally lovely sexual significance. When sex and religion are integrated into the realities of human sexuality, think of how much more fun and joy and celebration attending a wedding service will be. Instead of worrying about sexual sin and a God who forgives sin, you will find a new, loving God who equates human loving with the divinity. You will be able to release your natural eroticism, sing hymns to your sexual self, and discover that our real problem as interacting individuals, and as a nation, is that we refuse to recognize our basic interdependence, sexual, or otherwise.

"When that happens, we'll sing new hymns and Walt Whitman's poem, which was being written when the cornerstone of this church was being laid, will be etched on the front door of every church:

I too, following many and follow'd by many, inaugurate a
    new religion. . . .
Each is not for its own sake,
I say the whole earth and all the stars in the sky are for religion's sake,
I say no man has ever yet been half devout enough,
None has ever adored or worship'd half enough,
None has begun to think how divine he himself is, and how
    certain the future is.
My comrade . . . share with me two greatnesses, and a third one
    rising inclusive and more resplendent.

The greatness of Love and Democracy, and the greatness of
    Religion.
I say that the real and permanent grandeur of these States
    must be their Religion.

. . . Matt smiled at the numbed congregation. "Let's rebuild this monument
and prove to our forefathers that a Church of Love and Modern Moralities can
point the way to moral excellence. Thank you. We'll sing hymn #230 in the Blue
Book: 'Let Us Now Sing the Praises of Famous Men.' Appropriately, the words
are taken from Ecclesiasticus 41, one of the Apocryphal books of the Bible."